ATLAS HANDBOOK OF SURGICAL OPERATIONS

A Clinical Textbook Covering Step-by-Step Technique, Danger Zone Anatomy, and Perioperative Management for PGY Trainees

Ramon C. Henson, MD

Trademark Disclaimer

All brand names, product names, drug names, certification names, and registered trademarks mentioned in this textbook are the property of their respective owners. Their use in this publication does not imply endorsement, affiliation, or sponsorship by the trademark owner, nor does it imply that the trademark owner has reviewed, approved, or is in any way associated with this work. All trademarked names and registered marks appearing in this textbook are used solely for purposes of identification and educational reference, without any intent of trademark infringement.

Medical Disclaimer

This textbook is intended solely for educational and informational purposes and is designed to support the continuing professional development of licensed healthcare providers. The clinical content presented herein reflects information believed to be accurate and current at the time of publication; however, medicine evolves rapidly, and readers are advised that new research findings, updated clinical practice guidelines, and revised regulatory approvals may alter or supersede information contained in this work after its publication date.

Nothing in this publication constitutes medical advice, clinical guidance specific to any individual patient, or a substitute for the independent professional judgment of a licensed and qualified healthcare provider. No clinician-patient relationship is established, implied, or intended by the use of this textbook or any portion thereof. All clinical decisions, including but not limited to diagnosis, therapeutic selection, drug dosing, and patient monitoring, must be individualized based on thorough and direct assessment of the patient, the totality of current published evidence, applicable clinical practice guidelines, institutional protocols, and the informed professional judgment of the responsible clinician.

Drug information, dosages, treatment protocols, and therapeutic recommendations presented in this publication are offered for educational reference only and must be independently verified against current prescribing information, pharmacopeial references, and applicable regulatory approvals prior to clinical application. The author and publisher have made every reasonable effort to ensure the accuracy and completeness of the information presented; nevertheless, they expressly disclaim all liability for any adverse outcomes, clinical errors, patient harm, loss, or injury alleged to arise, directly or indirectly, from the use, misuse, or application of any information, recommendation, protocol, or clinical guidance contained in this publication.

TABLE OF CONTENT

PREFACE

Surgery is not learned from words alone. It is learned from the disciplined integration of anatomical knowledge, technical precision, and real-time clinical judgment — a synthesis that must happen under pressure, often with incomplete information, and always with consequences. This textbook exists because the gap between knowing a procedure intellectually and executing it safely has never been adequately bridged by a single resource.

Existing surgical references tend to serve one purpose well at the expense of another. The comprehensive atlases deliver outstanding visual step-by-step technique but remain largely silent on the critical question that haunts every trainee standing at the operating table: what can go wrong at this step, and what do I do about it? The dense operative textbooks teach clinical reasoning and decision logic but lack the visual immediacy that operative learning demands. The handbooks offer portability and quick reference but sacrifice the anatomical depth that safe surgery requires. No single volume has successfully combined atlas-quality visual instruction with the intraoperative decision scaffolding and danger-zone awareness that define the difference between a competent surgeon and a confident one.

The **Atlas Handbook of Surgical Operations** was designed to close that gap. Every chapter in this textbook is built around the same principle: operative technique is inseparable from operative anatomy, and operative anatomy is inseparable from the knowledge of what structures are most vulnerable at each step of each procedure. This is a textbook that not only shows you what to do but tells you where the danger lies and how to protect against it.

At the heart of this book is **the Operative Danger Zone Atlas** — a proprietary system embedded in every chapter. For each major procedure, branded Danger Zone callout blocks identify the specific anatomical structures at greatest risk during that operative step, describe the clinical consequences of injury, and prescribe the safe technical maneuver that protects the structure. These callout blocks are not supplementary. They are the operating logic of the book — the layer that transforms a reference text into an operative decision-support tool. At the back of this volume, the **Operative Danger Zone Master Atlas** consolidates every danger zone from every chapter into an indexed quick-reference organized by anatomical region, procedure, and structure at risk, so the reader can look up any danger zone in seconds before scrubbing in.

The scope of this textbook spans the full breadth of general surgical operations — from foundational operative principles and perioperative care through gastrointestinal, hepatobiliary, pancreatic, colorectal, breast, endocrine, vascular, thoracic, trauma, and specialty procedures. The twenty-five chapters follow a natural clinical progression, organized by organ system and operative domain, aligned with the American Board of Surgery In-Training Examination content blueprint and current ACGME general surgery milestones. Every chapter follows a standardized clinical architecture: learning objectives, core operative content with step-by-step technique, integrated Danger Zone callouts, clinical cases written as narrative scenarios with guided reasoning, clinical pearls and key points, evidence-based management standards, and a chapter-end Danger Zone Consolidation that synthesizes every danger zone introduced in the chapter into a scannable indexed reference.

The visual program reflects Enhanced Clinical imaging standards. Figures are drawn exclusively from the locked Visual Type Inventory for surgical operations — operative anatomy illustrations, step-by-step procedural diagrams, layer-by-layer dissection views, danger zone anatomy diagrams, intraoperative clinical photographs, diagnostic imaging examples, and patient positioning diagrams. Every figure carries a detailed image prompt specifying rendering style, anatomical labeling conventions, and structural labels only. Tables are rendered as native formatted tables, and clinical algorithms are rendered as structured numbered decision-tree prose — never as images.

This book is written for the general surgery resident preparing for tomorrow's case at the end of a long call day, for the surgical fellow operating outside their primary subspecialty, for the practicing community surgeon encountering an uncommon procedure, and for the medical student seeking to understand not just what happens in the operating room but why. The voice throughout is that of an experienced attending authoring a definitive reference — authoritative, mechanism-driven, and clinically precise.

Every recommendation in this textbook reflects current evidence-based surgical practice, aligned with the most recent guidelines from the American College of Surgeons, the Society of American Gastrointestinal and Endoscopic Surgeons, the American Association for the Surgery of Trauma, the Society for Vascular Surgery, and other relevant specialty societies. Drug dosing information is presented as reference ranges flagged for confirmation against current formulary. All content is originally written.

The operating room is unforgiving. It rewards preparation, anatomical awareness, and the discipline to recognize danger before it becomes injury. This textbook was built to deliver exactly that.

CHAPTER 1: PRINCIPLES OF SURGICAL TECHNIQUE AND OPERATIVE ANATOMY

Learning Objectives

1. Describe the principles of atraumatic tissue handling and the consequences of excessive mechanical trauma to surgical planes.
2. Explain the physiological basis of hemostatic techniques, including mechanical, thermal, and pharmacological methods of vascular control.
3. Compare suture materials by their absorption profiles, tensile strength retention, and appropriate tissue applications.
4. Differentiate the mechanisms of action, thermal spread profiles, and safety considerations of monopolar, bipolar, ultrasonic, and advanced bipolar energy devices.
5. Select appropriate wound closure techniques based on tissue layer, wound tension, contamination risk, and anatomical location.
6. Identify the biomechanical principles of patient positioning and their relationship to nerve injury, pressure injury, and optimal surgical exposure.

Tissue Handling and Dissection Principles

Atraumatic Technique and the No-Touch Principle

The foundation of safe operative surgery rests on the discipline of atraumatic tissue handling. Every grasp of a tissue forceps, every pass of a retractor, and every stroke of a dissecting instrument either preserves or destroys the tissue planes that define surgical anatomy. Excessive mechanical force causes cellular disruption, edema, and inflammatory infiltration, which in turn obscure tissue planes, increase bleeding, delay wound healing, and raise the risk of surgical site infection. The no-touch principle — handling tissue as little as possible, as gently as possible, and through defined anatomical planes — is the operational foundation that separates technically sound surgery from technically destructive surgery.

Grasping instruments are categorized by their crushing potential. Tissue forceps with teeth (Adson, Bonney, Debakey) are preferred for skin and fascia because they achieve a secure grip with minimal compression force, reducing the need for excessive squeeze. Smooth-jawed forceps are reserved for vascular and visceral tissues where serration marks would damage vessel intima or bowel serosa. Ring forceps (Babcock) distribute force over a wider surface area and are used for atraumatic retraction of tubular structures. Locking forceps (Kelly, Kocher) are reserved for tissue that is being permanently ligated or removed — never for retraction of viable tissue that must remain in situ.

Sharp Versus Blunt Dissection

Sharp dissection with a scalpel or scissors follows defined anatomical planes and produces clean tissue interfaces with minimal collateral injury. It is mandatory when dissecting near named neurovascular structures, when tissue planes are obscured by inflammation or scarring, and when precision of the dissection margin determines oncological adequacy. Cold sharp dissection (scalpel blade, Metzenbaum or Potts scissors) is the safest method for working within 5 mm of structures that cannot tolerate any thermal energy — the common bile duct during cholecystectomy, the recurrent laryngeal nerve during thyroidectomy, and the ureter during pelvic mobilization.

Blunt dissection — performed with a Kittner dissector, peanut sponge, or the surgeon's finger — is appropriate in loose areolar planes where tissue separates naturally along fascial interfaces. The critical error is using blunt dissection in dense, adherent, or inflamed tissue, where tearing replaces controlled division and creates unrecognized injuries to adjacent structures. In reoperative fields, the areolar planes that existed at the first operation have been replaced by fibrous scar that does not separate bluntly — attempts to recreate those planes with a finger or blunt instrument produce avulsion injuries to the bowel wall, mesenteric vessels, and retroperitoneal structures.

Retraction and Exposure Principles

Adequate exposure is the prerequisite for safe dissection, and the quality of retraction determines the quality of exposure. Self-retaining retractors (Bookwalter, Thompson, Omni) distribute retraction force across multiple blades and free the assistant's hands for counter-traction and suction, but they create continuous pressure on the tissue beneath each blade. Retractor blades positioned over the abdominal wall can compress the lateral femoral cutaneous nerve at the anterior superior iliac spine, producing postoperative meralgia paresthetica. Retractor blades placed deep in the pelvis can compress the femoral nerve beneath the inguinal ligament or the obturator nerve against the lateral pelvic wall. The operating surgeon must balance the exposure benefit of deep retraction against the neurovascular risk of sustained pressure, and retractors should be periodically released and repositioned during long procedures.

CLINICAL PEARL: When tissue planes are obliterated by prior surgery or inflammation, revert to sharp dissection under direct vision. Blunt finger dissection in scarred fields is the single most common cause of inadvertent enterotomy during adhesiolysis.

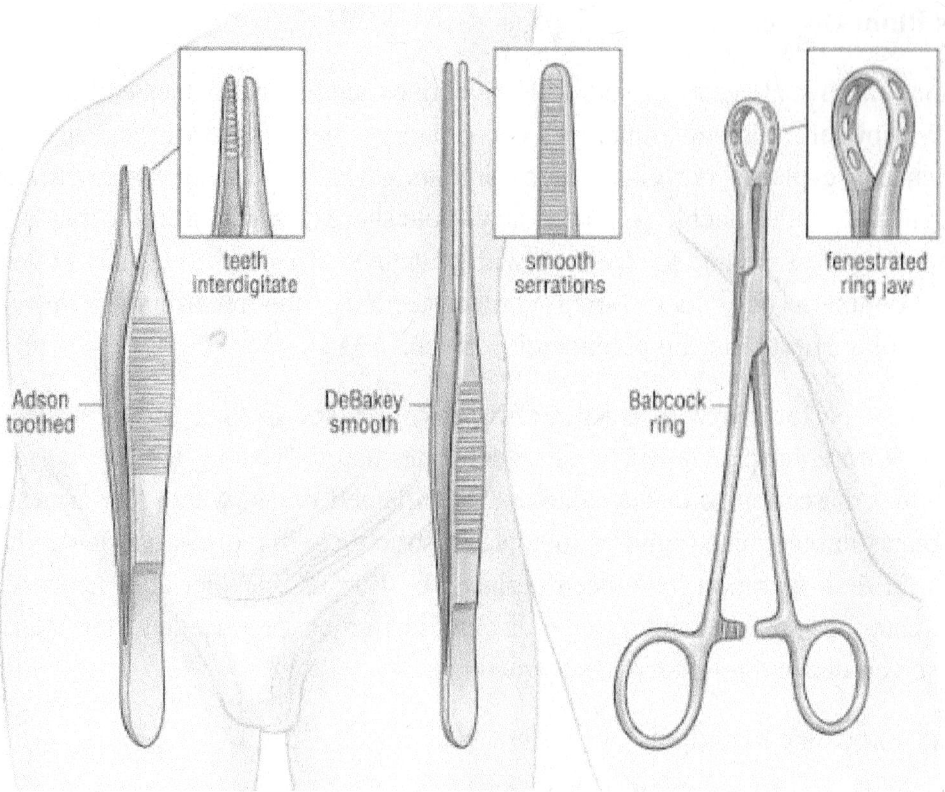

THE OPERATIVE DANGER ZONE ATLAS — Instrument-Related Tissue Injury

The Zone: Any dissection field where tissue forceps are applied directly to structures not intended for excision — particularly bowel serosa, vascular adventitia, and nerve epineurium.

The Structure at Risk: Small bowel serosa and mesenteric vessels during retraction; common bile duct wall during dissection in Calot triangle; ureter during pelvic mobilization. Each of these structures is vulnerable to crush injury from toothed forceps applied with excessive force.

The Consequence: Serosal crush injury leads to delayed perforation (manifesting 3 to 7 days postoperatively as peritonitis). Vascular adventitial injury leads to thrombosis or pseudoaneurysm. Nerve crush leads to neuropraxia or axonotmesis with motor and sensory deficit that may require months for recovery.

The Safe Maneuver: Use the appropriate forceps for the tissue: toothed for skin and fascia only; smooth (DeBakey) for vascular and visceral structures; Babcock or Penrose drain for atraumatic bowel retraction. Grasp adjacent mesentery or peritoneum rather than the visceral wall itself. Never clamp across unidentified tissue.

Hemostasis and Vascular Control

Principles of Surgical Hemostasis

Hemostasis is the prerequisite for every subsequent operative step. Uncontrolled bleeding obscures the surgical field, drives transfusion requirements, precipitates coagulopathy, and extends operative time — each of which independently increases morbidity and mortality. The hierarchy of hemostatic techniques proceeds from mechanical methods (direct pressure, clamping, ligation) through thermal methods (electrocautery, energy devices) to topical hemostatic agents and systemic pharmacological adjuncts, with the choice determined by the source vessel caliber, anatomical location, and urgency of control.

Mechanical Hemostasis

Direct pressure remains the most reliable first-response hemostatic technique. Sustained pressure with a laparotomy sponge for three to five minutes controls the majority of raw surface and small-vessel bleeding by permitting physiological clot formation. The common error is releasing pressure prematurely — removing the sponge after 30 to 60 seconds before a stable fibrin clot has formed, which strips the nascent clot and restarts the bleeding cycle. For named vessels, the clamp-cut-tie sequence remains the standard: the vessel is isolated, doubly clamped proximal and distal to the point of division, divided between clamps, and secured with suture ligation. Absorbable suture (polyglactin 910, 3-0 or 4-0) is preferred for most soft tissue vessel ligations; nonabsorbable suture (silk or polypropylene) is reserved for large-caliber vessels where long-term mechanical strength is required.

Topical Hemostatic Agents

When mechanical and thermal methods are insufficient — as occurs with diffuse parenchymal bleeding from the liver, spleen, or raw peritoneal surfaces — topical hemostatic agents provide a complementary layer of control. Oxidized regenerated cellulose provides a scaffold for platelet aggregation and is effective on low-flow venous ooze. Absorbable gelatin sponge swells on contact with blood and acts as a physical matrix for clot formation. Microfibrillar collagen activates platelet adhesion and aggregation directly and is effective on diffuse capillary bleeding surfaces. Fibrin sealants deliver preformed fibrinogen and thrombin to the wound surface and are useful for anastomotic reinforcement and splenic repair. Thrombin-soaked gelatin matrix combines the mechanical scaffold with active thrombin and is particularly effective in anticoagulated patients with coagulopathic parenchymal bleeding.

Agent	Mechanism	Indication	Key Consideration
Oxidized cellulose	Scaffold for platelet aggregation; low pH bactericidal effect	Venous ooze, raw surfaces	Swells — do not pack in closed spaces near nerves
Gelatin sponge	Physical matrix; absorbs 45x its weight in blood	Parenchymal bleeding, dental sockets	Absorbs in 4–6 weeks; avoid in infected fields

Microfibrillar collagen	Direct platelet adhesion and activation	Diffuse capillary bleeding	Ineffective in thrombocytopenia; do not wet before application
Fibrin sealant	Delivers fibrinogen plus thrombin	Anastomotic reinforcement, splenic repair	Contains bovine aprotinin — allergic risk on re-exposure
Thrombin-gelatin matrix	Active thrombin plus gelatin scaffold	Parenchymal bleeding in anticoagulated patients	Swells up to 20%; avoid near confined neural foramina

THE OPERATIVE DANGER ZONE ATLAS — Blind Clamping in a Bloody Field

The Zone: Any operative field where active hemorrhage has obscured anatomical landmarks — most critically the hepatoduodenal ligament, the retroperitoneum lateral to the aorta, and the deep pelvis near the iliac bifurcation.

The Structure at Risk: Common bile duct during hepatic pedicle hemorrhage; ureter during pelvic or retroperitoneal bleeding; iliac vein during iliac artery hemorrhage control attempts. Each of these lies within millimeters of the expected bleeding source and is indistinguishable from surrounding tissue when the field is obscured by blood.

The Consequence: Blind clamping of the common bile duct produces complete biliary obstruction requiring complex reconstruction (Roux-en-Y hepaticojejunostomy). Ureteral clamping produces ureteral transection or stricture requiring stenting or reimplantation. Iliac vein laceration from a misplaced clamp converts a controlled arterial injury into an uncontrolled venous hemorrhage with massive blood loss.

The Safe Maneuver: Apply direct pressure with a laparotomy sponge and pause. Suction the field clear. Identify the bleeding source under direct vision before placing any clamp. For hepatic pedicle hemorrhage, apply the Pringle maneuver (atraumatic clamp across the hepatoduodenal ligament en bloc) as a temporary inflow control measure while identifying the specific bleeding vessel. Never blindly clamp into a pool of blood.

Suturing and Knot-Tying Techniques

Suture Material Classification

Suture materials are classified along two independent axes: absorbable versus nonabsorbable, and monofilament versus braided. Absorbable sutures lose tensile strength over a defined time course through hydrolysis (synthetic) or enzymatic degradation (natural), and are used in tissues that heal rapidly enough to become self-supporting before suture strength is lost. Nonabsorbable sutures maintain tensile strength indefinitely and are used where permanent tissue approximation is required (fascial closure, vascular anastomosis, hernia mesh fixation) or where the suture will be removed (skin closure).

Monofilament sutures (polydioxanone, nylon, polypropylene) pass through tissue with minimal drag and resist bacterial harboring because they lack interstices, but they are less pliable and require more throws per knot to maintain security. Braided sutures (polyglactin 910, polyester, silk) handle smoothly, tie securely with fewer throws, and conform to irregular tissue surfaces, but their multifilament interstices can harbor bacteria and promote capillary wicking of fluid along the suture tract, which raises infection risk in contaminated fields. This distinction determines suture choice in contaminated wounds: monofilament suture is mandatory in Class III and IV wounds to minimize the foreign body burden available for bacterial colonization.

Suture	Type	Tensile Strength Retention	Common Application
Polyglactin 910 (Vicryl)	Absorbable, braided	75% at 2 weeks; 0% at 4–5 weeks	Subcutaneous closure, bowel anastomosis, vessel ligation
Poliglecaprone 25 (Monocryl)	Absorbable, monofilament	50–60% at 1 week; 0% at 3–4 weeks	Subcuticular skin closure, mucosal repair
Polydioxanone (PDS)	Absorbable, monofilament	70% at 2 weeks; 25% at 6 weeks	Fascial closure, tendon repair, pediatric cardiovascular
Nylon (Ethilon)	Nonabsorbable, monofilament	Permanent (degrades 15–20% per year)	Skin closure (interrupted), microsurgery
Polypropylene (Prolene)	Nonabsorbable, monofilament	Permanent (no degradation)	Vascular anastomosis, running fascial closure, hernia repair
Silk	Nonabsorbable, braided	Loses 50% by 1 year; effectively absorbed	Vessel ligation, drain fixation; avoid in contaminated fields

Knot-Tying Principles and Failure Modes

A correctly tied surgical knot converts linear suture tension into a stable friction lock. The minimum number of throws for knot security depends on the suture material: braided sutures achieve security with three square throws, while monofilament sutures require four to five throws because their smooth surface generates less interfiber friction. Every throw must be laid flat — crossing throws produces a granny knot that slips under tension. The most common knot-tying error among trainees is inconsistent tension across throws, which creates a loose first throw that permits tissue gapping before subsequent throws can compensate. The second most common error is cutting tails too short — knots under physiological tension require a minimum 3 mm tail for buried knots and 5 mm for skin knots to prevent slippage and unraveling.

KEY POINT: For monofilament sutures (Prolene, PDS, Monocryl), always tie a minimum of four square throws. Cut tails at 3 mm for buried knots and 5 mm for skin knots to prevent unraveling. Instrument ties are more secure than hand ties for deep knots because they permit controlled tension on each throw under direct vision.

Energy Devices and Tissue Sealing Technology

Monopolar Electrosurgery

Monopolar electrosurgery passes radiofrequency current from the active electrode (the pencil tip or spatula) through the patient to a dispersive return electrode (grounding pad). The current density at the small active electrode generates localized tissue heating sufficient for cutting (continuous waveform, high voltage, minimal lateral thermal damage) or coagulation (intermittent waveform, lower voltage, wider thermal spread). Because the current traverses the entire body, monopolar electrosurgery carries risk of thermal injury at sites distant from the operative field — most critically at the grounding pad (if improperly applied, producing a partial contact burn) and at sites where current is channeled through narrow tissue bridges (capacitive coupling in laparoscopic instruments, insulation failure along the shaft of reusable instruments).

Bipolar and Advanced Bipolar Devices

Bipolar electrosurgery confines the current path between two electrode tines separated by only a few millimeters, eliminating the risk of distant thermal injury. Standard bipolar forceps are effective for coagulation of small vessels (up to 2 mm) but do not reliably seal larger vessels. Advanced bipolar tissue-sealing devices apply controlled pressure and calibrated energy delivery to denature collagen and elastin in the vessel wall, creating a permanent transluminal seal reliable for vessels up to 7 mm in diameter. Seal failure occurs when the device is applied to vessels under tension (which prevents complete collagen denaturation), when tissue is too wet for adequate impedance, or when the device jaws do not fully encompass the vessel bundle. The burst pressure of a well-formed advanced bipolar seal exceeds 900 mmHg — well above physiological arterial pressure — but this strength is achieved only when the tissue is properly clamped and the full energy cycle completes.

Ultrasonic Devices

Ultrasonic coagulating shears produce tissue effects through mechanical vibration at 55,500 Hz rather than electrical current. The rapid blade oscillation generates frictional heat at the tissue interface, which denatures protein, coagulates vessels (reliable to 5 mm diameter), and cuts simultaneously. Because no electrical current passes through the patient, there is no risk of grounding pad injury or stray current burns. However, the active blade reaches temperatures of 150 to 300 degrees Celsius and retains heat after activation — placing the hot blade against adjacent tissue within three to five seconds of activation causes thermal injury. The lateral thermal spread of ultrasonic devices is approximately 1 to 3 mm, significantly less than monopolar electrosurgery (3 to 6 mm), which makes them safer for dissection near critical structures when adequate clearance is maintained.

THE OPERATIVE DANGER ZONE ATLAS — Thermal Spread from Energy Devices

The Zone: Any dissection within 5 mm of a critical structure — most dangerously the common bile duct during cholecystectomy, the recurrent laryngeal nerve during thyroidectomy, and the ureter during pelvic dissection.

The Structure at Risk: Common bile duct (thermal stricture), recurrent laryngeal nerve (neuropraxia or permanent palsy), ureter (delayed thermal necrosis with urinoma formation 5 to 10 days postoperatively), superior mesenteric artery (adventitial thermal injury during pancreatic dissection).

The Consequence: Thermal injuries to tubular structures produce delayed necrosis — the tissue appears intact intraoperatively but undergoes full-thickness wall necrosis over the following week, presenting as bile leak, urine leak, or delayed hemorrhage. These injuries are often more devastating than sharp transection injuries because the zone of thermal necrosis extends beyond the visible operative field and the injury declares itself days later.

The Safe Maneuver: Maintain a minimum 5 mm clearance between any energy device activation and critical structures. Use cold scissors or sharp dissection for the final millimeters of dissection adjacent to the common bile duct, recurrent laryngeal nerve, and ureter. After activating an ultrasonic device, wait a minimum of 5 seconds before allowing the blade to contact adjacent tissue. Use bipolar (not monopolar) when working in confined spaces near named structures.

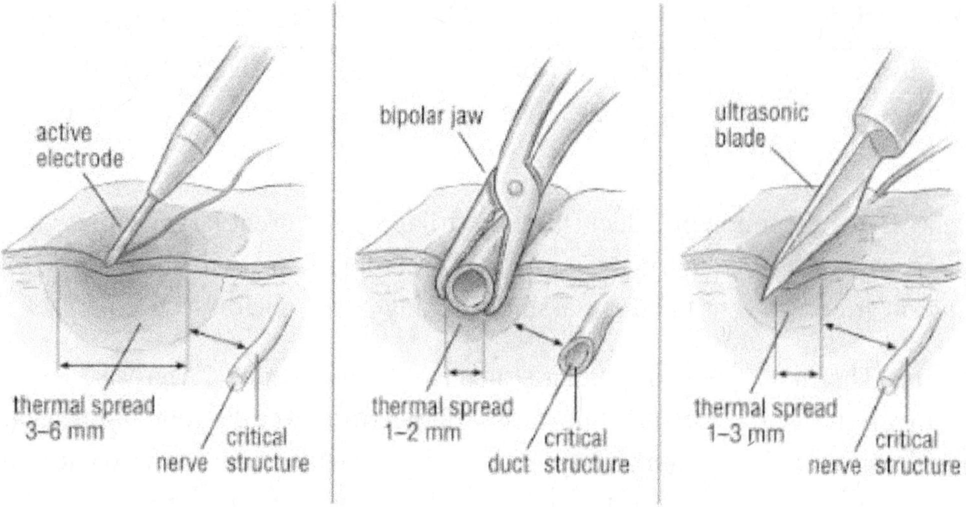

Wound Closure Principles and Materials

Layered Closure and Tension Distribution

Wound closure restores anatomical integrity by re-approximating tissue layers in sequence — peritoneum (when closed), posterior fascia, anterior fascia, subcutaneous tissue, and skin. Each layer contributes independently to wound strength, and failure to close a critical layer (particularly fascia) leaves the wound dependent on superficial layers that cannot withstand the forces of abdominal wall contraction, coughing, and Valsalva. Fascial closure is the load-bearing layer of the abdominal wall and is the single most important determinant of wound integrity.

The Israelsson principle of fascial closure requires a suture-length-to-wound-length ratio of at least 4:1 — meaning the total length of suture placed in the fascia must be at least four times the wound length. This is achieved by taking bites 5 to 8 mm from the fascial edge, spacing bites 5 mm apart, and using a running technique with consistent tension. A ratio below 4:1 is the strongest independent predictor of incisional hernia development. Bite size matters because large bites (greater than 10 mm from the edge) incorporate excessive tissue, create tissue ischemia under the suture, and paradoxically weaken the closure by strangulating the very tissue that must heal.

KEY POINT: Fascial closure with a suture-length-to-wound-length ratio of at least 4:1, using slowly absorbable monofilament suture (PDS or equivalent) with small bites (5 to 8 mm from edge, 5 mm apart), reduces incisional hernia rates to below 10% in prospective studies. This small-bite technique is the current evidence-based standard for midline laparotomy closure.

Closure by Wound Classification

Wound classification determines closure strategy. Clean wounds (Class I) are closed primarily in layers. Clean-contaminated wounds (Class II — controlled entry into a hollow viscus) are closed primarily with consideration of subcutaneous drain placement if the subcutaneous fat layer exceeds 2 cm. Contaminated wounds (Class III — open traumatic wounds, major breaks in sterile technique, gross spillage from a hollow viscus) may be closed primarily with close surveillance or managed with delayed primary closure at postoperative day 4 to 5 after the wound is confirmed to be free of infection. Dirty-infected wounds (Class IV — established infection, devitalized tissue, fecal peritonitis) are managed with open wound care and delayed closure or healing by secondary intention. The choice between primary closure and delayed primary closure in Class III and IV wounds is a risk-benefit calculation: primary closure restores tissue planes and eliminates the need for wound care, but it carries a surgical site infection rate of 15 to 30% in contaminated wounds; delayed primary closure adds 4 to 5 days of open wound management but reduces infection rates to below 5%.

Complications of Wound Closure

Wound complications follow a predictable temporal pattern. Hematoma and seroma develop within the first 48 hours and result from inadequate hemostasis of subcutaneous vessels or failure to obliterate dead space. Surgical site infection typically manifests between postoperative days 5 and 10 with erythema, induration, wound warmth, and purulent drainage — management is incision and drainage with wound culture, not antibiotics alone. Wound dehiscence — separation of the fascial closure — occurs between postoperative days 5 and 14, often heralded by serosanguinous drainage ('salmon-colored fluid') from the wound, and requires emergent operative reclosure. Incisional hernia is the late complication of fascial failure, developing months to years after the index operation, and is most commonly the consequence of technical factors at closure (suture-length-to-wound-length ratio below 4:1, too-large bites, absorbable suture in high-risk patients) rather than patient factors alone.

Patient Positioning and Surgical Exposure

Biomechanics of Surgical Positioning

Patient positioning determines surgical exposure, and every position creates a specific pattern of neurovascular vulnerability. The biomechanical principle is straightforward: nerves are injured by stretch, compression, or a combination of both, and the risk increases with duration of exposure and the presence of preexisting neuropathy, diabetes, peripheral vascular disease, or low body mass index (which reduces the soft tissue padding over bony prominences). Positioning injuries are among the most common preventable adverse events in surgery, and the majority are avoidable with systematic attention to padding, angle limitation, and periodic repositioning checks.

Standard Positions and Their Nerve Injury Profiles

Supine positioning is the default for most abdominal and lower extremity procedures. The brachial plexus is at risk when the arm is abducted beyond 90 degrees on an arm board, because traction on the plexus at the level of the costoclavicular space exceeds the elastic tolerance of the nerve trunks. The ulnar nerve is at risk at the medial epicondyle, where it rests in a shallow groove with minimal soft tissue coverage — external compression from the operating table edge or arm board produces neuropraxia (and occasionally axonotmesis) that manifests as fourth and fifth digit numbness and intrinsic hand weakness. Tucking the arms at the sides using a draw sheet and ensuring the forearm rests in neutral or slight supination protects both the brachial plexus and the ulnar nerve.

Lateral decubitus positioning, used for thoracic, renal, and adrenal procedures, creates dependent-side compression on the brachial plexus (from the axillary roll, which must be positioned caudal to the axilla, not in it), the common peroneal nerve at the fibular head of the dependent leg, and the dependent eye. Lithotomy positioning, used for colorectal, urological, and gynecological procedures, places the common peroneal nerve at risk from direct compression by stirrup posts at the lateral fibular head, and creates bilateral femoral nerve stretch if the hips are hyperflexed beyond 90 degrees. Prone positioning, used for posterior spine and certain anorectal procedures, creates risk of direct ocular pressure injury and brachial plexus stretch if the arms are abducted or extended on arm boards — chest rolls must be positioned lateral to the sternum to protect the abdomen from compression and must not extend superiorly to the level of the clavicle.

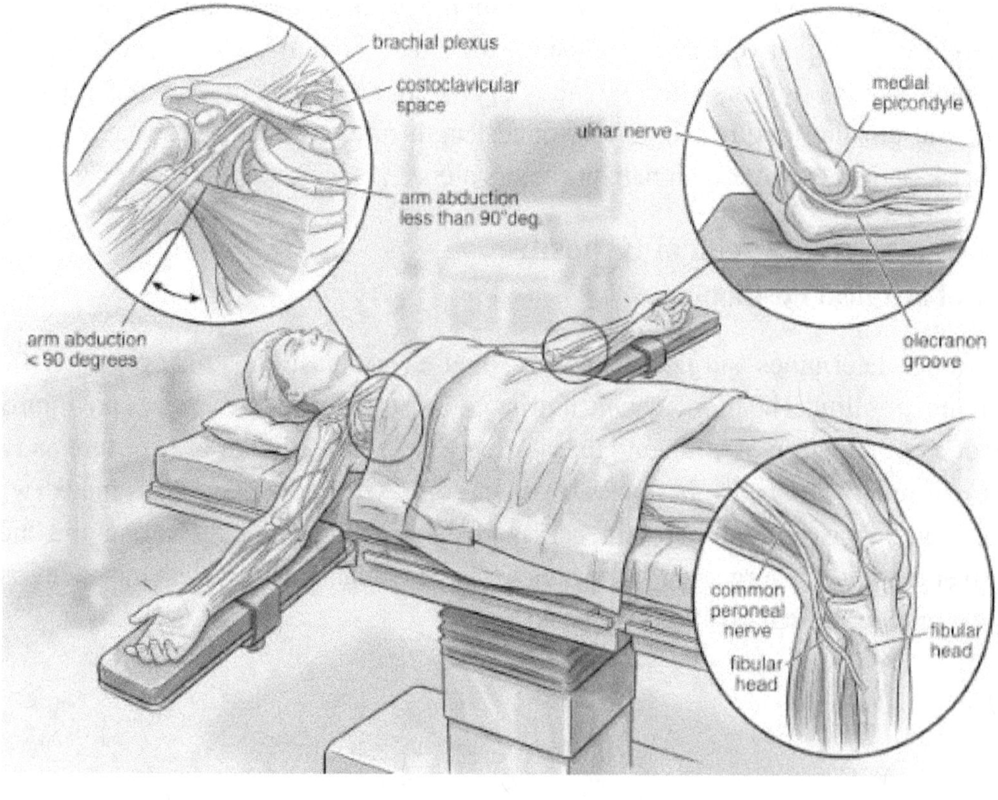

THE OPERATIVE DANGER ZONE ATLAS — Positioning-Related Nerve Injury

The Zone: Arm boards in supine position (brachial plexus, ulnar nerve); dependent axilla in lateral decubitus (brachial plexus); stirrup posts in lithotomy (common peroneal nerve); hyperflexed hips in lithotomy (femoral nerve); arm boards in prone position (brachial plexus stretch).

The Structure at Risk: Brachial plexus (upper trunk — C5, C6 most vulnerable to traction); ulnar nerve at medial epicondyle; common peroneal nerve at fibular head; femoral nerve under inguinal ligament; dependent eye in prone positioning (direct pressure causing ischemic optic neuropathy).

The Consequence: Brachial plexus injury produces upper extremity motor and sensory deficit (Erb palsy pattern for upper trunk — deltoid weakness, biceps weakness, shoulder external rotation loss). Ulnar neuropathy produces fourth and fifth digit numbness and intrinsic hand weakness (claw hand in severe cases). Common peroneal injury produces foot drop (ankle dorsiflexion and eversion weakness). Femoral neuropathy produces quadriceps weakness and anterior thigh numbness. Ischemic optic neuropathy produces irreversible visual loss.

The Safe Maneuver: Limit arm abduction to less than 90 degrees on arm boards. Pad the medial epicondyle with foam or gel and position the forearm in neutral or slight supination. Position the axillary roll caudal to (below) the axilla — never directly in the axilla. Pad lateral stirrup posts to prevent direct compression of the fibular head. Limit hip flexion in lithotomy to 90 degrees or less. In prone positioning, use gel headrests that eliminate direct ocular pressure and check eyes periodically during prolonged cases. Recheck positioning after any table tilt or repositioning during the case.

Principles of Minimally Invasive Surgery

Pneumoperitoneum and Its Physiological Effects

Laparoscopic surgery requires the creation of a pneumoperitoneum — insufflation of the peritoneal cavity with carbon dioxide to a target pressure of 12 to 15 mmHg — to generate the working space between the abdominal wall and viscera. This insufflation produces systemic physiological changes that the surgical team must anticipate and manage. Cardiovascular effects include decreased venous return (from caval compression), increased systemic vascular resistance, and transient reduction in cardiac output, which are exacerbated by steep Trendelenburg or reverse Trendelenburg positioning. Pulmonary effects include cephalad displacement of the diaphragm, reduced functional residual capacity, increased peak airway pressures, and CO2 absorption from the peritoneal surface producing hypercarbia if minute ventilation is not increased. Renal effects include decreased renal blood flow and urine output from both direct renal vein compression and activation of the renin-angiotensin-aldosterone system — these effects are reversible with desufflation and do not typically require pharmacological intervention.

Trocar Placement and Access Techniques

Safe peritoneal access is the first critical step of any laparoscopic procedure. Three access techniques are in common use: Veress needle followed by optical trocar insertion, open (Hasson) technique with direct cutdown to the peritoneum under vision, and direct optical entry with a bladed or bladeless trocar under laparoscopic visualization. The Hasson technique is the safest initial access method in patients with prior abdominal surgery, because it places the first trocar under direct vision rather than relying on blind needle or trocar passage through adhesion-bearing abdominal wall. Regardless of technique, the principles of safe access require elevation of the abdominal wall to maximize the distance between the anterior abdominal wall and the retroperitoneal great vessels, confirmation of intraperitoneal position (saline drop test, opening pressure below 10 mmHg for Veress), and controlled insufflation with continuous pressure monitoring.

Subsequent trocar placement follows the principle of triangulation — positioning the camera and working ports so that the instruments approach the target anatomy from different angles, creating a working triangle that permits bimanual dissection without instrument sword-fighting. Port sites should be placed at least 8 cm from the target anatomy and at least 5 cm apart from each other to prevent external handle collisions. In obese patients, port placement must account for the increased abdominal wall thickness, which effectively shortens the intra-abdominal working length of standard instruments and may require longer trocars or repositioned access points.

Conversion to Open Surgery

Conversion from laparoscopic to open surgery is a judgment call, not a failure. The indications for conversion include uncontrolled hemorrhage, inability to identify critical anatomy despite adequate dissection, dense adhesions precluding safe laparoscopic dissection, and any intraoperative finding that cannot be managed safely through the existing port access. The decision to convert should be made early — the most dangerous conversions are those made late, after significant bleeding or tissue injury has already occurred. The operating surgeon should establish a personal threshold for conversion before the case begins, based on the specific procedure and patient anatomy, and communicate this threshold to the operative team during the preoperative briefing.

CAUTION: Trocar insertion injuries to the aorta, vena cava, and iliac vessels account for approximately 50% of all major vascular injuries in laparoscopic surgery. The majority occur during initial access. Elevate the abdominal wall during Veress needle insertion, confirm intraperitoneal position with saline drop test and opening pressure below 10 mmHg, and direct the needle toward the pelvis (away from the aortic bifurcation) in thin patients.

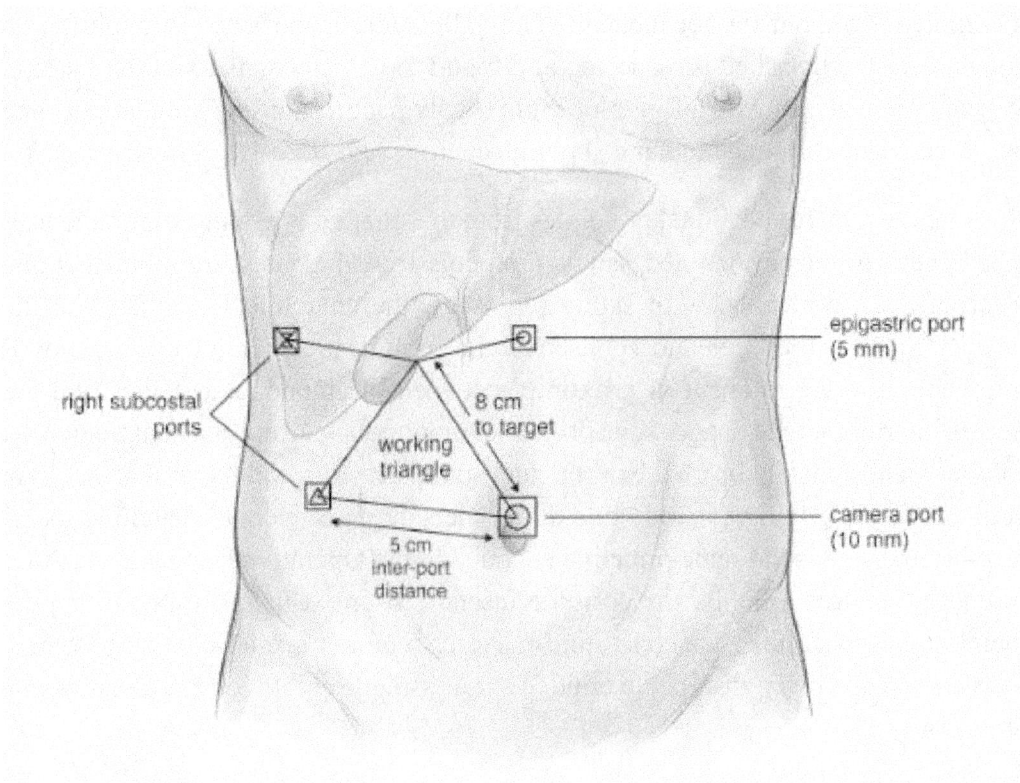

Clinical Case — Inadvertent Thermal Injury During Laparoscopic Cholecystectomy

A 54-year-old woman with a body mass index of 38 and two prior cesarean deliveries presents for elective laparoscopic cholecystectomy for symptomatic cholelithiasis. Her preoperative workup is unremarkable, and she is positioned supine with the right arm tucked and the left arm extended on an arm board. Pneumoperitoneum is established via Veress needle at the umbilicus with an opening pressure of 6 mmHg, confirming intraperitoneal placement, and insufflation proceeds to 15 mmHg. Initial inspection of the abdomen reveals omental adhesions to the anterior abdominal wall from the prior cesarean incisions but no adhesions in the right upper quadrant.

Dissection proceeds to the hepatocystic triangle. The cystic duct and cystic artery are identified and the critical view of safety is achieved with two structures — and only two structures — seen entering the gallbladder. The cystic artery is sealed and divided with an advanced bipolar vessel-sealing device. During dissection of the gallbladder from the liver bed, the resident uses monopolar electrosurgery on a coagulation setting to manage parenchymal bleeding from the hepatic surface. At one point, the monopolar hook is activated within 3 mm of the cystic duct stump while controlling an area of oozing on the medial gallbladder wall. The attending surgeon immediately halts the dissection and instructs the resident to switch to a cold Kittner dissector and blunt technique for the remaining dissection adjacent to the cystic duct stump, explaining that monopolar coagulation at that proximity risks thermal injury to the common bile duct through conductive heating of the clip on the cystic duct stump.

The case is completed without further incident. The gallbladder is extracted through the umbilical port site in a retrieval bag, the liver bed is inspected and found to be hemostatic, and the fascial defect at the 10 mm umbilical port is closed with a figure-of-eight 0 polyglactin suture to prevent port-site hernia. The skin incisions are closed with subcuticular 4-0 poliglecaprone and adhesive skin strips.

This case illustrates several foundational principles from this chapter operating simultaneously. The initial Veress needle access followed accepted safety protocols (opening pressure confirmation, appropriate insufflation target). The critical view of safety represents the anatomical identification discipline that prevents bile duct injury — the single most consequential complication of cholecystectomy. The attending surgeon's intervention at the moment of proximity between the monopolar device and the cystic duct stump applied the thermal spread danger zone principle: monopolar current at a coagulation setting spreads 3 to 6 mm laterally, and a metal clip on the cystic duct stump acts as a conductor that can transmit thermal energy directly to the underlying common bile duct. The safe maneuver — switching to cold dissection for the final millimeters — is the same principle encoded in the Operative Danger Zone Atlas for thermal spread from energy devices. Finally, the port-site fascial closure at the 10 mm site applies the wound closure principle that any fascial defect 10 mm or larger requires formal closure to prevent incisional hernia, and the choice of slowly absorbable braided suture is appropriate for this clean wound (Class I) at a non-load-bearing site.

CLINICAL PEARL: Metal clips on the cystic duct stump conduct monopolar current directly to the adjacent common bile duct. After clip application, all subsequent dissection within 5 mm of the clips should use cold technique (scissors, Kittner dissector) or bipolar energy only — never monopolar electrosurgery. This principle applies to any clipped structure adjacent to a critical duct, nerve, or vessel.

THE OPERATIVE DANGER ZONE ATLAS — Foundational Operative Dangers

Instrument-Related Tissue Injury: Toothed forceps applied to bowel serosa, bile duct wall, or vascular adventitia cause crush injury leading to delayed perforation (3 to 7 days), thrombosis, or neuropraxia. **Safe maneuver:** match forceps type to tissue — toothed for skin and fascia; smooth for viscera and vessels; ring forceps or Penrose drain for atraumatic bowel retraction.

Blind Clamping in a Bloody Field: Hemorrhage-obscured fields at the hepatoduodenal ligament, retroperitoneum, and pelvic sidewall create high risk of common bile duct, ureteral, and iliac vein injury from blind clamp placement. **Safe maneuver:** direct pressure first, suction to clear the field, visual identification before clamping; Pringle maneuver for hepatic pedicle hemorrhage.

Thermal Spread from Energy Devices: Monopolar electrosurgery spreads thermal injury 3 to 6 mm laterally; ultrasonic devices spread 1 to 3 mm but retain blade heat for 5 seconds after activation. Structures at risk: common bile duct, recurrent laryngeal nerve, ureter, superior mesenteric artery. **Safe maneuver:** maintain 5 mm clearance; use cold scissors for the final dissection adjacent to named structures; wait 5 seconds after ultrasonic activation before tissue contact.

Positioning-Related Nerve Injury: Brachial plexus (arm abduction beyond 90 degrees), ulnar nerve (medial epicondyle compression), common peroneal nerve (fibular head compression by stirrup posts), and femoral nerve (hip hyperflexion in lithotomy) are at risk from improper positioning. **Safe maneuver:** limit abduction to less than 90 degrees; pad bony prominences; position axillary roll caudal to the axilla; limit hip flexion to 90 degrees; recheck after repositioning.

Summary and Key Concepts

Atraumatic tissue handling with appropriate instrument selection preserves tissue planes, reduces inflammation, and minimizes the risk of delayed perforation and neuropraxia — match forceps type to tissue type and grasp adjacent connective tissue rather than visceral walls.

The hemostatic hierarchy proceeds from mechanical methods (pressure, ligation) to thermal methods (energy devices) to topical agents, with device selection determined by vessel caliber, anatomical proximity to critical structures, and urgency of control.

Suture selection is driven by tissue healing requirements: absorbable for self-supporting tissues, nonabsorbable for permanent load-bearing; monofilament for contaminated fields, braided for ease of handling in clean wounds; minimum four square throws for monofilament knot security.

Energy device safety requires understanding thermal spread profiles — maintain minimum 5 mm clearance from critical structures and use cold dissection for the final millimeters adjacent to named neurovascular and ductal structures; ultrasonic blades retain heat for 5 seconds after activation.

Fascial closure with a suture-length-to-wound-length ratio of at least 4:1 using slowly absorbable monofilament suture with small bites (5 to 8 mm from edge, 5 mm apart) is the strongest modifiable predictor of wound integrity and incisional hernia prevention.

Patient positioning determines nerve injury risk profiles — every position creates specific vulnerabilities that are preventable with proper padding, angle limitation, and pre-incision and post-repositioning neurovascular checks.

Safe laparoscopic access requires elevated abdominal wall, confirmed intraperitoneal position, and Hasson technique in patients with prior abdominal surgery; conversion from laparoscopic to open is a surgical judgment call that should be made early, not late.

CHAPTER 2: PREOPERATIVE ASSESSMENT AND PERIOPERATIVE CARE

Learning Objectives

1. Apply the Revised Cardiac Risk Index and American College of Surgeons Surgical Risk Calculator to stratify perioperative cardiac risk and determine the need for further cardiac workup.
2. Identify the surgeon's role in airway assessment and the clinical predictors of difficult intubation that must be communicated to the anesthesiology team before induction.
3. Select the appropriate antibiotic prophylaxis regimen by procedure type, time the dose correctly relative to incision, and identify the indications for extended prophylaxis.
4. Stratify venous thromboembolism risk using the Caprini score and implement pharmacological and mechanical thromboprophylaxis according to current guidelines.
5. Calculate perioperative fluid requirements using physiological principles and recognize the clinical consequences of both over-resuscitation and under-resuscitation.
6. Assess nutritional status preoperatively using validated screening tools and initiate nutritional optimization to reduce surgical site infection and anastomotic leak rates.

Preoperative Risk Stratification and Optimization

Cardiac Risk Assessment

Perioperative cardiac events remain the leading cause of non-surgical morbidity and mortality after major operations. The Revised Cardiac Risk Index identifies six independent predictors of major adverse cardiac events: high-risk surgery (intraperitoneal, intrathoracic, or suprainguinal vascular), history of ischemic heart disease, history of congestive heart failure, history of cerebrovascular disease, preoperative treatment with insulin for diabetes mellitus, and preoperative serum creatinine above 2.0 mg/dL (177 micromol/L). Each predictor contributes one point; patients with zero predictors carry a major cardiac event rate below 1%, while patients with three or more predictors face event rates exceeding 10%. The American College of Surgeons National Surgical Quality Improvement Program Surgical Risk Calculator integrates 21 preoperative variables into procedure-specific risk estimates for mortality, morbidity, cardiac events, pneumonia, surgical site infection, urinary tract infection, venous thromboembolism, renal failure, and readmission — and is the preferred tool for patient-specific risk counseling and informed consent documentation.

Pulmonary Risk Assessment

Postoperative pulmonary complications — atelectasis, pneumonia, respiratory failure, and prolonged mechanical ventilation — occur in 5 to 10% of patients undergoing major abdominal surgery and carry a 30-day mortality of 10 to 20% when they occur. The strongest risk factors are patient-related (COPD, current smoking, functional dependence, ASA class III or higher) and procedure-related (upper abdominal or thoracic incision, operative time exceeding three hours, general anesthesia versus regional or neuraxial). Preoperative spirometry does not improve risk prediction beyond clinical assessment and is not routinely recommended; however, it is indicated when the degree of obstructive or restrictive physiology is unclear or when lung resection is planned and the predicted postoperative FEV1 must be calculated. Smoking cessation for a minimum of four weeks before elective surgery reduces pulmonary complication rates by approximately 50%, and every additional week of cessation further improves mucociliary clearance and reduces airway hyperreactivity.

Optimization of Modifiable Risk Factors

Preoperative optimization targets the modifiable predictors of surgical morbidity. Glycemic control in diabetic patients aims for a hemoglobin A1c below 8% and perioperative glucose of 140 to 180 mg/dL (7.8 to 10.0 mmol/L) — tighter perioperative glucose targets increase hypoglycemic episodes without reducing surgical site infection rates. Anemia correction addresses preoperative hemoglobin below 13 g/dL in men and 12 g/dL in women through iron supplementation (oral or intravenous) or, when the timeline permits, erythropoiesis-stimulating agents — preoperative transfusion to a target hemoglobin is reserved for patients with symptomatic anemia or hemoglobin below 7 g/dL. Functional capacity is assessed using the Duke Activity Status Index or metabolic equivalent (MET) estimation: patients unable to achieve 4 METs of activity (climbing a flight of stairs, walking two blocks at normal pace) warrant further investigation before intermediate- or high-risk surgery.

KEY POINT: A patient who cannot climb one flight of stairs or walk two blocks on level ground without stopping has a functional capacity below 4 METs. This threshold, combined with a Revised Cardiac Risk Index of 2 or more, triggers consideration for preoperative pharmacological stress testing or echocardiography per current ACC/AHA perioperative cardiovascular guidelines.

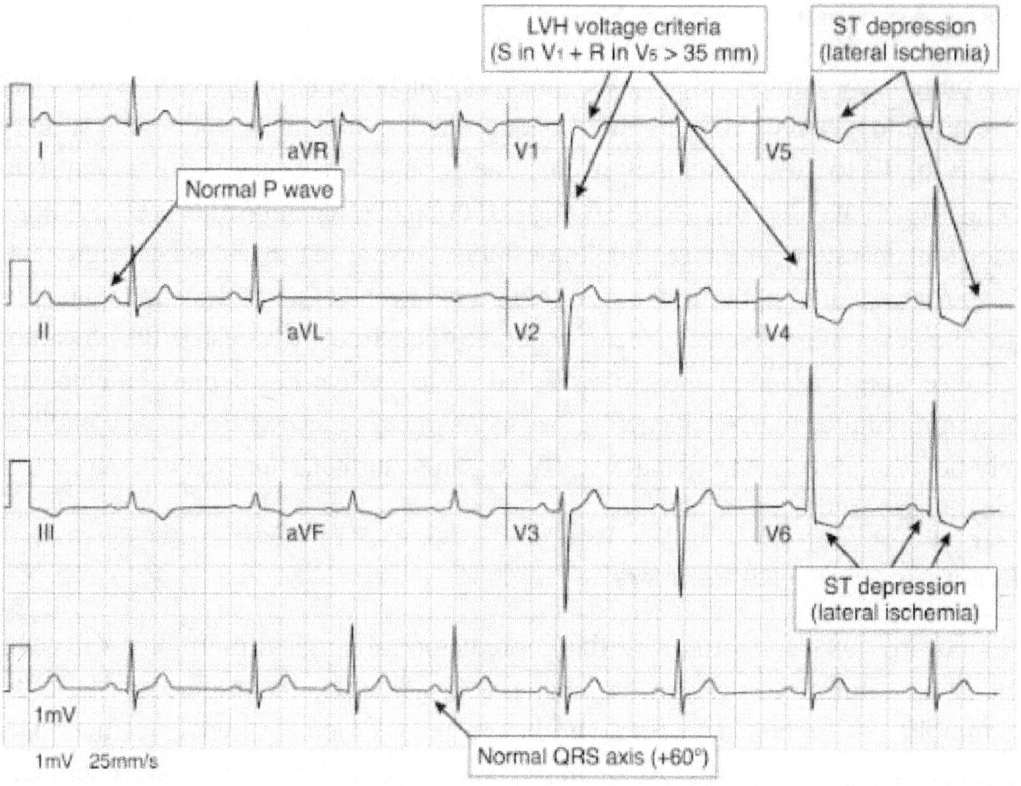

THE OPERATIVE DANGER ZONE ATLAS — Unrecognized Perioperative Cardiac Risk

The Zone: The preoperative assessment period for any patient with two or more Revised Cardiac Risk Index predictors undergoing intermediate- or high-risk surgery — the window where unrecognized ischemic heart disease can be identified before surgical stress triggers a perioperative myocardial infarction.

The Structure at Risk: Coronary arterial supply to the myocardium. Perioperative demand ischemia occurs when surgical stress (catecholamine surge, tachycardia, hypovolemia, anemia) increases myocardial oxygen demand beyond the supply capacity of stenotic coronary vessels that were asymptomatic at baseline.

The Consequence: Perioperative myocardial infarction carries a 30-day mortality of 15 to 25% — five to ten times the mortality of non-perioperative MI — because the competing demands of the surgical wound (anticoagulation risk, hemodynamic instability, reoperation risk) preclude standard interventional management. Most perioperative MIs are type 2 (supply-demand mismatch), not type 1 (plaque rupture).

The Safe Maneuver: Apply the RCRI systematically to every preoperative patient. For patients with RCRI 2 or more and functional capacity below 4 METs, obtain pharmacological stress testing or echocardiography. Continue beta-blockers in patients already taking them — abrupt perioperative withdrawal doubles the risk of atrial fibrillation and MI. Do NOT initiate beta-blockers de novo on the day of surgery.

Anesthetic Considerations for the Surgeon

Airway Assessment and Communication

Although airway management is the primary domain of the anesthesiologist, the surgeon bears responsibility for identifying airway risk factors during the preoperative visit and communicating them to the anesthesia team before the patient arrives in the operating room. The Mallampati classification (Class I: full visibility of the soft palate, fauces, uvula, and tonsillar pillars; Class IV: hard palate only) correlates with the ease of laryngoscopy but is an imperfect predictor in isolation. Additional predictors of difficult intubation include thyromental distance less than 6 cm (three fingerbreadths), limited mouth opening (inter-incisor gap less than 3 cm), limited cervical extension (cervical arthritis, prior fusion, ankylosing spondylitis), short thick neck, prominent upper incisors, and history of head and neck radiation or surgery. The surgeon must recognize these findings because a difficult airway may require an awake fiberoptic intubation or surgical airway — and in emergent situations, the surgeon may be called upon to perform a cricothyrotomy.

Anesthesia Type and Surgical Implications

The choice between general, regional, and neuraxial anesthesia influences operative exposure, patient hemodynamics, postoperative pain management, and complication risk. General anesthesia with endotracheal intubation is required for all intraperitoneal, intrathoracic, and head-and-neck procedures and for any operation requiring muscle relaxation or controlled ventilation. Neuraxial anesthesia (spinal or epidural) provides excellent analgesia and reduces the stress response for lower abdominal, pelvic, and lower extremity operations; thoracic epidural analgesia as a supplement to general anesthesia for major abdominal surgery reduces postoperative opioid requirements, improves pulmonary function, and accelerates return of bowel function. Regional nerve blocks (transversus abdominis plane block, rectus sheath block, paravertebral block) are increasingly used as components of enhanced recovery after surgery protocols to reduce systemic opioid exposure.

Perioperative Medication Management

The surgeon must review the patient's medication list and issue specific instructions for perioperative management. Beta-blockers and statins should be continued through the perioperative period because abrupt withdrawal of either increases the risk of perioperative myocardial ischemia — beta-blocker withdrawal doubles the incidence of atrial fibrillation and MI, and statin withdrawal produces a rebound inflammatory state that destabilizes coronary plaque. Angiotensin-converting enzyme inhibitors and angiotensin receptor blockers are generally held on the morning of surgery because they potentiate intraoperative hypotension, particularly during induction. Oral hypoglycemic agents and non-insulin injectables are held on the day of surgery, and insulin regimens are adjusted (typically basal insulin at 50 to 80% of the usual dose the evening before or morning of surgery, with short-acting insulin held). Antiplatelet agents require nuanced management: aspirin is continued for most surgical procedures (the cardiac protection outweighs the marginal increase in surgical bleeding), while clopidogrel, prasugrel, and ticagrelor are held 5 to 7 days before elective surgery to allow platelet function recovery — except in patients with recent coronary stents, where the thrombotic risk of discontinuation exceeds the surgical bleeding risk and the operation should be delayed if possible.

Antibiotic Prophylaxis and Infection Prevention

Timing and Selection of Prophylactic Antibiotics

Surgical antibiotic prophylaxis prevents surgical site infection by ensuring bactericidal tissue concentrations at the time of incision and throughout the operative period. The dose must be administered within 60 minutes before skin incision — earlier administration allows tissue levels to fall below effective concentrations, and post-incision administration arrives after bacterial contamination has already occurred. Vancomycin and fluoroquinolones require a 120-minute infusion window because of their infusion-related adverse effects and slower tissue distribution. Redosing is required for procedures exceeding two half-lives of the prophylactic agent (cefazolin: redose at 4 hours) or for operations with significant blood loss exceeding 1,500 mL.

Agent selection is determined by the expected bacterial flora at the operative site. Clean cases (skin, soft tissue, hernia without mesh — though mesh cases typically receive prophylaxis) require coverage of skin flora: cefazolin 2 g IV (3 g if patient weight exceeds 120 kg) is the standard agent. Clean-contaminated cases involving the gastrointestinal tract require additional anaerobic coverage: cefazolin plus metronidazole, or cefoxitin alone. Biliary procedures require coverage of enteric gram-negative organisms: cefazolin alone is adequate for low-risk biliary surgery, while cefoxitin or ampicillin-sulbactam is preferred when acute cholecystitis or choledocholithiasis raises the contamination burden. For patients with a documented beta-lactam allergy producing anaphylaxis, clindamycin plus gentamicin provides alternative coverage, or vancomycin can substitute for gram-positive coverage.

Skin Preparation and Surgical Site Infection Bundle

Chlorhexidine-alcohol skin preparation is superior to povidone-iodine for reducing surgical site infection rates across clean and clean-contaminated procedures and is the current standard for all operative skin preparation unless the surgical site involves mucous membranes (where aqueous chlorhexidine or povidone-iodine is used) or the eyes (where povidone-iodine is preferred). The preparation is applied in concentric circles from the incision site outward and must dry completely before draping to achieve its full bactericidal effect and to eliminate the ignition risk of alcohol-based solutions in contact with electrosurgical devices. Preoperative chlorhexidine bathing (the night before and morning of surgery) further reduces skin bacterial load and is a standard element of surgical site infection prevention bundles.

CAUTION: Chlorhexidine-alcohol skin preparation is flammable. The solution must dry completely before draping, and pooling beneath the patient (in skin folds, under the drape, or on the operating table surface) must be eliminated. Ignition by monopolar electrosurgery on prep-soaked drapes has caused severe intraoperative burns.

Procedure Category	Recommended Agent	Dose	Redose Interval
Clean (hernia, breast, soft tissue)	Cefazolin	2 g IV (3 g if >120 kg)	Every 4 hours
Clean-contaminated (GI, biliary — low risk)	Cefazolin	2 g IV	Every 4 hours
Clean-contaminated (GI — colorectal)	Cefazolin + metronidazole	2 g IV + 500 mg IV	Cefazolin every 4 hours
Clean-contaminated (biliary — acute cholecystitis)	Cefoxitin or ampicillin-sulbactam	2 g IV or 3 g IV	Every 2 hours (cefoxitin)
Beta-lactam allergy (anaphylactic)	Clindamycin + gentamicin	900 mg IV + 5 mg/kg IV	Clindamycin every 6 hours

THE OPERATIVE DANGER ZONE ATLAS — Prophylactic Antibiotic Timing Failure

The Zone: The 60-minute window before skin incision — the interval during which prophylactic antibiotic tissue concentration must reach bactericidal levels. Failure to administer within this window negates the entire prophylactic strategy.

The Structure at Risk: The surgical wound and any implanted prosthetic material (mesh, vascular graft, joint prosthesis). Contamination with skin flora (Staphylococcus aureus, coagulase-negative staphylococci) and enteric organisms (Escherichia coli, Bacteroides fragilis) occurs within seconds of incision.

The Consequence: Surgical site infection rates double when prophylaxis is administered more than 60 minutes before incision or after incision has already been made. Deep surgical site infection involving mesh or prosthetic material may require explantation, prolonged antibiotic therapy, and staged reconstruction — converting an elective procedure into a months-long recovery.

The Safe Maneuver: Confirm antibiotic administration on the preoperative checklist (WHO Surgical Safety Checklist) before allowing incision to proceed. Verify the specific agent, dose, and time of administration. For procedures exceeding two drug half-lives, set a timer for redosing (cefazolin: 4 hours). The surgeon — not the circulating nurse alone — confirms prophylaxis at the pre-incision time-out.

Thromboprophylaxis and Anticoagulation Management

Venous Thromboembolism Risk Stratification

Venous thromboembolism — deep vein thrombosis and pulmonary embolism — is a preventable cause of postoperative death. The Caprini Risk Assessment Model scores patient-specific and procedure-specific risk factors to assign a cumulative VTE risk score: scores of 0 to 1 (very low risk) require early ambulation only; scores of 2 (low risk) warrant mechanical prophylaxis (intermittent pneumatic compression devices); scores of 3 to 4 (moderate risk) require pharmacological prophylaxis (low-molecular-weight heparin or unfractionated heparin) plus mechanical prophylaxis; scores of 5 or higher (high risk) require pharmacological prophylaxis plus mechanical prophylaxis with consideration for extended prophylaxis (4 weeks) after discharge for major abdominal or pelvic cancer surgery.

Mechanical Prophylaxis and Implementation

Intermittent pneumatic compression devices are the cornerstone of mechanical thromboprophylaxis and are indicated for virtually all surgical patients regardless of pharmacological prophylaxis status. IPC devices enhance venous return from the lower extremities and stimulate endogenous fibrinolysis through the release of tissue plasminogen activator from the venous endothelium. To be effective, devices must be applied before induction of anesthesia and remain in place continuously until the patient is ambulating independently — intermittent application (removing devices for transport, nursing care, or patient comfort) eliminates the fibrinolytic benefit and converts the intervention from prophylactic to decorative. Graduated compression stockings provide passive venous compression but are less effective than IPC devices as monotherapy and carry risk of skin breakdown, tourniquet effect from rolling, and posterior tibial nerve compression in patients with peripheral arterial disease — they should not be used in patients with an ankle-brachial index below 0.8.

Management of Chronic Anticoagulation

Patients on chronic anticoagulation for atrial fibrillation, mechanical heart valves, or prior venous thromboembolism require a structured bridging plan. Warfarin is held 5 days before surgery to allow the INR to fall below 1.5. Bridging with therapeutic-dose low-molecular-weight heparin is indicated for patients with high thrombotic risk (mechanical mitral valve, CHA2DS2-VASc score of 7 or higher, recent VTE within 3 months) and is held 24 hours before surgery with the last dose at 50% of therapeutic. Direct oral anticoagulants (rivaroxaban, apixaban, dabigatran) are held 48 to 72 hours before surgery depending on renal function and procedure bleeding risk — bridging is generally NOT required for DOACs because of their short half-lives and rapid offset. Resumption of anticoagulation postoperatively is a risk-benefit decision: the general principle is to resume pharmacological prophylaxis-dose anticoagulation 12 to 24 hours after hemostasis is achieved, transitioning to therapeutic dosing over the subsequent 48 to 72 hours.

Caprini Score	Risk Level	VTE Incidence (without prophylaxis)	Recommended Prophylaxis
0–1	Very low	Less than 0.5%	Early ambulation only
2	Low	1.5%	Intermittent pneumatic compression (IPC)
3–4	Moderate	3.0%	LMWH or UFH + IPC
5 or higher	High	6.0% or higher	LMWH or UFH + IPC; extended prophylaxis (4 weeks) for cancer surgery

Fluid and Electrolyte Management

Perioperative Fluid Physiology

Perioperative fluid management balances two competing harms: hypovolemia (reduced cardiac output, organ hypoperfusion, acute kidney injury) and hypervolemia (interstitial edema, pulmonary edema, anastomotic edema with impaired healing, prolonged ileus). The traditional approach of aggressive crystalloid resuscitation (so-called liberal fluid strategy of 10 to 15 mL/kg/hour intraoperatively) has been supplanted by goal-directed fluid therapy, which uses dynamic hemodynamic parameters (stroke volume variation, pulse pressure variation, cardiac output monitoring) to titrate fluid boluses to individual physiological need. Restrictive fluid strategies (less than 5 mL/kg/hour maintenance) reduce postoperative complications in major abdominal surgery, including surgical site infection, pneumonia, and anastomotic leak, compared with liberal strategies.

Crystalloid Versus Colloid Selection

Balanced crystalloid solutions (lactated Ringer solution, Plasma-Lyte) are the preferred perioperative resuscitation fluids because they approximate plasma electrolyte composition and avoid the hyperchloremic metabolic acidosis produced by large-volume normal saline (0.9% sodium chloride) infusions. Normal saline contains 154 mEq/L of chloride — 40% above plasma chloride concentration — and volumes exceeding 2 liters produce a dose-dependent non-anion-gap metabolic acidosis that can confound the interpretation of arterial blood gases and lactate clearance during resuscitation. Albumin (5% solution) is an effective volume expander for patients with hypoalbuminemia and is used in hepatic resection, liver transplantation, and large-volume paracentesis, but offers no survival advantage over crystalloid for routine perioperative resuscitation. Hydroxyethyl starch solutions are avoided because of their association with acute kidney injury and coagulopathy.

Perioperative Electrolyte Correction

Electrolyte abnormalities are common in surgical patients and must be corrected before elective surgery proceeds. Hypokalemia below 3.5 mEq/L (3.5 mmol/L) predisposes to cardiac arrhythmias under general anesthesia and impairs gastrointestinal motility postoperatively; replacement targets a serum potassium of 4.0 mEq/L or higher before induction, with intravenous potassium chloride administered at rates not exceeding 20 mEq/hour through a peripheral line (40 mEq/hour through a central line with cardiac monitoring). Hypomagnesemia below 1.8 mg/dL (0.74 mmol/L) frequently accompanies hypokalemia and renders potassium replacement ineffective until the magnesium deficit is corrected — the renal tubular potassium-sparing mechanism is magnesium-dependent, and patients with concurrent hypomagnesemia waste potassium in the urine despite aggressive replacement. Hypocalcemia and hyperkalemia are particularly dangerous in the perioperative setting because of their direct effects on cardiac conduction and must be corrected before the hemodynamic stress of induction and surgical manipulation.

CLINICAL PEARL: Intraoperative urine output of 0.5 mL/kg/hour is the traditional adequacy target, but it is an unreliable marker of volume status under general anesthesia — ADH secretion, sympathetic tone, and pneumoperitoneum all reduce urine output independent of intravascular volume. Dynamic parameters (stroke volume variation greater than 12% predicts fluid responsiveness) are more reliable for guiding intraoperative fluid boluses.

Nutritional Assessment and Optimization

Screening for Malnutrition

Malnutrition is present in 30 to 50% of surgical patients and is an independent predictor of surgical site infection, anastomotic leak, wound dehiscence, prolonged hospitalization, and mortality. The American Society for Parenteral and Enteral Nutrition (ASPEN) defines malnutrition using two or more of the following criteria: insufficient energy intake, weight loss, loss of muscle mass, loss of subcutaneous fat, localized or generalized fluid accumulation that may mask weight loss, and diminished functional status. Preoperative serum albumin below 3.0 g/dL is the single strongest biochemical predictor of postoperative morbidity and 30-day mortality across all surgical specialties — the NSQIP database consistently demonstrates a stepwise increase in complication rates for every 0.5 g/dL decrement in preoperative albumin below 3.5 g/dL.

Validated screening tools allow rapid identification of at-risk patients. The Nutritional Risk Screening 2002 (NRS-2002) combines nutritional status (weight loss, BMI, food intake) with disease severity (surgical stress grading) into a single score: patients scoring 3 or higher are at nutritional risk and require formal nutritional assessment and intervention. The Subjective Global Assessment (SGA) classifies patients as well-nourished, moderately malnourished, or severely malnourished based on history of weight change, dietary intake, functional capacity, and physical examination findings (subcutaneous fat loss, muscle wasting, ankle edema). Both tools have been validated in surgical populations and should be applied within 24 hours of admission for all patients undergoing major elective surgery.

Preoperative Nutritional Optimization

For elective surgery, patients identified as severely malnourished (albumin below 3.0 g/dL, weight loss exceeding 10% in 6 months, or BMI below 18.5) benefit from 7 to 14 days of preoperative nutritional supplementation before proceeding to operation. The preferred route is enteral (oral nutritional supplements or enteral tube feeding) because enteral nutrition maintains gut mucosal integrity, supports the gut-associated lymphoid tissue, and reduces the risk of bacterial translocation. Total parenteral nutrition is reserved for patients who cannot tolerate enteral feeding (complete bowel obstruction, high-output fistula, severe ileus) and should be initiated 7 to 10 days before surgery when the enteral route is not feasible. Immunonutrition — enteral formulas supplemented with arginine, omega-3 fatty acids, and nucleotides — reduces infectious complications and length of stay in malnourished patients undergoing major gastrointestinal surgery.

THE OPERATIVE DANGER ZONE ATLAS — Nutritional Depletion and Anastomotic Failure

The Zone: Any gastrointestinal anastomosis constructed in a patient with preoperative serum albumin below 3.0 g/dL or unrecognized severe malnutrition — the tissue healing environment where collagen synthesis and wound tensile strength are insufficient to maintain anastomotic integrity.

The Structure at Risk: The anastomotic suture or staple line — the weakest point of any gastrointestinal reconstruction. Collagen deposition at the anastomosis requires adequate protein substrate, vitamin C for hydroxylation, and zinc for metalloproteinase regulation, all of which are depleted in malnourished patients.

The Consequence: Anastomotic leak produces peritoneal contamination, sepsis, and fistula formation with mortality rates of 10 to 30% for colorectal anastomoses and up to 50% for esophageal anastomoses. Even when survived, anastomotic failure converts a curative resection into a prolonged recovery with diversion, drainage, and months of nutritional support.

The Safe Maneuver: Check serum albumin before every elective operation involving gastrointestinal anastomosis. For albumin below 3.0 g/dL, delay elective surgery 7 to 14 days for nutritional optimization (enteral preferred, parenteral if enteral is not feasible). When emergency surgery precludes optimization, consider proximal diversion (protective ileostomy or colostomy) rather than relying on primary anastomotic healing in the malnourished patient.

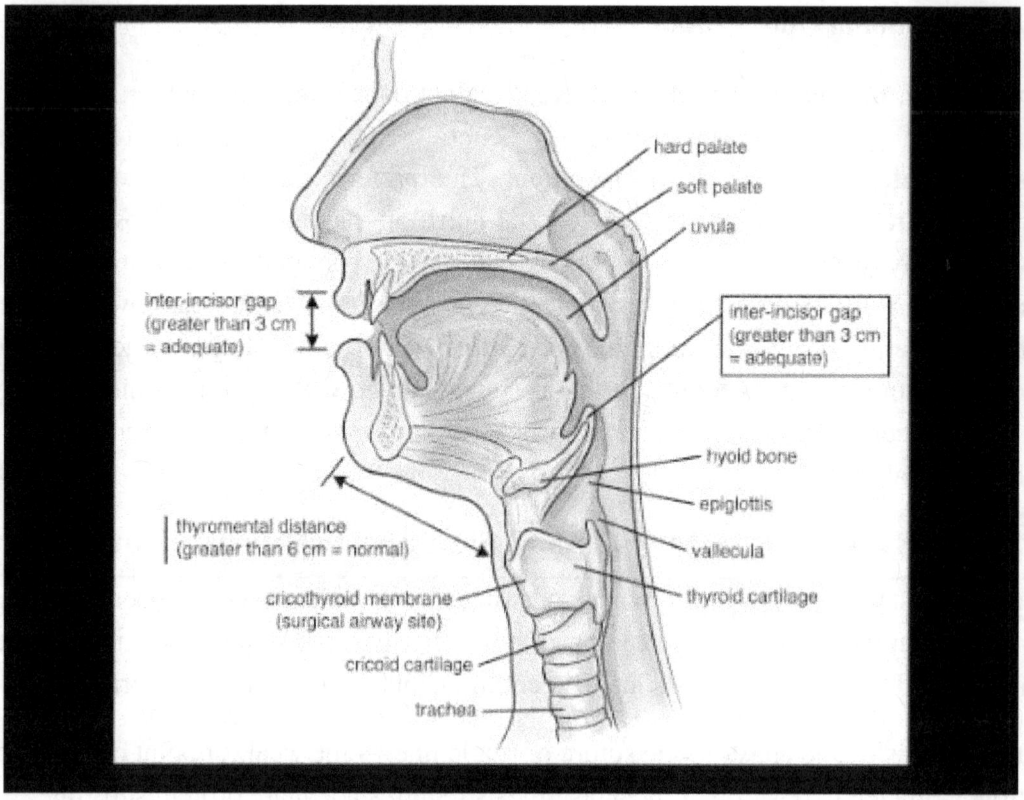

Postoperative Care and Complication Surveillance

Enhanced Recovery After Surgery Principles

Enhanced Recovery After Surgery (ERAS) protocols represent the systematic application of evidence-based perioperative interventions designed to reduce the surgical stress response, maintain physiological function, and accelerate recovery. Core ERAS elements include preoperative carbohydrate loading (clear liquid containing 50 g of complex carbohydrates 2 hours before induction), avoidance of routine mechanical bowel preparation for colorectal surgery, goal-directed intraoperative fluid therapy, multimodal opioid-sparing analgesia (acetaminophen, NSAIDs, gabapentinoids, regional blocks), early postoperative mobilization (out of bed within 6 hours of surgery), and early enteral nutrition (clear liquids on postoperative day 0, regular diet by postoperative day 1). ERAS protocols reduce length of stay by 1 to 3 days and lower complication rates by 30 to 50% across major abdominal surgical procedures when implemented with high compliance.

Postoperative Complication Surveillance

Systematic postoperative surveillance detects complications at the stage where intervention is most effective. The Clavien-Dindo classification provides a standardized grading system: Grade I (any deviation from normal course not requiring pharmacological, surgical, endoscopic, or radiological intervention); Grade II (requiring pharmacological treatment, including blood transfusion and total parenteral nutrition); Grade IIIa (requiring surgical, endoscopic, or radiological intervention not under general anesthesia); Grade IIIb (intervention under general anesthesia); Grade IV (life-threatening complication requiring ICU management); Grade V (death). Daily postoperative assessment must include systematic evaluation for the five most common surgical complications: surgical site infection (wound erythema, drainage, fever), venous thromboembolism (calf swelling, tachycardia, hypoxia), pulmonary complications (atelectasis, pneumonia — incentive spirometry compliance, oxygen saturation trend), urinary retention (bladder scan after catheter removal), and anastomotic leak (tachycardia, fever, abdominal pain disproportionate to expected postoperative course).

KEY POINT: Tachycardia (heart rate exceeding 100 bpm) on postoperative days 3 to 7 is the most sensitive early sign of anastomotic leak — it often precedes fever, leukocytosis, and peritoneal signs by 12 to 24 hours. Any unexplained tachycardia in this window after gastrointestinal surgery warrants CT with oral and IV contrast.

Postoperative Fever Evaluation

Postoperative fever follows a temporal pattern that guides the differential diagnosis. Fever within the first 48 hours is most commonly atelectasis-related (though the causal relationship between atelectasis and fever is debated, pulmonary toilet remains the primary intervention) or a response to the systemic inflammatory response to tissue injury. Fever on postoperative days 3 to 5 raises concern for urinary tract infection (especially after catheterization), catheter-related bloodstream infection, and early surgical site infection. Fever after postoperative day 5 suggests deep surgical site infection, anastomotic leak, abscess formation, Clostridium difficile colitis (particularly after antibiotic exposure), and venous thromboembolism. The traditional mnemonic 'Wind, Water, Wound, Walking, Wonder drugs' (atelectasis, UTI, SSI, DVT/PE, drug fever) remains a useful framework for systematic evaluation, though it oversimplifies the overlapping temporal windows. Each fever episode warrants directed investigation — chest radiograph, urinalysis with culture, wound inspection, lower extremity examination, and review of medication timing — rather than reflexive broad-spectrum antibiotic escalation.

Postoperative Ileus and Early Feeding

Postoperative ileus — the temporary cessation of coordinated bowel motility after abdominal surgery — is a physiological response to operative manipulation, anesthetic agents, opioid administration, and the inflammatory cascade at the operative site. Small bowel motility typically returns within 6 to 12 hours, gastric motility within 24 to 48 hours, and colonic motility within 48 to 72 hours. Prolonged ileus beyond 72 hours is pathological and warrants investigation for intra-abdominal complications (anastomotic leak, abscess, hematoma) and correction of contributing factors (hypokalemia, hypomagnesemia, ongoing opioid use). ERAS protocols have demonstrated that early enteral feeding (beginning on postoperative day 0) does not increase the incidence of ileus or aspiration and may in fact accelerate the return of bowel function by stimulating the gastrocolic reflex and maintaining enterocyte integrity. Alvimopan, a peripherally acting mu-opioid receptor antagonist, reduces the duration of ileus after open bowel surgery by blocking opioid-mediated inhibition of gut motility without reversing systemic analgesia.

THE OPERATIVE DANGER ZONE ATLAS — Failure to Rescue from Postoperative Complications

The Zone: The postoperative surveillance period from day 0 to discharge — the window in which early signs of major complications (anastomotic leak, pulmonary embolism, postoperative hemorrhage, sepsis) are subtle and can be missed by routine vital sign assessment alone.

The Structure at Risk: Patient survival. Failure to rescue — defined as death after a treatable postoperative complication — is the metric that separates high-performing surgical centers from low-performing ones. The complication RATE is similar across institutions; the MORTALITY after complications diverges dramatically based on surveillance rigor and escalation speed.

The Consequence: Delayed recognition of anastomotic leak converts a manageable Grade IIIa complication (percutaneous drainage) into a Grade IV septic shock requiring ICU admission, vasopressors, and reoperation with diversion — increasing mortality from below 5% to 15 to 30%. Delayed recognition of pulmonary embolism allows hemodynamic collapse from a treatable event.

The Safe Maneuver: Institute systematic twice-daily complication surveillance rounds using a checklist: heart rate trend (tachycardia as leak sentinel), wound inspection (erythema, drainage), pulmonary status (oxygen saturation trend, incentive spirometry volumes), lower extremity examination (calf asymmetry), and urine output. Escalate any unexplained tachycardia, fever, or clinical deterioration with imaging — CT with contrast for suspected leak, CT pulmonary angiography for suspected PE — within 4 hours of recognition.

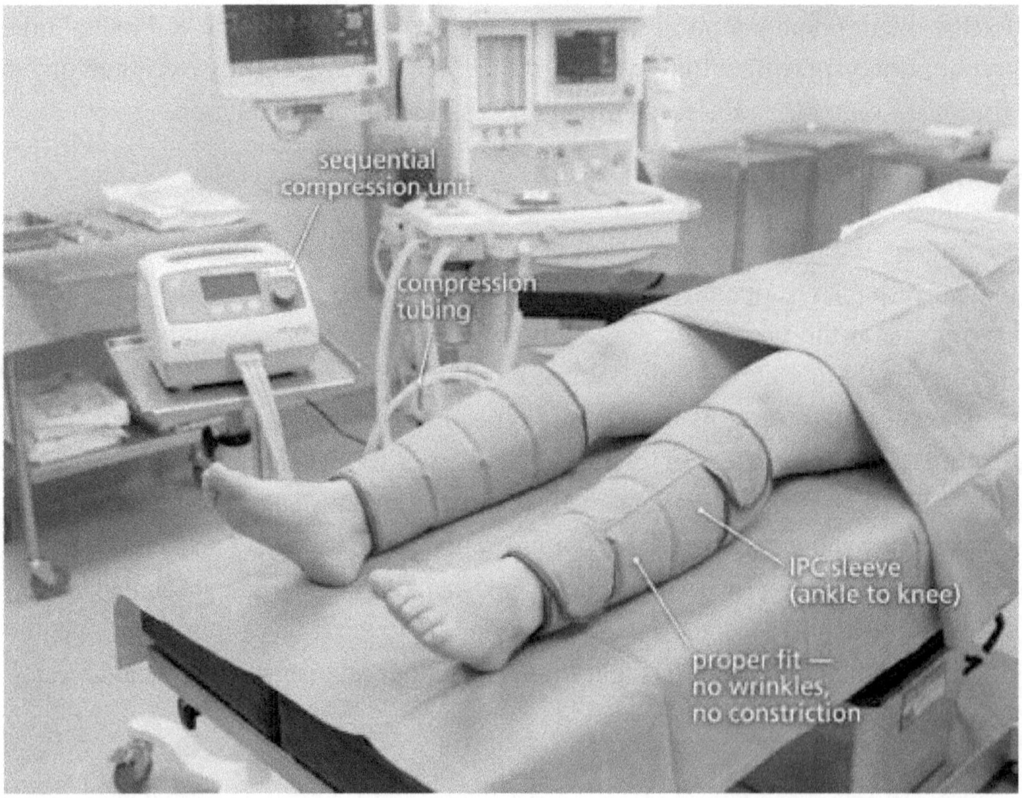

Clinical Case — Perioperative Cardiac Event After Inadequate Risk Stratification

A 68-year-old man with a history of type 2 diabetes requiring insulin, hypertension, and a remote transient ischemic attack presents for elective open sigmoid colectomy for recurrent diverticulitis. His preoperative evaluation notes 'cardiac history: negative' and he is cleared for surgery without further cardiac workup. His Revised Cardiac Risk Index, however, scores 3 points (intraperitoneal surgery, insulin-dependent diabetes, cerebrovascular disease), placing him in a high-risk category. His functional capacity is limited — he reports becoming dyspneic after walking one block — corresponding to fewer than 4 METs. No stress test is performed.

On postoperative day 2, the patient develops sustained tachycardia to 115 bpm, mild hypotension to 90/55 mmHg, and diaphoresis. A 12-lead ECG shows new ST depression in leads V4 through V6. Troponin I returns at 2.8 ng/mL (reference range below 0.04). Cardiology is consulted and diagnoses a type 2 perioperative myocardial infarction — demand ischemia driven by the surgical stress response in the setting of unrecognized coronary artery disease. Medical management with beta-blockade, antiplatelet therapy (aspirin only — dual antiplatelet therapy is held because of the fresh surgical wound), and hemodynamic optimization is initiated. Percutaneous intervention is deferred given the operative site bleeding risk. The patient recovers but requires an additional 5 days of monitored care.

This case demonstrates the consequence of failing to apply a systematic risk stratification tool. Had the RCRI been calculated preoperatively, the score of 3 combined with functional capacity below 4 METs would have triggered pharmacological stress testing per ACC/AHA guidelines. A positive stress test would have prompted coronary evaluation and optimization — potentially medical optimization with beta-blockade started 7 days before surgery, or coronary intervention before the elective colectomy. The Operative Danger Zone Atlas entry for perioperative cardiac risk encodes exactly this principle: the safe maneuver is systematic RCRI application, functional capacity assessment, and appropriate stress testing before committing the patient to the physiological stress of major surgery.

THE OPERATIVE DANGER ZONE ATLAS — Perioperative Safety Arcs

Unrecognized Perioperative Cardiac Risk: Patients with RCRI of 2 or more and functional capacity below 4 METs face perioperative MI rates exceeding 10%. Perioperative MI carries 15 to 25% 30-day mortality because interventional management is limited by the surgical wound. **Safe maneuver:** systematic RCRI scoring, functional capacity assessment, pharmacological stress testing when indicated, and continuation (never abrupt withdrawal) of chronic beta-blockade.

Prophylactic Antibiotic Timing Failure: Surgical site infection rates double when prophylaxis is given outside the 60-minute pre-incision window. Deep SSI involving mesh or prosthetic material may require explantation and staged reconstruction. **Safe maneuver:** verify agent, dose, and administration time at the pre-incision time-out; redose at two half-lives (cefazolin: every 4 hours); the surgeon personally confirms prophylaxis.

Nutritional Depletion and Anastomotic Failure: Serum albumin below 3.0 g/dL is the strongest biochemical predictor of anastomotic leak, wound dehiscence, and 30-day mortality. Collagen synthesis at the anastomosis requires adequate protein substrate. **Safe maneuver:** check albumin before all elective GI anastomoses; delay surgery 7 to 14 days for nutritional optimization when feasible; consider proximal diversion when emergency surgery precludes optimization.

Failure to Rescue from Postoperative Complications: Complication rates are similar across surgical centers — mortality after complications diverges based on surveillance rigor. Delayed leak recognition converts a Grade IIIa event into Grade IV sepsis with 15 to 30% mortality. **Safe maneuver:** twice-daily surveillance rounds using a complication checklist; treat unexplained postoperative tachycardia as leak until proven otherwise; escalate with imaging within 4 hours of recognition.

Summary and Key Concepts

Perioperative cardiac risk stratification using the Revised Cardiac Risk Index and functional capacity assessment (4 MET threshold) identifies patients who require further workup before intermediate- or high-risk surgery — perioperative MI carries 15 to 25% mortality because standard interventional management is limited by surgical wound considerations.

Antibiotic prophylaxis must be administered within 60 minutes before incision, with agent selection matched to expected wound flora (cefazolin for clean cases, cefazolin plus metronidazole or cefoxitin for GI cases), and redosing timed at two half-lives for prolonged procedures.

Venous thromboembolism prophylaxis is stratified by Caprini score: mechanical prophylaxis alone for low risk, combined pharmacological and mechanical for moderate and high risk, with extended 4-week prophylaxis for major abdominal cancer surgery.

Goal-directed fluid therapy using dynamic hemodynamic parameters replaces fixed-volume crystalloid protocols and reduces postoperative complications; balanced crystalloid solutions are preferred over normal saline to avoid hyperchloremic acidosis.

Preoperative serum albumin below 3.0 g/dL is the strongest biochemical predictor of postoperative morbidity — severely malnourished patients undergoing elective surgery benefit from 7 to 14 days of preoperative nutritional supplementation before proceeding.

Enhanced Recovery After Surgery protocols reduce length of stay and complication rates through systematic application of evidence-based perioperative interventions — multimodal analgesia, early mobilization, early nutrition, and goal-directed fluid management.

Postoperative tachycardia between days 3 and 7 after gastrointestinal surgery is the most sensitive early sign of anastomotic leak and warrants urgent CT with contrast — failure to rescue from treatable complications is the metric that separates high-performing from low-performing surgical centers.

CHAPTER 3: INGUINAL AND FEMORAL HERNIA REPAIR

Learning Objectives

1. Describe the layered anatomy of the inguinal canal, the boundaries of the myopectineal orifice, and the anatomical distinction between direct, indirect, and femoral hernias.
2. Perform the key operative steps of the Lichtenstein tension-free mesh repair, including identification and protection of the ilioinguinal and iliohypogastric nerves.
3. Compare the totally extraperitoneal (TEP) and transabdominal preperitoneal (TAPP) laparoscopic approaches with respect to mesh placement, peritoneal integrity, and anatomical landmarks.
4. Identify the Triangle of Doom and the Triangle of Pain in the preperitoneal space and describe the structures at risk from tack fixation in each zone.
5. Select the appropriate repair strategy for recurrent inguinal hernia based on the index repair approach and the anterior-posterior principle.
6. Describe the operative approach to femoral hernia repair and the anatomical rationale for avoiding lateral dissection at the femoral ring.

Anatomy of the Inguinal Region and Myopectineal Orifice

Layers of the Anterior Abdominal Wall

The inguinal canal is a 4 cm oblique passage through the anterior abdominal wall that transmits the spermatic cord in males and the round ligament in females. Understanding the layered anatomy is essential because each layer contributes a fascial covering to the cord structures, and the surgeon must recognize each layer during dissection to avoid entering the wrong plane. From superficial to deep, the layers are: skin, Camper fascia (superficial fatty layer of superficial fascia), Scarpa fascia (deep membranous layer of superficial fascia), external oblique aponeurosis, internal oblique muscle, transversus abdominis muscle, transversalis fascia, preperitoneal fat, and peritoneum. The external oblique aponeurosis forms the anterior wall of the inguinal canal and is the first major fascial layer encountered in an anterior open repair. The internal oblique and transversus abdominis muscles form the superior wall (roof) of the canal, and the transversalis fascia forms the posterior wall (floor) — the site of direct inguinal hernias.

The Myopectineal Orifice of Fruchaud

The myopectineal orifice is the conceptual framework that unifies all groin hernias under a single anatomical construct. Described by Fruchaud, it is the area of the abdominal wall bounded superiorly by the internal oblique and transversus abdominis muscles, inferiorly by the pectineal (Cooper) ligament and the superior pubic ramus, medially by the rectus abdominis muscle and its sheath, and laterally by the iliopsoas muscle. The inguinal ligament bisects this orifice: indirect inguinal hernias protrude through the deep inguinal ring (lateral to the inferior epigastric vessels) in the superior compartment; direct inguinal hernias protrude through the floor of Hesselbach triangle (medial to the inferior epigastric vessels) in the superior compartment; femoral hernias protrude through the femoral ring in the inferior compartment. This unified concept explains why laparoscopic preperitoneal mesh repairs (TEP and TAPP) are effective for all three hernia types — a single mesh placed in the preperitoneal space covers the entire myopectineal orifice.

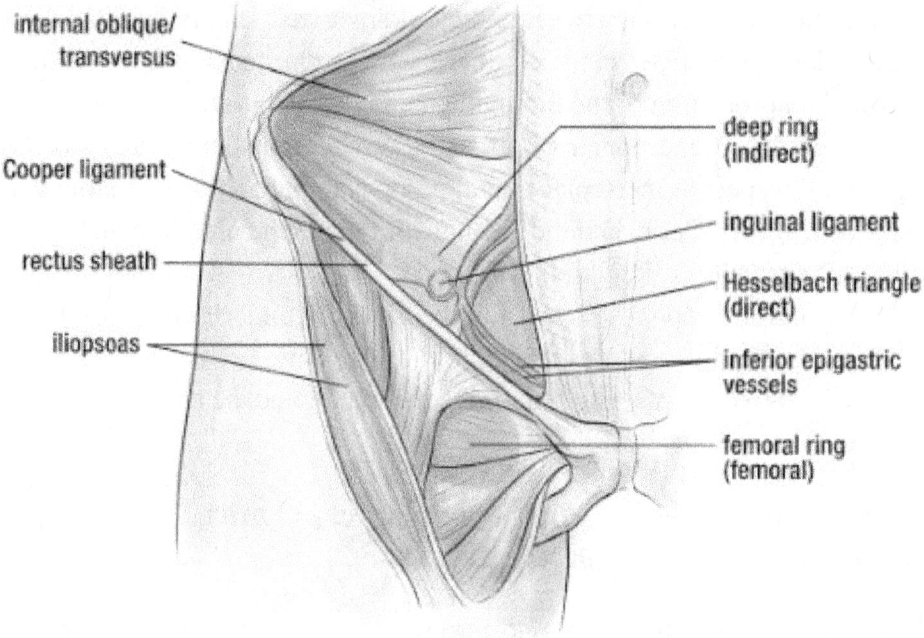

Epidemiology and Classification

Groin hernias are the most common condition requiring surgical intervention worldwide, with an estimated 20 million repairs performed annually. Inguinal hernias account for approximately 75% of all abdominal wall hernias, with a lifetime risk of 27% in men and 3% in women. The male predominance reflects the anatomical weakness created by testicular descent through the inguinal canal during fetal development — the processus vaginalis, which normally obliterates after descent, persists as a patent peritoneal conduit in indirect inguinal hernias. Indirect hernias are the most common type overall (accounting for roughly two-thirds of inguinal hernias), are more frequent in younger patients, and arise lateral to the inferior epigastric vessels through a congenitally patent or acquired deep ring. Direct hernias arise medial to the inferior epigastric vessels through an attenuated transversalis fascia floor and are associated with aging, collagen degradation, and chronic increases in intra-abdominal pressure (obesity, chronic cough, constipation, prostatism). Femoral hernias account for 3 to 5% of groin hernias but carry the highest rate of incarceration and strangulation.

Nyhus Type	Description	Characteristics
Type I	Indirect — normal deep ring	Pediatric indirect hernias with a patent processus vaginalis; deep ring not dilated
Type II	Indirect — dilated deep ring	Deep ring enlarged but posterior wall (Hesselbach triangle floor) intact; sac does not extend to the scrotum
Type III-A	Direct inguinal hernia	Posterior wall deficiency in Hesselbach triangle; transversalis fascia attenuated or absent
Type III-B	Indirect — massive deep ring	Deep ring so enlarged it encroaches on the posterior wall; includes pantaloon (combined direct and indirect) hernias and sliding hernias
Type III-C	Femoral hernia	Protrusion through the femoral ring below the inguinal ligament
Type IV	Recurrent hernia	Any recurrent hernia — subclassified as IV-A (direct), IV-B (indirect), IV-C (femoral), IV-D (combined)

Open Anterior Inguinal Hernia Repair (Lichtenstein Technique)

Operative Steps and Mesh Placement

The Lichtenstein tension-free mesh repair is the gold standard for open inguinal hernia repair. A 5 to 6 cm oblique incision is made 2 cm above and parallel to the inguinal ligament, centered over the deep inguinal ring. The external oblique aponeurosis is opened through the external ring, and the superior and inferior flaps are mobilized to expose the inguinal canal floor. The spermatic cord is mobilized circumferentially with a Penrose drain and elevated. For indirect hernias, the sac is identified arising from the deep ring, dissected free from the cord structures, and either reduced into the preperitoneal space (large sacs) or ligated and excised at the deep ring (small to moderate sacs). For direct hernias, the attenuated transversalis fascia is inverted with an absorbable suture. A polypropylene mesh (approximately 7.5 x 15 cm) is trimmed to fit the inguinal floor, secured medially to the pubic tubercle and inferiorly to the inguinal ligament with running nonabsorbable suture, and tailed around the spermatic cord at the deep ring to create a new, reinforced internal ring.

Nerve Identification and Preservation

Three nerves traverse the inguinal canal and are at risk during open repair. The ilioinguinal nerve (L1) runs between the external and internal oblique muscles, emerges through the external ring, and provides sensation to the ipsilateral medial thigh, mons pubis, and scrotum or labium majus — it is the nerve most commonly injured during anterior inguinal hernia repair and the most common cause of chronic postoperative inguinal pain. The iliohypogastric nerve (T12-L1) runs between the internal oblique and transversus abdominis, emerging through the internal oblique to provide sensation to the suprapubic region — it is at risk during superior flap dissection of the external oblique aponeurosis. The genital branch of the genitofemoral nerve (L1-L2) enters the inguinal canal through the deep ring, runs on the surface of the spermatic cord, and innervates the cremaster muscle and provides sensation to the scrotum — it is at risk during cord mobilization and deep ring reconstruction. The operative principle is 'see it and preserve it, or see it and resect it' — a nerve that is identified and intentionally divided produces predictable numbness but not pain, while a nerve that is partially injured or entrapped in mesh or suture produces chronic post-herniorrhaphy inguinodynia.

KEY POINT: Chronic post-herniorrhaphy inguinodynia (pain persisting beyond 3 months after repair) occurs in 10 to 12% of patients and is most commonly caused by nerve entrapment in mesh or suture rather than nerve transection. Deliberate neurectomy during the index repair is preferable to inadvertent partial nerve injury — a cleanly divided nerve produces numbness, not pain.

Outcomes and Evidence Base

The Lichtenstein repair achieves recurrence rates of 1 to 2% in experienced hands, a result attributable to the tension-free mesh principle — the mesh bridges the defect without approximating tissues under tension, which was the primary failure mechanism of older tissue-based repairs (Bassini, Shouldice, McVay). Multiple randomized controlled trials and meta-analyses confirm that mesh repair reduces recurrence by 50 to 75% compared to non-mesh techniques, regardless of hernia type. The Shouldice repair (a four-layer imbrication of the transversalis fascia and conjoint tendon using continuous nonabsorbable suture) remains the best-performing non-mesh technique, with recurrence rates of 1 to 4% in specialized centers, and is reserved for patients with mesh contraindications (active infection, contaminated field, strangulated hernia requiring bowel resection) or young patients who prefer to avoid permanent prosthetic material. Lightweight large-pore polypropylene mesh has largely replaced heavyweight small-pore mesh because it induces less foreign body reaction, less chronic pain, and better abdominal wall compliance without increasing recurrence.

EVIDENCE: The HerniaSurge Group international guideline (2018) recommends the Lichtenstein technique as the gold standard for open inguinal hernia repair and laparoscopic TEP or TAPP for bilateral and recurrent hernias. Watchful waiting is an acceptable alternative for men with minimally symptomatic inguinal hernias — the risk of acute incarceration in watchful waiting cohorts is approximately 0.2% per year.

THE OPERATIVE DANGER ZONE ATLAS — Ilioinguinal Nerve Injury During Anterior Repair

The Zone: The dissection plane between the external oblique aponeurosis and the internal oblique muscle during superior flap mobilization — the plane where the ilioinguinal nerve emerges from beneath the internal oblique and courses superficially toward the external ring.

The Structure at Risk: Ilioinguinal nerve (L1). The nerve lies directly beneath the external oblique aponeurosis and can be divided, crushed, or entrapped during aponeurotic opening, flap mobilization, or mesh fixation suture placement along the inguinal ligament.

The Consequence: Partial injury or mesh entrapment produces chronic post-herniorrhaphy inguinodynia — burning pain radiating to the medial thigh and scrotum or labium that persists beyond 3 months and may require reoperation with neurectomy and mesh explantation. This complication affects quality of life more severely than the index hernia.

The Safe Maneuver: Identify the ilioinguinal nerve immediately after opening the external oblique aponeurosis. Mobilize it off the inguinal canal floor with a vessel loop. Place mesh fixation sutures with the nerve under direct vision. If the nerve is inadvertently injured or cannot be preserved without compromising the repair, perform deliberate proximal neurectomy and bury the stump beneath the internal oblique to prevent neuroma formation.

Open Preperitoneal Inguinal Hernia Repair

Indications and Operative Approach

The open preperitoneal approach places the mesh behind the transversalis fascia in the preperitoneal space — the same plane used by laparoscopic TEP and TAPP repairs. This approach is indicated primarily for recurrent hernias after a prior anterior repair (the anterior-posterior principle: if the first repair was anterior, the recurrence is approached posteriorly), for femoral hernias (the preperitoneal space provides direct access to the femoral ring), and for bilateral inguinal hernias when laparoscopic repair is not feasible. The Stoppa (giant prosthetic reinforcement of the visceral sac) technique uses a large mesh placed bilaterally in the preperitoneal space to cover both myopectineal orifices through a lower midline incision. The Nyhus posterior approach accesses the preperitoneal space through a transverse incision above the inguinal canal, dividing the external and internal oblique muscles and the transversus abdominis to enter the preperitoneal plane.

Key Anatomical Landmarks in the Preperitoneal Space

The preperitoneal space contains vascular and neural structures that are invisible from an anterior approach but must be identified and protected during posterior repair. The inferior epigastric vessels course along the medial edge of the deep inguinal ring and serve as the landmark dividing direct (medial) from indirect (lateral) hernias. The external iliac artery and vein lie deep in the preperitoneal space, running laterally and inferiorly toward the femoral canal beneath the inguinal ligament. Cooper ligament — the dense periosteal condensation on the superior pubic ramus — is the key fixation point for mesh in posterior repairs and is exposed by sweeping the preperitoneal fat medially off the pubic symphysis. The corona mortis (aberrant obturator artery arising from the inferior epigastric or external iliac artery) crosses the superior pubic ramus between the external iliac vessels and the obturator foramen and is at risk of laceration during Cooper ligament exposure.

Laparoscopic Totally Extraperitoneal (TEP) Repair

Access and Dissection Technique

TEP repair accesses the preperitoneal space without entering the peritoneal cavity. A 1.5 cm infraumbilical incision is made, the anterior rectus sheath is opened, and the rectus muscle is retracted laterally to expose the posterior rectus sheath. A balloon dissector is inserted along the posterior rectus sheath toward the pubic symphysis and inflated to create the preperitoneal working space. Carbon dioxide insufflation to 12 mmHg maintains the space, and additional trocars are placed in the midline between the umbilicus and pubic symphysis. Dissection proceeds laterally to identify the inferior epigastric vessels (the medial-lateral hernia landmark), Cooper ligament inferiorly, the cord structures crossing into the deep ring, and the iliopubic tract (the laparoscopic equivalent of the inguinal ligament). A lightweight polypropylene or polyester mesh (at least 10 x 15 cm) is placed to cover the entire myopectineal orifice, overlapping the hernia defect by at least 3 cm in all directions.

Mesh Fixation and the Zones of Safe Tacking

Mesh fixation in TEP repair — whether by absorbable tacks, fibrin glue, or self-gripping mesh — must respect two anatomical danger zones defined by their contents. The Triangle of Doom is bounded medially by the vas deferens, laterally by the spermatic vessels, and contains the external iliac artery and vein — tack or staple fixation within this triangle risks life-threatening vascular injury. The Triangle of Pain is bounded medially by the spermatic vessels, laterally by the iliopubic tract, and contains the lateral femoral cutaneous nerve, the femoral branch of the genitofemoral nerve, and the femoral nerve — fixation in this zone risks chronic neuropathic pain. Safe fixation zones include Cooper ligament medially and the transversus abdominis aponeurotic arch superiorly, both of which are well away from the danger triangles.

Perioperative Considerations and Complication Prevention

Preoperative antibiotic prophylaxis is not routinely recommended for elective laparoscopic hernia repair in low-risk patients — meta-analytic evidence shows no significant reduction in surgical site infection rates with prophylaxis in clean laparoscopic groin hernia cases. Peritoneal tears during TEP dissection are the most common intraoperative complication, occurring in 5 to 10% of cases, and cause carbon dioxide escape into the peritoneal cavity with loss of the preperitoneal working space. Small peritoneal tears are managed by placing a Veress needle into the peritoneal cavity to vent the pneumoperitoneum while maintaining preperitoneal insufflation pressure. Larger tears may necessitate conversion to TAPP technique (using the peritoneal defect as the access point) or open repair. Seroma formation in the hernia sac space is the most common postoperative finding after laparoscopic repair, occurring in up to 25% of large hernias, and is generally self-limiting — aspiration is avoided because it introduces infection risk and does not accelerate resolution. Urinary retention after groin hernia repair under general anesthesia occurs in 3 to 5% of patients and is more frequent in older men with baseline obstructive symptoms.

THE OPERATIVE DANGER ZONE ATLAS — Triangle of Doom — Vascular Injury During Laparoscopic Hernia Repair

The Zone: The triangular space bounded medially by the vas deferens and laterally by the spermatic (gonadal) vessels, with its apex at the deep inguinal ring — visible during TEP and TAPP dissection deep to the peritoneal flap.

The Structure at Risk: External iliac artery and external iliac vein. Both vessels traverse the floor of this triangle as they course from the retroperitoneum toward the femoral canal beneath the inguinal ligament.

The Consequence: Tack, staple, or suture fixation through the iliac vein wall produces immediate hemorrhage that is extremely difficult to control laparoscopically because the vessel retracts into the retroperitoneum. Iliac artery injury risks distal limb ischemia. Either injury may require emergency open conversion with vascular control.

The Safe Maneuver: Never place tacks, staples, or sutures within the Triangle of Doom. Identify the vas deferens and gonadal vessels as boundaries before any fixation. Secure mesh medially to Cooper ligament and superiorly to the transversus aponeurotic arch — both safe fixation points well outside the triangle. If fixation is needed laterally, apply it only above the iliopubic tract.

Laparoscopic Transabdominal Preperitoneal (TAPP) Repair

Peritoneal Flap Development and Mesh Placement

TAPP repair enters the peritoneal cavity first and then creates a preperitoneal space by incising the peritoneum superior to the hernia defect. Three trocars are placed — a 10 mm umbilical camera port and two 5 mm working ports at the level of the umbilicus lateral to the rectus muscles. The peritoneum is incised from the anterior superior iliac spine to the medial umbilical ligament, creating a peritoneal flap that is dissected inferiorly to expose the preperitoneal space, the hernia defect, and the same anatomical landmarks as TEP (inferior epigastric vessels, Cooper ligament, cord structures, iliopubic tract, Triangle of Doom, Triangle of Pain). Mesh placement and fixation follow the same principles as TEP. The critical additional step unique to TAPP is closure of the peritoneal flap over the mesh — this prevents mesh contact with intraperitoneal contents, which reduces the risk of adhesion formation, bowel adhesion to mesh, and mesh erosion into viscera.

TAPP Versus TEP — Comparative Considerations

Both TEP and TAPP achieve equivalent long-term recurrence rates (1 to 2%) and are equally effective for unilateral and bilateral repairs. TEP offers the advantage of avoiding peritoneal entry and its associated complications (adhesion formation, port-site hernias at 10 mm trocar sites, rare small bowel obstruction from peritoneal flap defects), but it provides a smaller working space and has a steeper learning curve. TAPP provides superior visualization because the intraperitoneal vantage point allows direct identification of the hernia defect and contralateral exploration, and it is technically easier in patients with prior preperitoneal surgery or large inguinoscrotal hernias where space development is difficult. The choice between TEP and TAPP is primarily determined by surgeon experience and the specific clinical scenario.

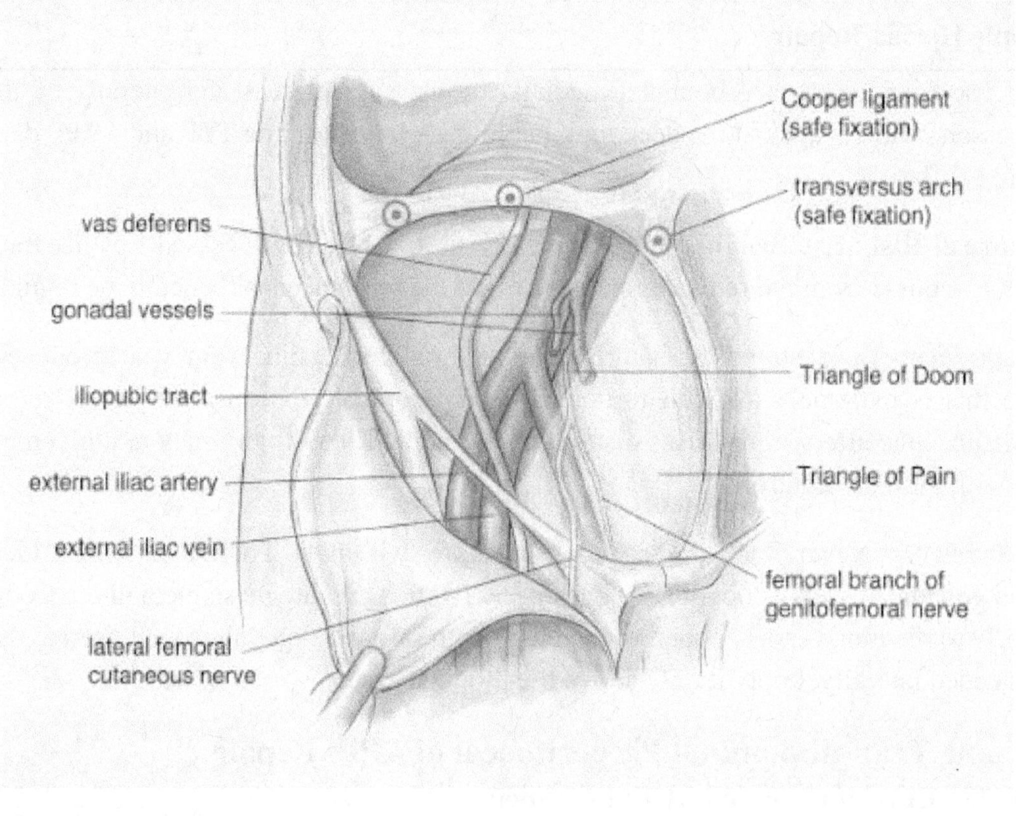

Femoral Hernia Repair

Anatomy of the Femoral Canal

Femoral hernias protrude through the femoral ring — the most medial compartment of the femoral sheath, bounded anteriorly by the inguinal ligament, posteriorly by Cooper ligament, medially by the lacunar ligament, and laterally by the femoral vein. The femoral canal normally contains lymphatic tissue (the node of Cloquet) and loose areolar fat. Femoral hernias account for only 3 to 5% of groin hernias overall but are disproportionately represented in emergency presentations because their rigid fascial boundaries make incarceration and strangulation common — up to 40% of femoral hernias present with incarceration at diagnosis. They are more common in women than men, and a femoral hernia should always be suspected in any woman presenting with a groin hernia, even when an inguinal hernia appears more likely on initial examination.

Operative Approach

Three approaches are available for femoral hernia repair: the infrainguinal (low) approach, the inguinal (Lotheissen-McVay) approach, and the preperitoneal approach (including laparoscopic TEP or TAPP). The infrainguinal approach provides direct access to the femoral canal through an incision below the inguinal ligament, the sac is reduced or excised, and the femoral ring is closed by approximating the inguinal ligament to Cooper ligament with interrupted nonabsorbable sutures or a mesh plug. The McVay repair closes the femoral ring as part of a comprehensive posterior wall reconstruction by suturing the transversus abdominis aponeurotic arch to Cooper ligament medially (closing the femoral canal) and transitioning to the inguinal ligament laterally. The preperitoneal approach (TEP or TAPP) is preferred when expertise is available because a single mesh covering the entire myopectineal orifice addresses both the femoral defect and any occult inguinal hernia simultaneously.

Special Populations and Emergency Presentation

In women, femoral hernias are nearly as common as inguinal hernias, and a careful examination of the femoral canal should accompany every groin hernia evaluation in female patients — a femoral hernia misdiagnosed as an inguinal hernia and repaired through an anterior approach alone leaves the femoral defect unaddressed and the patient at continued risk of incarceration. In emergency presentations with suspected bowel strangulation (signs of peritonitis, leukocytosis, lactate elevation, CT evidence of pneumatosis or portal venous gas), the surgical approach must provide access for bowel resection if nonviable bowel is found at reduction. A preperitoneal or inguinal approach with the option of extending to a lower midline laparotomy provides the necessary access. Use of prosthetic mesh in contaminated or potentially contaminated fields (bowel resection, gross contamination, fecal spillage) is contraindicated because of the risk of mesh infection — in these situations, the femoral ring is closed with a tissue repair (McVay or Cooper ligament repair) and mesh-based reinforcement is deferred to an elective interval procedure.

THE OPERATIVE DANGER ZONE ATLAS — Femoral Vein Injury During Femoral Ring Closure

---

The Zone: The lateral border of the femoral ring — the 1 to 2 mm interval between the femoral canal (containing the hernia) and the femoral vein (lying immediately lateral within the femoral sheath).

The Structure at Risk: Femoral vein. The vein forms the immediate lateral boundary of the femoral ring and is separated from the hernia sac by only the thin lateral wall of the femoral canal. During reduction of an incarcerated femoral hernia and closure of the ring, the vein is at direct risk of laceration, compression, or suture entrapment.

The Consequence: Femoral vein laceration produces immediate hemorrhage in a confined space that is difficult to control. Suture stenosis of the femoral vein increases the risk of postoperative deep vein thrombosis and chronic venous insufficiency in the ipsilateral limb. Complete vein ligation (if required for hemorrhage control) creates immediate venous outflow obstruction.

The Safe Maneuver: Visualize the femoral vein before placing any closure sutures. Place sutures through Cooper ligament and the inguinal ligament only — never blindly lateral to the reduced sac. Palpate the femoral artery pulse as a lateral landmark (the vein lies immediately medial to the artery). If placing a mesh plug in the femoral ring, size it to fit the canal snugly without compressing the vein. During laparoscopic repair, the vein is under direct vision; use tack fixation only at Cooper ligament, medial to the vein.

Recurrent Inguinal Hernia Management

The Anterior-Posterior Principle

Recurrent inguinal hernia after primary repair occurs in 1 to 4% of tension-free mesh repairs and reflects either technical failure (inadequate mesh overlap, mesh migration, missed hernia) or patient-related factors (connective tissue disorders, obesity, chronic cough, prostatism). The operative strategy for recurrence follows the anterior-posterior principle: if the primary repair was an anterior approach (Lichtenstein), the recurrence should be repaired through a posterior approach (laparoscopic TEP or TAPP, or open preperitoneal) to operate through virgin tissue planes rather than through the scar and mesh of the prior repair. Conversely, if the primary repair was a laparoscopic posterior approach, the recurrence should be repaired through an anterior approach. This principle minimizes the risk of injury to cord structures and nerves that are encased in scar tissue from the prior dissection, and it allows mesh placement in the undissected tissue plane for optimal incorporation.

Operative Considerations in the Reoperative Field

Reoperation in a previously repaired groin carries elevated risk of testicular ischemia (from spermatic cord devascularization during re-dissection through scar), chronic pain (from repeated nerve manipulation), and mesh infection (from contact with prior mesh material). When an anterior approach is used for recurrence after anterior repair (violating the anterior-posterior principle, sometimes necessary for patient or surgeon-specific reasons), the cord structures are identified proximal and distal to the scar and the prior mesh is partially excised only where necessary to identify the recurrent defect — complete mesh removal is avoided unless mesh infection is present. Testicular atrophy from ischemic orchitis occurs in 1 to 2% of reoperative inguinal hernia repairs and results from thrombosis of the pampiniform plexus and testicular artery due to excessive cord manipulation in a scarred field.

Chronic Post-Herniorrhaphy Pain — Evaluation and Management

Chronic post-herniorrhaphy inguinodynia (persistent groin pain beyond 3 months after repair) is the most significant long-term morbidity of inguinal hernia surgery, reported in 10 to 12% of patients across all repair techniques. The etiology is multifactorial: neuropathic pain from nerve entrapment or injury (ilioinguinal, iliohypogastric, or genital branch of the genitofemoral nerve), nociceptive pain from mesh-related foreign body reaction or mesh contraction, and inflammatory pain from mesh fixation devices or periostitis at the pubic tubercle. Evaluation begins with a careful history to characterize the pain quality (burning and radiating suggests neuropathic origin; deep aching suggests nociceptive or mesh-related causes) and a targeted physical examination including the pinch-roll test over the inguinal region (reproducing sharp, lancinating pain suggests cutaneous nerve entrapment). Diagnostic injection of local anesthetic at the suspected nerve entrapment site provides both diagnostic confirmation and temporary relief. Conservative management includes neuropathic pain medications (gabapentin, pregabalin, tricyclic antidepressants), targeted nerve blocks, and pulsed radiofrequency ablation. Surgical management — reserved for refractory cases after at least 6 to 12 months of conservative therapy — involves triple neurectomy (division of the ilioinguinal, iliohypogastric, and genital branch of the genitofemoral nerve) with or without mesh removal, and achieves pain relief in 70 to 80% of patients.

THE OPERATIVE DANGER ZONE ATLAS — Cord Devascularization During Reoperative Hernia Repair

The Zone: The spermatic cord within the inguinal canal during reoperative anterior repair — the segment where the cord structures (testicular artery, pampiniform venous plexus, vas deferens) are encased in scar tissue from the prior dissection and mesh.

The Structure at Risk: Testicular artery and pampiniform venous plexus. Both are incorporated into scar tissue around the prior mesh and cannot be distinguished from fibrotic tissue during re-dissection without meticulous technique.

The Consequence: Thrombosis of the pampiniform plexus and testicular artery produces ischemic orchitis (presenting as painful, swollen testicle 2 to 5 days postoperatively) leading to testicular atrophy in 1 to 2% of reoperative repairs. Once ischemic orchitis is established, no intervention reverses the atrophy.

The Safe Maneuver: Follow the anterior-posterior principle — approach the recurrence from the opposite side of the prior repair to operate through undissected planes. If anterior re-repair is unavoidable, identify the cord proximal and distal to the scar, minimize dissection of the cord off the mesh, and accept partial mesh preservation rather than risking complete cord devascularization through aggressive mesh removal.

Clinical Case — Incarcerated Femoral Hernia Presenting as Small Bowel Obstruction

A 72-year-old woman presents to the emergency department with 24 hours of crampy abdominal pain, nausea, vomiting, and obstipation. She has no prior surgical history. Abdominal examination reveals distension and diffuse tenderness without peritoneal signs. A CT scan of the abdomen and pelvis demonstrates dilated small bowel loops with a transition point at a right groin mass consistent with an incarcerated femoral hernia containing a loop of small bowel (Richter hernia). The incarcerated bowel wall shows mural thickening and adjacent fat stranding but no pneumatosis or portal venous gas.

The patient is taken urgently to the operating room for inguinal exploration and femoral hernia repair. Through an infrainguinal approach, the femoral canal is exposed and the incarcerated bowel loop is identified. The lacunar ligament is carefully divided medially to widen the femoral ring and permit atraumatic reduction of the incarcerated bowel — the division is performed away from the femoral vein laterally to avoid vascular injury. The reduced bowel loop shows serosal contusion and venous congestion but has a palpable mesenteric pulse, and the antimesenteric wall is intact without signs of full-thickness necrosis. After wrapping the segment in warm saline-soaked laparotomy sponges for 10 minutes, peristalsis resumes and the bowel color improves — criteria consistent with bowel viability. The femoral ring is closed with interrupted sutures between the inguinal ligament and Cooper ligament, reinforced with a mesh plug.

This case illustrates several key principles. Femoral hernias disproportionately present with incarceration because of the rigid, unyielding boundaries of the femoral ring. A Richter hernia involves only the antimesenteric wall of the bowel, so small bowel obstruction may be partial or intermittent — the lumen is not completely occluded, and the classic obstructive pattern may be incomplete on imaging. The decision to divide the lacunar ligament medially rather than the inguinal ligament superiorly is anatomically driven by the position of the femoral vein — the vein lies immediately lateral, making medial release the only safe direction for ring widening. Bowel viability assessment requires a combination of visual appearance (color, peristalsis), Doppler assessment of mesenteric pulse, and observation over 10 minutes — if viability remains indeterminate, bowel resection with primary anastomosis is safer than returning questionable bowel to the abdomen.

THE OPERATIVE DANGER ZONE ATLAS — Inguinal and Femoral Hernia Repair Dangers

Ilioinguinal Nerve Injury During Anterior Repair: The ilioinguinal nerve lies directly beneath the external oblique aponeurosis and is at risk during flap mobilization and mesh fixation. Partial injury or entrapment produces chronic post-herniorrhaphy inguinodynia in 10 to 12% of patients. **Safe maneuver:** identify the nerve immediately after opening the aponeurosis; protect with a vessel loop; if injured, perform deliberate neurectomy and bury the stump.

Triangle of Doom — Vascular Injury During Laparoscopic Repair: The triangle bounded by the vas deferens and gonadal vessels contains the external iliac artery and vein. Tack or staple fixation within this zone risks life-threatening hemorrhage from iliac vessel injury. **Safe maneuver:** never fix mesh within the Triangle of Doom; use Cooper ligament medially and the transversus arch superiorly as safe fixation points.

Femoral Vein Injury During Femoral Ring Closure: The femoral vein forms the immediate lateral boundary of the femoral ring. Sutures placed lateral to the hernia sac risk vein laceration or stenosis. **Safe maneuver:** visualize the vein; suture only through Cooper ligament and inguinal ligament; widen the ring medially (lacunar ligament) rather than laterally.

Cord Devascularization During Reoperative Repair: Spermatic cord structures are encased in scar tissue after prior repair. Aggressive re-dissection produces testicular ischemia and atrophy in 1 to 2% of reoperations. **Safe maneuver:** follow the anterior-posterior principle — approach recurrence from the opposite side; minimize cord dissection in scarred fields.

Summary and Key Concepts

The myopectineal orifice of Fruchaud unifies all groin hernias under a single anatomical framework — indirect inguinal (lateral to inferior epigastric vessels), direct inguinal (medial to inferior epigastric vessels), and femoral (below inguinal ligament) — and explains why preperitoneal mesh covering the entire orifice addresses all three hernia types.

The Lichtenstein tension-free mesh repair requires identification and preservation of the ilioinguinal, iliohypogastric, and genital branch of the genitofemoral nerves — chronic post-herniorrhaphy pain occurs in 10 to 12% of patients and is caused by nerve entrapment rather than nerve transection.

The Triangle of Doom (vas deferens and gonadal vessels bounding the iliac vessels) and the Triangle of Pain (gonadal vessels and iliopubic tract bounding the lateral cutaneous and genitofemoral nerves) define the zones where mesh fixation during TEP and TAPP repair must never be placed.

Femoral hernias present with incarceration in up to 40% of cases because of the rigid unyielding boundaries of the femoral ring — femoral hernia should be suspected in any woman presenting with a groin hernia, and repair should widen the ring medially (lacunar ligament) to protect the femoral vein laterally.

Recurrent inguinal hernia management follows the anterior-posterior principle — if the index repair was anterior, the recurrence is best approached posteriorly, and vice versa — to minimize cord devascularization, nerve injury, and mesh infection in the reoperative field.

Bowel viability assessment during incarcerated hernia repair requires visual inspection (color, peristalsis), Doppler mesenteric pulse assessment, and 10-minute warm saline observation — indeterminate viability warrants resection rather than reduction of questionable bowel.

CHAPTER 4: VENTRAL, INCISIONAL, AND COMPLEX ABDOMINAL WALL HERNIA REPAIR

Learning Objectives

1. Describe the layered anatomy of the anterior abdominal wall, including the rectus sheath and its anterior and posterior components above and below the arcuate line.
2. Perform primary repair of umbilical and epigastric hernias and identify the criteria for mesh reinforcement based on defect size and patient risk factors.
3. Execute an open retrorectus (Rives-Stoppa) mesh repair for incisional hernia, including posterior rectus sheath closure and mesh placement.
4. Compare intraperitoneal onlay mesh (IPOM) repair with retrorectus mesh placement regarding mesh-tissue interface, adhesion risk, and recurrence outcomes.
5. Describe the operative steps and anatomical plane of the robotic transversus abdominis release (rTAR) and identify the neurovascular structures at risk during lateral dissection.
6. Differentiate anterior component separation (external oblique release) from posterior component separation (transversus abdominis release) and select the appropriate technique based on defect size and contamination status.

Abdominal Wall Anatomy and Fascial Layers

Rectus Sheath Composition and the Arcuate Line

The anterior abdominal wall is a layered musculofascial structure whose understanding is essential for hernia repair because every repair technique is defined by the plane in which the mesh is placed. From superficial to deep, the layers are: skin, subcutaneous fat (Camper and Scarpa fascia), anterior rectus sheath, rectus abdominis muscle, posterior rectus sheath, transversalis fascia, preperitoneal fat, and peritoneum. The rectus sheath is formed by the aponeuroses of the three lateral abdominal wall muscles (external oblique, internal oblique, and transversus abdominis) and changes composition at the arcuate line (semicircular line of Douglas), located approximately one-third of the distance from the umbilicus to the pubic symphysis. Above the arcuate line, the anterior rectus sheath is formed by the external oblique aponeurosis and the anterior lamella of the internal oblique aponeurosis, while the posterior rectus sheath is formed by the posterior lamella of the internal oblique aponeurosis and the transversus abdominis aponeurosis. Below the arcuate line, all three aponeuroses pass anterior to the rectus muscle — the posterior rectus sheath is absent, and the rectus muscle rests directly on the transversalis fascia. This transition explains why incisional hernias in the infraumbilical midline have less fascial support for repair and why retrorectus mesh placement below the arcuate line requires the surgeon to develop the preperitoneal plane.

The Lateral Abdominal Wall Muscles and Their Neurovascular Supply

The three lateral abdominal wall muscles — external oblique, internal oblique, and transversus abdominis — provide dynamic support to the abdominal wall through their concentric contraction and aponeurotic contributions to the linea alba and rectus sheath. The segmental neurovascular supply to these muscles and to the rectus abdominis runs between the internal oblique and transversus abdominis muscles (the neurovascular plane) and consists of the lower thoracic intercostal nerves (T7 through T12) and the subcostal vessels. These nerves and vessels enter the lateral abdominal wall posteriorly, course anteriorly in the neurovascular plane, and penetrate the posterior rectus sheath to supply the rectus muscle. During component separation techniques, preserving these segmental neurovascular bundles is essential — denervation of the rectus muscle produces atrophy and functional weakness that can predispose to hernia recurrence despite technically successful fascial closure.

The Linea Alba and Incisional Hernia Pathophysiology

The linea alba is the midline fibrous raphe formed by the decussation of the aponeuroses of the three lateral muscles. It extends from the xiphoid process to the pubic symphysis and is the site of midline laparotomy incisions — and, consequently, the most common location for incisional hernias. Incisional hernias develop in 10 to 20% of patients after midline laparotomy, with the highest incidence occurring within the first 3 years. Risk factors include surgical site infection (which increases incisional hernia risk three- to fivefold), obesity, emergency surgery, midline incisions longer than 18 cm, connective tissue disorders (Ehlers-Danlos syndrome, Marfan syndrome), chronic corticosteroid use, and fascial closure technique. Current evidence supports a small-bite continuous closure technique using a slowly absorbable suture (such as polydioxanone) with a suture-to-wound-length ratio of at least 4:1 to minimize fascial ischemia and reduce incisional hernia rates.

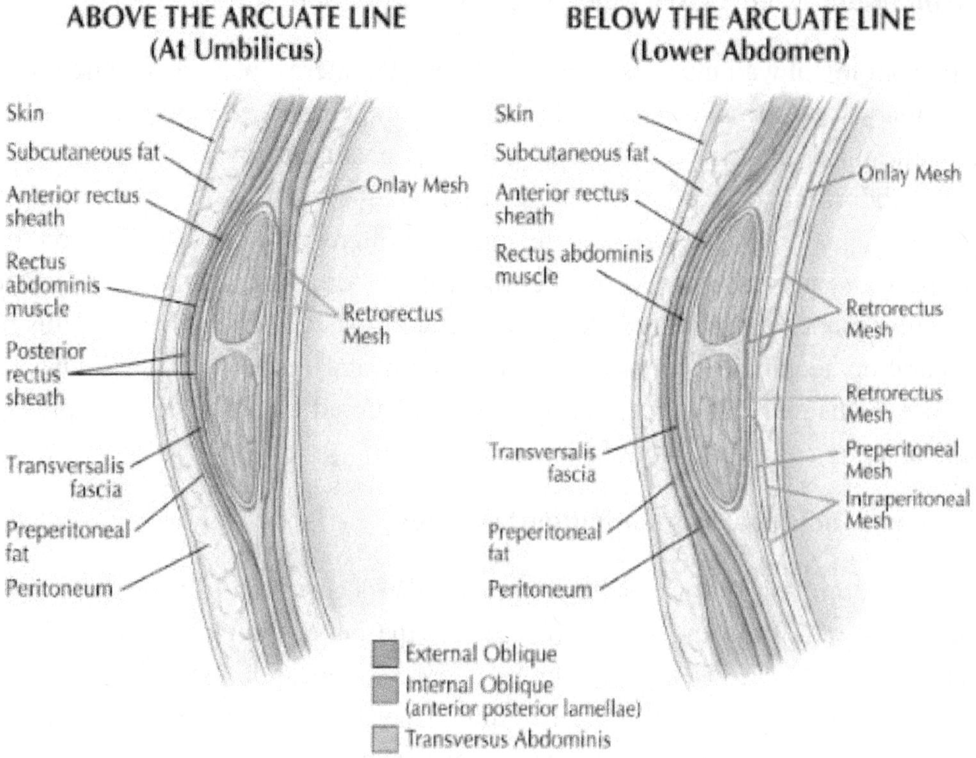

Primary Umbilical and Epigastric Hernia Repair

Indications and Operative Technique

Umbilical hernias in adults are acquired defects at the umbilical ring caused by progressive fascial weakening from obesity, pregnancy, ascites, or chronic intra-abdominal pressure elevation. Epigastric hernias are defects in the linea alba between the xiphoid process and the umbilicus through which preperitoneal fat herniates, often producing localized pain disproportionate to the small defect size. Both are repaired electively when symptomatic. Small defects (less than 2 cm) may be closed primarily with interrupted nonabsorbable sutures in a figure-of-eight or horizontal mattress pattern, placing the sutures through the fascial edges with a 1 cm bite. However, primary suture repair of umbilical hernias carries recurrence rates of 10 to 30%, and current evidence supports mesh reinforcement even for small umbilical hernias — a randomized controlled trial demonstrated a reduction in recurrence from 11% with suture repair to 1% with mesh reinforcement. Mesh placement may be in the onlay position (superficial to the anterior rectus sheath), the sublay/retrorectus position, or the preperitoneal position. For defects larger than 2 cm, mesh reinforcement is considered the standard of care.

Mesh Selection and Plane of Placement

The plane of mesh placement determines the biomechanical behavior of the repair and the risk of mesh-related complications. The onlay position (mesh placed superficial to the anterior fascia) provides the simplest technical approach but requires creation of subcutaneous lipocutaneous flaps, which increases the risk of seroma and surgical site infection. The retrorectus (sublay) position places the mesh between the rectus muscle and the posterior rectus sheath — this plane is preferred because intra-abdominal pressure pushes the mesh against the abdominal wall (Pascal principle), the mesh is separated from the subcutaneous space (reducing wound complication risk), and it is separated from the peritoneal cavity (eliminating visceral adhesion risk). For small umbilical repairs where retrorectus access is impractical, a preperitoneal mesh placed through the hernia defect and spread flat behind the fascia provides a similar advantage with less dissection.

Open Incisional Hernia Repair With Mesh

Retrorectus (Rives-Stoppa) Repair — Operative Steps

The retrorectus (Rives-Stoppa) repair is the gold standard for open incisional hernia repair. The prior midline incision scar is excised, skin and subcutaneous flaps are raised to expose the anterior rectus sheath bilaterally, and the hernia sac and its contents are reduced. The anterior rectus sheath is incised along the medial edge of each rectus muscle, and the rectus muscles are elevated off the posterior rectus sheath using a combination of blunt and electrocautery dissection. This creates the retrorectus space — the plane between the posterior surface of the rectus muscle and the anterior surface of the posterior rectus sheath. The dissection extends laterally to the semilunar line on each side (the lateral border of the rectus sheath, where the lateral muscle aponeuroses converge). Perforating segmental neurovascular bundles entering the rectus muscle from the posterior sheath are identified and preserved during lateral dissection. The posterior rectus sheath edges are then re-approximated in the midline with a running absorbable suture to reconstitute the posterior layer and create a closed retrorectus pocket. A large polypropylene or polyester mesh (with at least 5 cm of overlap beyond the hernia defect in all directions) is placed flat in the retrorectus space, and the anterior rectus sheath edges are re-approximated in the midline over the mesh. Closed suction drains are typically placed in the retrorectus space superficial to the mesh.

Outcomes and Recurrence Prevention

The Rives-Stoppa repair achieves recurrence rates of 5 to 10% in long-term follow-up, significantly superior to primary suture repair without mesh (which carries recurrence rates of 30 to 50% for incisional hernias). The biomechanical advantage of retrorectus mesh placement is the Pascal principle: intra-abdominal pressure acts uniformly on the mesh and pushes it against the abdominal wall musculature, converting the pressure that caused the hernia into the force that keeps the mesh in place. This is the same principle that makes preperitoneal mesh effective in inguinal hernia repair. Adequate mesh overlap (at least 5 cm beyond the defect edges in all directions) is the single most important modifiable technical factor in preventing recurrence — studies consistently demonstrate that inadequate overlap is the primary cause of mesh-related hernia recurrence.

KEY POINT: The retrorectus (Rives-Stoppa) space is the preferred plane for mesh placement in incisional hernia repair. It separates the mesh from the subcutaneous space (reducing wound infection risk) and from the peritoneal cavity (eliminating visceral adhesion risk), while harnessing intra-abdominal pressure to maintain the mesh in position against the musculature.

THE OPERATIVE DANGER ZONE ATLAS — Segmental Neurovascular Injury During Retrorectus Dissection

The Zone: The lateral extent of the retrorectus dissection along the posterior rectus sheath — the zone where the segmental intercostal neurovascular bundles (T7 through T12) penetrate the posterior sheath to enter the rectus muscle from its deep surface.

The Structure at Risk: Segmental intercostal nerves and accompanying vessels entering the rectus abdominis muscle through the posterior rectus sheath. These bundles run in the neurovascular plane between the internal oblique and transversus abdominis muscles before penetrating the posterior sheath at or near the semilunar line.

The Consequence: Division of segmental neurovascular bundles produces denervation of the corresponding rectus muscle segment, leading to muscle atrophy, abdominal wall bulging, and functional weakness. Bilateral extensive denervation can produce a thin, atonic abdominal wall that predisposes to hernia recurrence despite technically successful fascial closure and mesh placement.

The Safe Maneuver: During retrorectus dissection, extend laterally only to the semilunar line unless additional space is required. Identify perforating neurovascular bundles as they enter the posterior surface of the rectus muscle and preserve them by developing the retrorectus space superficial to (anterior to) each bundle. If a bundle must be divided for adequate mesh placement, limit the number of sacrificed bundles to maintain functional innervation of the majority of the muscle.

Laparoscopic Ventral Hernia Repair (IPOM)

Intraperitoneal Onlay Mesh Technique

Laparoscopic intraperitoneal onlay mesh (IPOM) repair places mesh directly on the peritoneal surface of the abdominal wall, covering the hernia defect from within the peritoneal cavity. The patient is positioned supine, and trocar placement is determined by the hernia location — typically placed as far laterally as possible to maximize the working angle and avoid the hernia defect. Adhesiolysis is performed to free the abdominal wall of all omental and bowel adhesions in the planned mesh coverage area. The hernia sac contents are reduced, and the defect is measured intracorporeally. A composite or barrier-coated mesh (with an antiadhesive surface facing the viscera and a tissue-integrating surface facing the abdominal wall) is introduced through the largest trocar and positioned to overlap the defect by at least 5 cm in all directions. The mesh is secured with a combination of transfascial sutures placed through the abdominal wall at the four quadrants and absorbable tacks around the perimeter.

Mesh Selection and Adhesion Prevention

The critical distinction in IPOM repair is the requirement for a barrier-coated or composite mesh rather than an uncoated polypropylene mesh. Uncoated polypropylene placed in direct contact with the visceral peritoneum produces dense adhesions to the bowel in virtually 100% of cases, creating the risk of bowel obstruction, fistula formation, and mesh erosion into the intestinal lumen. Barrier coatings (expanded polytetrafluoroethylene, oxidized regenerated cellulose, sodium hyaluronate-carboxymethylcellulose, collagen-polyethylene glycol, or omega-3 fatty acid coating) reduce but do not eliminate adhesion formation — no currently available barrier coating provides permanent adhesion protection. This limitation is the primary argument favoring retrorectus and preperitoneal mesh placement (where the mesh never contacts the viscera) over IPOM when technically feasible. The IPOM-Plus technique, which adds primary fascial closure of the defect before mesh placement, has emerged as a modification that improves outcomes by restoring the linea alba anatomy and reducing seroma formation beneath the mesh.

CAUTION: Uncoated polypropylene mesh must never be placed in direct contact with the visceral peritoneum. Dense visceral adhesions to uncoated mesh develop in virtually all cases and can produce bowel obstruction, enterocutaneous fistula, and mesh erosion into the intestinal lumen — complications that require complex reoperation with mesh explantation and potential bowel resection.

THE OPERATIVE DANGER ZONE ATLAS — Inadvertent Enterotomy During Adhesiolysis for Ventral Hernia Repair

---

The Zone: The interface between bowel loops or omentum and the anterior abdominal wall within and surrounding the hernia defect — the adhesion plane encountered during initial lysis to clear the mesh target area.

The Structure at Risk: Small bowel serosa and full-thickness wall, particularly loops adherent to the prior incision, mesh from a prior repair, or the hernia sac itself. The loops most at risk are those directly adherent to the fascial edges of the defect, where the plane between bowel and fascia may be obliterated.

The Consequence: Unrecognized enterotomy during adhesiolysis produces peritoneal contamination. If prosthetic mesh is placed over an unrecognized bowel injury, the resulting peritonitis leads to mesh infection, enterocutaneous fistula, sepsis, and the need for mesh explantation, bowel resection, and temporary diversion. Recognized enterotomy precludes the use of permanent synthetic mesh, converting a planned definitive repair into a contaminated-field operation.

The Safe Maneuver: Use sharp dissection close to the abdominal wall (rather than the bowel) when lysing adhesions. Avoid energy devices on bowel-to-wall adhesions — thermal spread can produce delayed perforation that manifests 3 to 7 days postoperatively. Inspect the entire length of freed bowel for serosal injuries after adhesiolysis is complete. If an enterotomy is recognized, repair the bowel, irrigate the peritoneal cavity, and convert to a biologic mesh repair or primary suture repair with delayed mesh placement at a second stage.

Robotic Transversus Abdominis Release (rTAR)

Operative Technique and Anatomical Plane

Robotic transversus abdominis release (rTAR) is a minimally invasive approach to posterior component separation that replicates the open transversus abdominis release (TAR) through a robotic platform. The procedure accesses the retrorectus space via a lateral trocar arrangement (typically four robotic ports placed along the left or right flank), enters the retrorectus space through the ipsilateral posterior rectus sheath, and extends the dissection across the midline to the contralateral semilunar line. The transversus abdominis muscle is then divided along its medial border just lateral to the semilunar line, entering the plane between the transversus abdominis muscle and the transversalis fascia — this is the transversus abdominis release itself. The release allows the posterior rectus sheath and transversalis fascia to advance medially, enabling midline posterior closure even for wide defects (up to 12 to 15 cm). A large uncoated polypropylene mesh is placed in this sublay position (retrorectus-preperitoneal plane) with wide overlap, and the posterior layer (posterior rectus sheath and transversalis fascia) is closed over the mesh to exclude it from the peritoneal cavity.

Advantages and Patient Selection

The rTAR approach offers several advantages over the open TAR: reduced surgical site complications (wound infection, seroma, surgical site occurrences) because the anterior abdominal wall soft tissue is not dissected through a large midline incision, shorter hospital stay, less postoperative pain, and equivalent recurrence rates in early comparative series. The robotic platform provides three-dimensional high-definition visualization and wristed instrument articulation that facilitates the precise lateral dissection required for transversus abdominis division and neurovascular bundle identification. Patient selection for rTAR includes moderate to large incisional hernias (defect width 6 to 15 cm), patients with loss of domain (hernia contents that chronically reside outside the abdominal cavity), and patients who have failed prior laparoscopic IPOM repair. Relative contraindications include extensive prior lateral abdominal wall surgery, hostile abdomen with dense adhesions precluding safe lateral port placement, and defects requiring combined flap coverage.

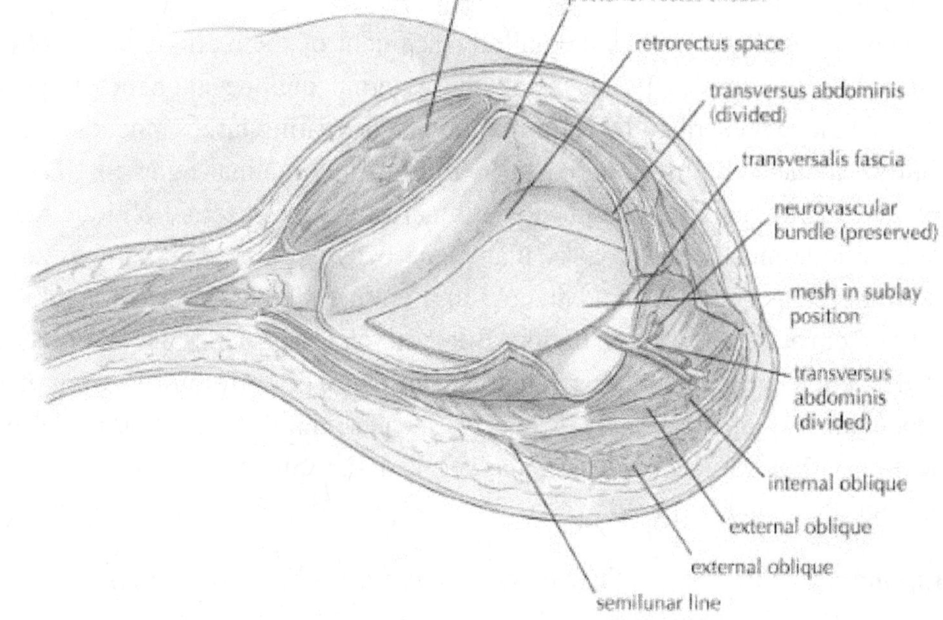

THE OPERATIVE DANGER ZONE ATLAS — Neurovascular Bundle Injury During Transversus Abdominis Release

---

The Zone: The lateral dissection plane during transversus abdominis release at the semilunar line — where the division of the transversus abdominis muscle passes immediately adjacent to the segmental intercostal neurovascular bundles running in the neurovascular plane between the internal oblique and transversus abdominis muscles.

The Structure at Risk: Segmental intercostal nerves (T7 through T12) and their accompanying arteries and veins. These bundles run in the plane between the internal oblique and transversus abdominis — the same plane that is entered when the transversus is divided at its medial border.

The Consequence: Division of multiple segmental neurovascular bundles during lateral release produces ipsilateral rectus denervation with muscle atrophy and abdominal wall bulge. Arterial branch injury causes bleeding in the neurovascular plane that can be difficult to control and compromises the blood supply to the rectus muscle. Bilateral extensive denervation produces a functionally incompetent abdominal wall.

The Safe Maneuver: Divide the transversus abdominis muscle at its medial border close to the linea semilunaris, staying medial to the neurovascular bundles. Identify each bundle as it courses from lateral to medial in the neurovascular plane and dissect the transversus fibers off each bundle individually rather than dividing the muscle in a single sweep. The robotic platform's wristed instruments and magnified three-dimensional visualization facilitate this precise dissection around each bundle.

Component Separation Techniques (Anterior and Posterior)

Anterior Component Separation — External Oblique Release

Anterior component separation achieves medial advancement of the rectus-internal oblique-transversus abdominis musculofascial complex by releasing the external oblique aponeurosis lateral to the linea semilunaris. The technique, described by Ramirez, involves creating large lipocutaneous flaps to expose the external oblique aponeurosis from the costal margin to the inguinal ligament. The external oblique aponeurosis is incised 2 cm lateral to the linea semilunaris, and the external oblique muscle is separated from the internal oblique muscle in the avascular plane between them. This release allows the rectus-internal oblique-transversus complex to advance 3 to 5 cm per side at the waist level, 5 to 10 cm at the umbilicus, and 1 to 3 cm at the suprapubic region. Bilateral release provides a total of 6 to 20 cm of medial advancement, sufficient to close many large incisional hernias. The perforator-sparing modification limits the extent of lipocutaneous flap creation by preserving the periumbilical perforator vessels, which reduces wound complications (skin flap necrosis, seroma, surgical site infection) — the major limitation of the classic open anterior component separation.

Posterior Component Separation — Transversus Abdominis Release (TAR)

Posterior component separation releases the transversus abdominis muscle at its medial border to achieve medial advancement of the posterior rectus sheath and transversalis fascia. The technique, described by Novitsky, accesses the retrorectus space as in the Rives-Stoppa repair, then extends the dissection lateral to the semilunar line by dividing the transversus abdominis fibers off the transversalis fascia. This releases the posterior layer and allows it to advance medially for midline closure, while creating a large retromuscular-preperitoneal pocket for mesh placement. TAR provides 6 to 10 cm of medial advancement per side and has largely replaced anterior component separation for large defects because the mesh is placed in a sublay position (retrorectus-preperitoneal), the anterior abdominal wall skin and soft tissues are not undermined (reducing wound complications), and uncoated macroporous mesh can be used (avoiding the adhesion concerns of IPOM). TAR is particularly advantageous for contaminated or potentially contaminated cases because the retromuscular plane can accept biologic or biosynthetic mesh when permanent synthetic mesh is contraindicated.

Technique	Release Plane	Advancement (per side)	Mesh Position	Key Advantage
Anterior (Ramirez)	External oblique aponeurosis lateral to semilunar line	5–10 cm at umbilicus	Onlay or retrorectus	Technically straightforward; wide advancement
Posterior (TAR)	Transversus abdominis muscle at medial border	6–10 cm per side	Retromuscular-preperitoneal (sublay)	No anterior flap dissection; sublay mesh; usable in

				contaminated fields
Rives-Stoppa (no release)	Retrorectus space only	3–5 cm per side	Retrorectus (sublay)	No muscle division; preserved muscle function; lower complexity

Complex Abdominal Wall Reconstruction

Loss of Domain and Preoperative Planning

Loss of domain describes the condition in which a substantial proportion of the abdominal viscera has chronically herniated outside the abdominal cavity, such that the abdominal cavity has contracted and cannot accommodate the reduction of the herniated contents without a dangerous elevation in intra-abdominal pressure. Loss of domain is defined radiographically when the hernia sac volume exceeds 20 to 25% of the total peritoneal volume (calculated by CT volumetry). Reduction of the hernia contents and fascial closure in a patient with loss of domain produces abdominal compartment syndrome — sustained intra-abdominal pressure exceeding 20 mmHg with associated organ dysfunction (renal failure from renal vein compression, respiratory failure from diaphragmatic splinting, mesenteric ischemia from venous outflow obstruction). Preoperative strategies to expand abdominal domain include progressive pneumoperitoneum (serial injection of air or carbon dioxide into the peritoneal cavity over 2 to 4 weeks to stretch the abdominal wall and re-expand the cavity), preoperative botulinum toxin injection into the lateral abdominal wall muscles (producing chemical paralysis and muscle lengthening of 2 to 3 cm per side), and weight loss optimization.

Contaminated and Infected Fields

Complex abdominal wall reconstruction frequently involves contaminated or infected operative fields (enterocutaneous fistula takedown, stoma reversal, infected mesh explantation, concomitant bowel resection). Permanent synthetic mesh (polypropylene, polyester) is contraindicated in frankly contaminated or infected fields because bacteria colonize the mesh interstices and produce chronic mesh infection requiring subsequent mesh explantation. Biologic mesh (acellular dermal matrix derived from human, porcine, or bovine dermis) and biosynthetic mesh (poly-4-hydroxybutyrate, TIGR matrix) serve as alternatives in these settings — biologic mesh is gradually remodeled and replaced by native tissue (with variable quality of the resulting neo-fascia), while biosynthetic mesh provides temporary scaffold support during tissue integration and is slowly absorbed. Neither biologic nor biosynthetic mesh achieves the durability and recurrence rates of permanent synthetic mesh in clean fields, so their use is reserved specifically for contaminated cases where permanent mesh is unsafe. A staged approach — initial hernia reduction and biologic mesh placement in the contaminated field, followed by definitive repair with permanent synthetic mesh in a clean field 6 to 12 months later — is an alternative strategy for patients at highest risk of recurrence.

CLINICAL PEARL: Preoperative progressive pneumoperitoneum (serial instillation of 500 to 1000 mL of air into the peritoneal cavity every 2 to 3 days for 2 to 4 weeks via a percutaneous catheter) and botulinum toxin injection into the lateral abdominal wall muscles are complementary techniques that can expand abdominal domain by 3 to 5 cm per side, converting an otherwise impossible primary fascial closure into a feasible reconstruction.

THE OPERATIVE DANGER ZONE ATLAS — Abdominal Compartment Syndrome After Hernia Reduction in Loss of Domain

---

The Zone: The closed abdominal cavity immediately following reduction of herniated viscera and fascial closure in a patient with loss of domain — the period when intra-abdominal pressure rises acutely as a large volume of viscera is returned to a contracted cavity.

The Structure at Risk: Renal veins (compression produces acute renal failure), diaphragm (cephalad displacement produces respiratory failure from reduced tidal volume and elevated airway pressures), mesenteric veins (compression produces intestinal ischemia), and inferior vena cava (compression reduces venous return and cardiac output).

The Consequence: Abdominal compartment syndrome — sustained intra-abdominal pressure exceeding 20 mmHg with progressive organ dysfunction: oliguria and anuria from renal vein compression, ventilatory failure from diaphragmatic splinting, intestinal ischemia from mesenteric venous congestion, and cardiovascular collapse from impaired venous return. Unrecognized abdominal compartment syndrome is rapidly fatal.

The Safe Maneuver: Measure bladder pressure (as a surrogate for intra-abdominal pressure) intraoperatively after provisional fascial closure and in the early postoperative period. If bladder pressure exceeds 20 mmHg or peak airway pressures rise above 40 cm H2O after closure, accept a bridged repair (mesh spanning the defect without fascial closure) or leave the abdomen open with a temporary abdominal closure device and plan staged reconstruction. Preoperative domain expansion with progressive pneumoperitoneum and botulinum toxin injection reduces the risk.

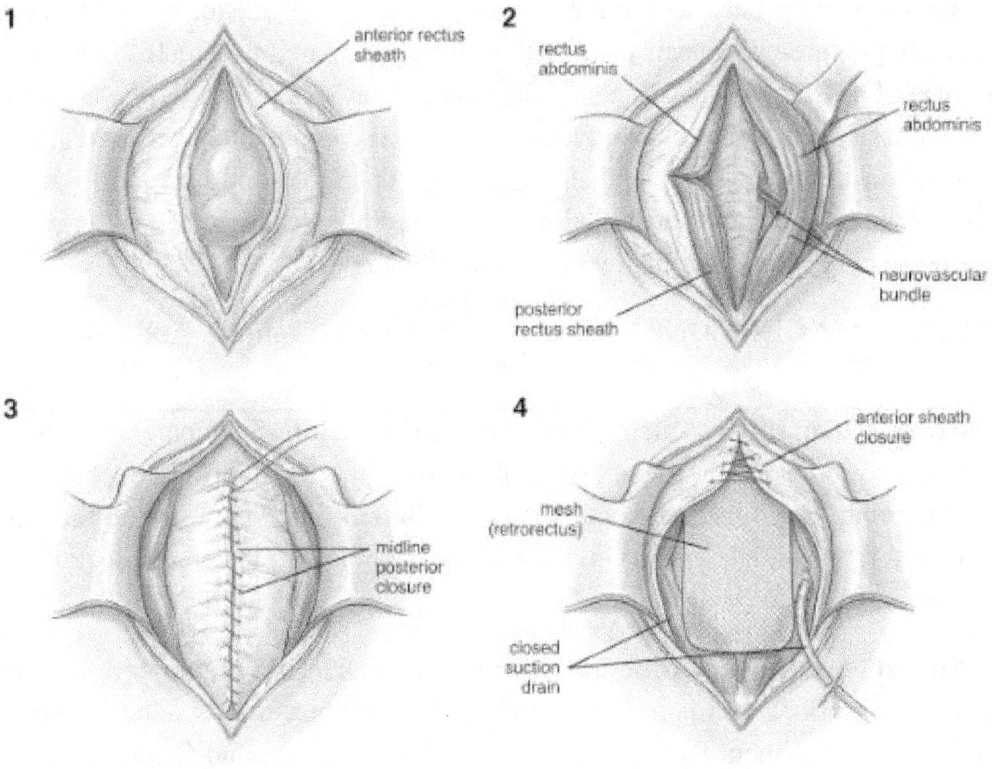

Clinical Case — Recurrent Incisional Hernia After Failed Primary Repair

A 58-year-old man with a BMI of 38, type 2 diabetes, and a history of open colectomy for diverticulitis 4 years prior presents with a large symptomatic midline incisional hernia. He had undergone primary suture repair of an incisional hernia 2 years ago, which recurred within 6 months. CT of the abdomen and pelvis demonstrates a 12 cm wide fascial defect with herniation of omentum and transverse colon into a large subcutaneous sac. CT volumetry estimates the hernia sac volume at 18% of total peritoneal volume — below the 20 to 25% threshold for loss of domain but approaching it. There is no evidence of mesh from the prior suture repair.

After medical optimization (hemoglobin A1c reduction to 7.5%, weight loss of 8 kg, smoking cessation for 6 weeks, and preoperative nutritional supplementation), the patient undergoes open transversus abdominis release (TAR) with retrorectus mesh placement. Through a midline incision excising the prior scar, the hernia contents are reduced, and the retrorectus space is developed bilaterally. Segmental neurovascular bundles are identified entering the rectus muscle and preserved. Because the defect width exceeds the advancement achievable with retrorectus dissection alone, bilateral transversus abdominis release is performed — the transversus muscle is divided at its medial border just lateral to the semilunar line, releasing the posterior layer to advance medially. The posterior rectus sheath and transversalis fascia are closed in the midline with running absorbable suture, and a 30 x 30 cm lightweight polypropylene mesh is placed in the retromuscular-preperitoneal pocket with wide overlap. The anterior rectus sheath is closed over the mesh, and two closed suction drains are left in the retrorectus space.

This case illustrates why primary suture repair without mesh is inadequate for incisional hernias — recurrence rates after suture-only repair exceed 30 to 50%, compared to 5 to 10% with mesh-reinforced repair. The choice of TAR over anterior component separation was driven by the defect width (12 cm) and the patient's obesity and diabetes (risk factors for wound complications with the lipocutaneous flap dissection required in anterior component separation). Preoperative optimization — glycemic control, weight loss, smoking cessation, and nutritional status — directly reduces the risk of surgical site infection, which is the strongest predictor of hernia recurrence after repair.

THE OPERATIVE DANGER ZONE ATLAS — Ventral and Complex Abdominal Wall Repair Dangers

---

Segmental Neurovascular Injury During Retrorectus Dissection: Segmental intercostal nerves (T7–T12) penetrate the posterior rectus sheath at the semilunar line to supply the rectus muscle. Division produces muscle atrophy and functional wall weakness. **Safe maneuver:** develop the retrorectus space anterior to each perforating bundle, preserving as many as possible; limit lateral dissection to the semilunar line unless release is required.

Inadvertent Enterotomy During Adhesiolysis for Ventral Hernia Repair: Bowel adherent to the fascial defect edges or prior mesh is at risk of full-thickness injury during adhesiolysis. Unrecognized enterotomy with mesh placement leads to peritonitis, mesh infection, and fistula. **Safe maneuver:** use sharp dissection close to the abdominal wall; avoid energy devices on bowel-wall adhesions; inspect all freed bowel before mesh placement.

Neurovascular Bundle Injury During Transversus Abdominis Release: Intercostal neurovascular bundles run in the plane between internal oblique and transversus abdominis — the plane entered during TAR. Division causes rectus denervation and atrophy. **Safe maneuver:** divide the transversus at its medial border, dissecting around each bundle individually; use robotic magnification to identify and preserve each bundle.

Abdominal Compartment Syndrome After Hernia Reduction in Loss of Domain: Reduction of a large volume of chronically herniated viscera into a contracted cavity produces sustained intra-abdominal hypertension with renal failure, respiratory failure, mesenteric ischemia, and cardiovascular collapse. **Safe maneuver:** measure bladder pressure after closure; accept bridged repair or temporary abdominal closure if pressure exceeds 20 mmHg; expand domain preoperatively with pneumoperitoneum and botulinum toxin.

Summary and Key Concepts

The rectus sheath changes composition at the arcuate line — all three lateral muscle aponeuroses pass anterior to the rectus below this line, leaving the posterior wall as transversalis fascia alone, which explains the vulnerability of the infraumbilical midline to incisional hernia development.

The retrorectus (Rives-Stoppa) space is the preferred plane for mesh placement in incisional hernia repair because intra-abdominal pressure holds the mesh against the musculature (Pascal principle), and the mesh is separated from both the subcutaneous space and the peritoneal cavity.

Intraperitoneal onlay mesh (IPOM) requires barrier-coated or composite mesh to prevent visceral adhesions — uncoated polypropylene in contact with the peritoneal surface produces dense bowel adhesions in virtually all cases, risking obstruction, fistula, and mesh erosion.

Transversus abdominis release (TAR) achieves posterior component separation by dividing the transversus muscle at its medial border, creating a retromuscular-preperitoneal plane for mesh placement while preserving the anterior abdominal wall soft tissues and the segmental neurovascular bundles.

Loss of domain (hernia sac volume exceeding 20 to 25% of total peritoneal volume) requires preoperative domain expansion with progressive pneumoperitoneum and botulinum toxin injection to prevent abdominal compartment syndrome after visceral reduction and fascial closure.

Complex abdominal wall reconstruction in contaminated fields uses biologic or biosynthetic mesh instead of permanent synthetic mesh — permanent mesh in infected or contaminated fields produces chronic mesh infection requiring explantation.

Anterior component separation (external oblique release) advances the rectus complex 5 to 10 cm per side at the umbilical level, while posterior component separation (TAR) advances the posterior layer 6 to 10 cm per side, with lower wound complication rates because the anterior soft tissues are not undermined.

CHAPTER 5: OPERATIONS OF THE ESOPHAGUS

Learning Objectives

1. Describe the surgical anatomy of the esophagus, including its blood supply, lymphatic drainage, lack of serosa, and the anatomical relationships at the gastroesophageal junction that define the antireflux barrier.
2. Perform the key operative steps of laparoscopic Nissen (360-degree) and Toupet (270-degree posterior partial) fundoplication for gastroesophageal reflux disease, including crural closure and short gastric vessel division.
3. Differentiate the types of paraesophageal hernia, identify the indications for surgical repair, and describe the operative technique including sac excision, crural closure, and fundoplication.
4. Describe the operative steps of Heller myotomy for achalasia, including the extent of myotomy and the rationale for combining it with a partial fundoplication.
5. Compare the Ivor Lewis and McKeown esophagectomy approaches with respect to conduit selection, anastomotic location, and the anatomy of the thoracic duct at risk during mediastinal dissection.
6. Apply the management algorithm for esophageal perforation based on the timing, location, and degree of contamination of the perforation.

Surgical Anatomy of the Esophagus and Gastroesophageal Junction

Esophageal Structure and the Absence of Serosa

The esophagus is a 25 cm muscular tube extending from the cricopharyngeus muscle at the level of the sixth cervical vertebra to the gastroesophageal junction at approximately the eleventh thoracic vertebra. It is divided into cervical (5 cm), thoracic (20 cm), and abdominal (2 to 4 cm) segments. The wall consists of four layers: mucosa (stratified squamous epithelium transitioning to columnar epithelium at the squamocolumnar junction or Z-line), submucosa (containing the submucosal venous plexus and Meissner plexus), muscularis propria (inner circular and outer longitudinal layers with Auerbach myenteric plexus between them), and adventitia. The esophagus is the only segment of the alimentary tract that lacks a serosal covering — this absence has two critical surgical implications: anastomoses are inherently weaker and more prone to leakage because they rely on the submucosa for holding strength rather than the serosa, and esophageal perforations lack the containment that serosa provides, allowing rapid contamination of the mediastinum and pleural cavities.

Blood Supply and Lymphatic Drainage

The esophageal blood supply is segmental and relatively sparse compared to other portions of the gastrointestinal tract. The cervical esophagus is supplied by branches of the inferior thyroid artery, the thoracic esophagus by direct branches from the aorta (bronchial arteries and small esophageal branches), and the abdominal esophagus by the left gastric artery and branches of the left inferior phrenic artery. Venous drainage is via the submucosal venous plexus into the azygos system (thoracic esophagus), the inferior thyroid veins (cervical esophagus), and the left gastric (coronary) vein (abdominal esophagus) — the left gastric vein drains into the portal system, which is why esophageal varices develop at the gastroesophageal junction in portal hypertension. Lymphatic drainage follows a longitudinal pattern with extensive submucosal lymphatic interconnections, meaning that lymph node metastases from esophageal cancer can be present several centimeters from the primary tumor in any direction — this explains the requirement for extensive lymphadenectomy and wide surgical margins during esophagectomy for malignancy.

The Antireflux Barrier

The gastroesophageal junction is the zone where the antireflux barrier prevents retrograde flow of gastric contents into the esophagus. This barrier is not a single structure but a composite of several anatomical elements working in concert: the lower esophageal sphincter (a zone of tonically contracted circular muscle fibers 2 to 4 cm in length that generates a resting pressure of 10 to 30 mmHg above gastric baseline), the crural diaphragm (the right crus of the diaphragm forms a sling around the esophagus at the hiatus and provides extrinsic compression during inspiration), the phrenoesophageal membrane (a fibroelastic ligament connecting the esophageal adventitia to the diaphragmatic hiatus that anchors the gastroesophageal junction in its intra-abdominal position), the angle of His (the acute angle at which the esophagus enters the stomach, creating a flap-valve mechanism), and the gastric sling fibers (oblique muscle fibers at the cardia that reinforce the sphincter mechanism). Disruption of any of these elements contributes to gastroesophageal reflux disease and forms the anatomical rationale for antireflux procedures.

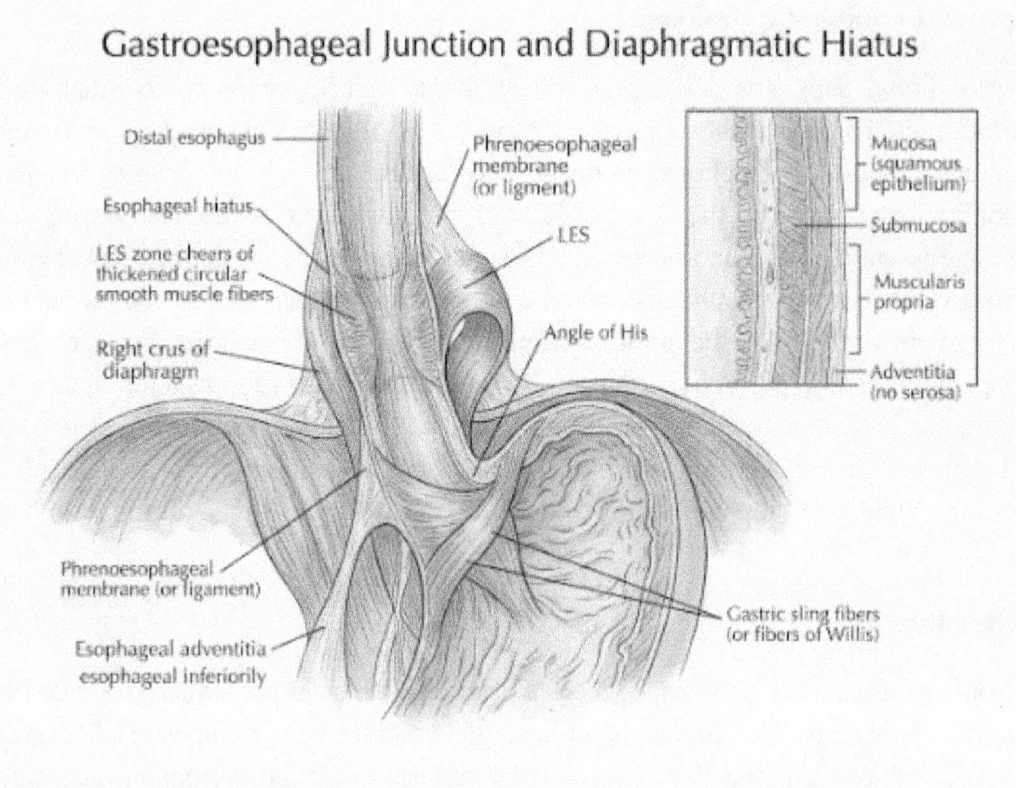

Laparoscopic Nissen and Toupet Fundoplication

Indications and Preoperative Evaluation

Fundoplication is indicated for patients with gastroesophageal reflux disease (GERD) refractory to maximal medical therapy, those who prefer surgical treatment over lifelong proton pump inhibitor (PPI) therapy, and patients with complications of reflux (erosive esophagitis, peptic stricture, Barrett esophagus). Preoperative workup includes upper endoscopy (to assess mucosal injury, rule out Barrett esophagus, and exclude malignancy), 24-hour ambulatory pH monitoring (to document pathologic acid exposure, particularly in patients with atypical symptoms or a normal endoscopy), high-resolution esophageal manometry (to assess peristaltic function and lower esophageal sphincter pressure, and to rule out achalasia and other motility disorders), and a barium swallow (to evaluate esophageal length and identify a hiatal hernia). Manometry is essential because it determines the type of fundoplication: patients with normal esophageal body peristalsis receive a full 360-degree (Nissen) wrap, while patients with impaired peristalsis (distal esophageal amplitude less than 30 mmHg or greater than 30% failed peristalsis) are better served by a partial 270-degree posterior (Toupet) wrap, which produces less dysphagia and a lower rate of wrap failure.

Operative Steps — Nissen Fundoplication

The patient is positioned in reverse Trendelenburg, and five ports are placed. The gastrohepatic ligament is opened to expose the right crus of the diaphragm, and the phrenoesophageal membrane is divided to enter the mediastinum and mobilize the distal esophagus. Both the right and left crura are dissected to fully expose the hiatus. The esophagus is mobilized circumferentially, and a Penrose drain is placed around it for retraction. Sufficient esophageal mobilization is critical to achieve at least 2 to 3 cm of intra-abdominal esophageal length — if the esophagus is foreshortened (a common finding in large hiatal hernias and longstanding GERD), an esophageal lengthening procedure (Collis gastroplasty) may be required. The short gastric vessels along the greater curvature of the fundus are divided to fully mobilize the fundus and create a tension-free wrap. The crura are approximated posteriorly with interrupted nonabsorbable sutures to reduce the hiatal hernia and restore the hiatal aperture to normal. The fundus is passed behind the esophagus and wrapped 360 degrees around the distal esophagus over a 56 to 60 French bougie dilator, creating a 2 to 3 cm floppy wrap secured with three interrupted nonabsorbable sutures incorporating the esophageal wall to prevent wrap migration.

Toupet (Posterior Partial) Fundoplication

The Toupet fundoplication follows the same initial steps as the Nissen — hiatal dissection, esophageal mobilization, crural closure, and short gastric vessel division. The fundus is passed behind the esophagus, but instead of completing a 360-degree wrap, it is secured to each side of the esophagus at the 4 o'clock and 8 o'clock positions, creating a 270-degree posterior partial wrap that leaves the anterior esophagus uncovered. The partial wrap produces less outflow obstruction at the gastroesophageal junction and is associated with lower rates of postoperative dysphagia, gas-bloat syndrome, and inability to belch compared to the Nissen. The trade-off is a slightly higher rate of persistent reflux compared to the Nissen. The Toupet is the preferred fundoplication after Heller myotomy for achalasia, where the myotomy inherently reduces lower esophageal sphincter pressure, and a full wrap would risk excessive outflow obstruction in a patient with already impaired esophageal body peristalsis.

CLINICAL PEARL: A floppy, short (2 to 3 cm) Nissen wrap constructed over a bougie dilator without tension is essential to prevent postoperative dysphagia. A wrap that is too tight, too long, or constructed under tension because of inadequate fundal mobilization (failure to divide the short gastric vessels) is the most common technical error leading to severe postoperative dysphagia requiring reoperation.

THE OPERATIVE DANGER ZONE ATLAS — Vagal Trunk Injury During Esophageal Mobilization

The Zone: The posterior surface of the distal esophagus at the hiatus — the plane where the posterior vagal trunk (arising from the right vagus) lies against the esophageal muscularis propria, often embedded in the periesophageal areolar tissue during circumferential esophageal mobilization.

The Structure at Risk: Posterior vagal trunk. The posterior vagus courses along the posterior esophageal wall and provides the criminal nerve of Grassi (the first branch of the posterior vagus to the gastric fundus) and the hepatic and celiac branches. The anterior vagal trunk lies on the anterior esophageal surface and is also at risk during dissection.

The Consequence: Vagal trunk injury disrupts gastric motility and acid secretion. Posterior vagal trunk injury produces delayed gastric emptying (gastroparesis) from loss of motor innervation to the antrum, dumping syndrome, and post-vagotomy diarrhea. Anterior vagal trunk injury similarly impairs gastric function. Bilateral vagal injury produces severe gastroparesis that may require pyloroplasty or gastric pacing.

The Safe Maneuver: Identify the posterior vagal trunk on the posterior esophageal surface before circumferential mobilization and preserve it throughout the dissection. Use blunt dissection close to the esophageal wall in the posterior plane, keeping the vagal trunk with the esophagus (not the crura). If the posterior vagus is seen in the crural closure suture line, reposition the sutures to exclude it. The anterior vagus is identified during anterior esophageal mobilization and similarly preserved.

Paraesophageal Hernia Repair

Classification and Indications

Hiatal hernias are classified into four types. Type I (sliding) involves axial herniation of the gastroesophageal junction through the hiatus — this is the most common type and is managed medically unless associated with GERD refractory to PPI therapy. Type II (true paraesophageal) involves herniation of the gastric fundus through the hiatus alongside a normally positioned gastroesophageal junction — the fundus rolls superiorly into the posterior mediastinum while the gastroesophageal junction remains fixed. Type III (mixed) combines elements of Types I and II — both the gastroesophageal junction and the fundus herniate through the hiatus, and this is the most common type of paraesophageal hernia. Type IV involves herniation of other abdominal organs (colon, spleen, omentum) in addition to the stomach through a large hiatal defect. Types II, III, and IV carry the risk of gastric volvulus (organoaxial or mesenteroaxial rotation of the herniated stomach producing obstruction and ischemia) and should be repaired electively when diagnosed, even in minimally symptomatic patients.

Operative Technique

Laparoscopic repair of paraesophageal hernia follows a systematic sequence. The hernia sac is dissected off the crura and mediastinal structures and completely excised — complete sac excision reduces recurrence by eliminating the peritoneal lining that serves as a lead point for re-herniation. The esophagus is mobilized to achieve at least 2 to 3 cm of intra-abdominal length (extensive mediastinal esophageal mobilization is often necessary for large hernias with esophageal foreshortening). The crura are closed posteriorly with interrupted nonabsorbable sutures. The use of mesh reinforcement of the crural closure remains debated — mesh may reduce short-term recurrence rates but carries the risk of mesh erosion into the esophagus, a devastating complication that is difficult to manage. A fundoplication (typically Nissen or Toupet) is added to prevent postoperative GERD and to anchor the gastroesophageal junction below the repaired hiatus. An anterior gastropexy (suturing the anterior stomach wall to the anterior abdominal wall) may be added for additional fixation in patients at high risk of recurrence.

CAUTION: Mesh reinforcement of the crural closure during paraesophageal hernia repair carries a risk of mesh erosion into the esophagus — a complication that produces dysphagia, mediastinitis, and may require esophagectomy for definitive management. If mesh reinforcement is used, biologic mesh is preferred over synthetic mesh, and the mesh should be placed as a buttress over the crural sutures, not in direct contact with the esophageal wall.

THE OPERATIVE DANGER ZONE ATLAS — Esophageal Perforation During Paraesophageal Hernia Sac Dissection

The Zone: The posterior mediastinum at the interface between the hernia sac and the esophageal wall — the plane where the peritoneal hernia sac is densely adherent to the esophageal adventitia, particularly at the gastroesophageal junction and along the left side of the esophagus.

The Structure at Risk: Esophageal wall — specifically the muscular wall and mucosa of the distal esophagus at the gastroesophageal junction. The absence of a serosal layer means the muscularis propria is the outermost layer, and it can be entered directly during sac dissection.

The Consequence: Esophageal perforation during hiatal dissection produces mediastinal contamination with saliva and gastric contents. An unrecognized perforation leads to mediastinitis, sepsis, empyema, and potentially fatal mediastinal necrosis. Even a recognized perforation requires intraoperative repair and significantly increases morbidity.

The Safe Maneuver: Dissect the hernia sac off the esophagus under direct vision, keeping the dissection plane on the sac (not the esophageal wall). If the sac is densely adherent to the esophagus, leave a small cuff of sac on the esophageal wall rather than risk perforation with aggressive dissection. After sac excision, inspect the entire circumference of the distal esophagus for mucosal violations. If a perforation is identified, repair it with interrupted absorbable sutures and reinforce with a fundoplication wrap placed directly over the repair.

Heller Myotomy for Achalasia

Pathophysiology and Diagnostic Workup

Achalasia is a primary esophageal motility disorder characterized by failure of the lower esophageal sphincter to relax in response to swallowing and absent esophageal body peristalsis. The underlying pathology is degeneration of the inhibitory neurons (nitric oxide-producing and vasoactive intestinal peptide-producing neurons) in the myenteric (Auerbach) plexus of the distal esophagus, leading to unopposed excitatory cholinergic drive, sustained sphincter contraction, and functional obstruction. Diagnosis is established by high-resolution manometry, which demonstrates elevated integrated relaxation pressure (IRP greater than 15 mmHg) and absent or spastic esophageal body peristalsis. The Chicago Classification (version 4.0) subclassifies achalasia into three types based on esophageal body contraction patterns: Type I (classic achalasia with absent peristalsis), Type II (panesophageal pressurization), and Type III (spastic achalasia with premature contractions). Type II has the best surgical outcomes, while Type III has the poorest response to myotomy alone. Endoscopy is mandatory to rule out pseudoachalasia from a tumor at the gastroesophageal junction, particularly in older patients with recent-onset dysphagia and significant weight loss.

Operative Steps of Laparoscopic Heller Myotomy

The patient is positioned in reverse Trendelenburg with five laparoscopic ports. The gastrohepatic ligament is divided, and the anterior surface of the esophagus and gastroesophageal junction is exposed. The anterior fat pad at the gastroesophageal junction is excised to clearly identify the longitudinal muscle fibers of the esophagus and the transition to the gastric wall. The myotomy is performed on the anterior esophageal surface at the 11 to 12 o'clock position. Using a hook electrocautery at low power or a sharp dissector, the longitudinal muscle fibers are divided first, then the circular muscle fibers are divided separately, exposing the intact submucosal plane. The myotomy extends at least 6 cm proximal on the esophagus and 2 to 3 cm distal onto the gastric cardia — the distal extension onto the cardia is essential to completely divide the lower esophageal sphincter fibers, which extend onto the stomach. The gastric extension must be limited to 2 to 3 cm to avoid disrupting the sling fibers of the cardia and producing iatrogenic gastroesophageal reflux. The edges of the myotomy are separated from the underlying submucosa to prevent re-healing. Mucosal integrity is confirmed by insufflation of the esophagus with air under saline irrigation — any mucosal perforation is repaired immediately with fine absorbable sutures. A partial fundoplication (Dor anterior 180-degree or Toupet posterior 270-degree) is then performed to prevent postoperative reflux and to buttress the exposed esophageal mucosa at the myotomy site.

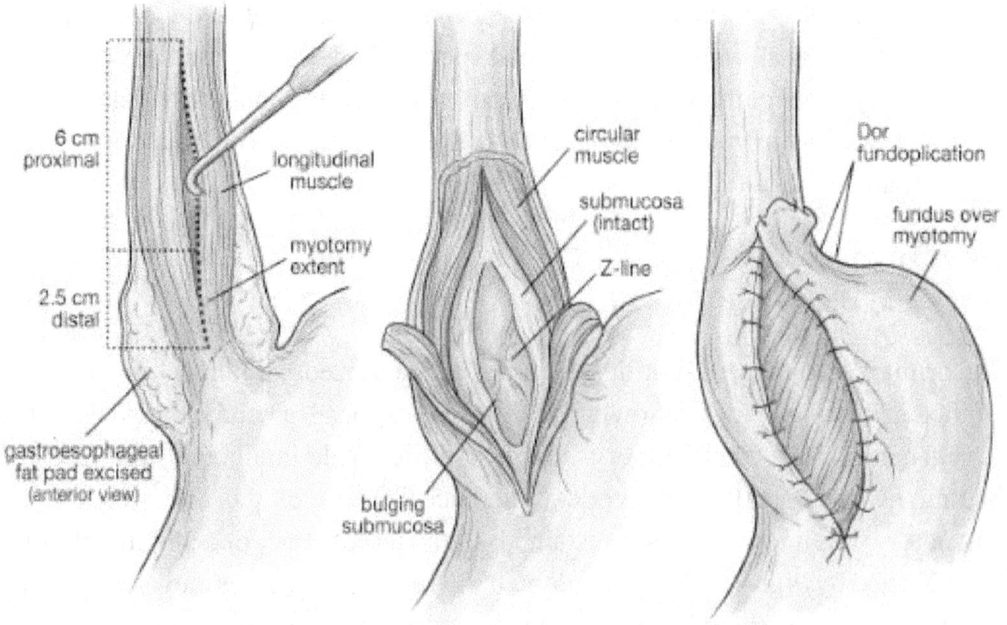

Heller Myotomy: Initial Muscle Division

Completed Myotomy: Exposure of Submucosa

Dor Anterior Fundoplication: Covering Myotomy

THE OPERATIVE DANGER ZONE ATLAS — Mucosal Perforation During Heller Myotomy

The Zone: The myotomy plane at the gastroesophageal junction — specifically the distal extent where the esophageal circular muscle fibers transition to the oblique sling fibers of the gastric cardia, and the muscle layer is thinnest and most intimately adherent to the submucosa.

The Structure at Risk: Esophageal and gastric mucosa at the gastroesophageal junction. The submucosa is the only layer separating the myotomy dissection from the mucosal lumen, and it is thinnest at the gastroesophageal junction where the muscle changes fiber orientation.

The Consequence: Mucosal perforation at the myotomy site, if unrecognized, produces mediastinal and peritoneal contamination with saliva and gastric contents, leading to mediastinitis, peritonitis, and sepsis. Even a recognized perforation, while repairable, increases the risk of postoperative leak and abscess.

The Safe Maneuver: Divide the muscle layers sequentially — longitudinal first, then circular — rather than through both layers simultaneously. Use blunt spreading to separate the circular fibers off the submucosa rather than cutting directly. Perform the myotomy under direct vision with the submucosal plane clearly exposed. Test mucosal integrity by insufflating the esophagus with air under saline irrigation (submerge the myotomy site and look for air bubbles). If a perforation is identified, repair immediately with interrupted 4-0 absorbable sutures and buttress with a Dor fundoplication draped over the repair.

Esophagectomy (Ivor Lewis and McKeown Approaches)

Indications and Conduit Selection

Esophagectomy is performed primarily for esophageal cancer (squamous cell carcinoma and adenocarcinoma), high-grade dysplasia in Barrett esophagus refractory to endoscopic management, and end-stage benign disease (caustic stricture, failed antireflux surgery with a destroyed esophagus). The gastric conduit (tubularized stomach constructed along the greater curvature, preserving the right gastroepiploic arcade as the primary blood supply) is the preferred conduit because it reaches the neck without tension, has a reliable vascular pedicle, and requires only one anastomosis. The colon interposition (using the left or transverse colon on its primary vascular pedicle) and jejunal interposition are reserved for cases where the stomach is unavailable (prior gastrectomy, extensive gastric disease, or conduit failure). Preoperative assessment includes staging endoscopic ultrasound with fine-needle aspiration of suspicious lymph nodes, PET-CT, and nutritional optimization. Neoadjuvant chemoradiation (CROSS protocol) is standard for locally advanced esophageal cancer (cT2-T4a or node-positive) before esophagectomy.

Ivor Lewis Esophagectomy

The Ivor Lewis approach is a two-phase operation: an abdominal phase (laparoscopic or open) for gastric mobilization and conduit creation, followed by a right thoracic phase (thoracoscopic or thoracotomy) for esophageal mobilization, lymphadenectomy, and intrathoracic esophagogastric anastomosis. During the abdominal phase, the stomach is mobilized by dividing the short gastric vessels, the left gastric artery (at its origin from the celiac axis), and the gastrohepatic and gastrocolic ligaments while preserving the right gastroepiploic artery and the right gastric artery. The stomach is tubularized along the greater curvature using a linear stapler, creating a 4 to 5 cm wide gastric conduit. During the right thoracic phase, the esophagus is mobilized from the thoracic inlet to the hiatus, the thoracic duct is identified and ligated, and a two-field lymphadenectomy (abdominal and mediastinal) is performed. The esophagogastric anastomosis is created in the upper thorax, typically using a circular stapler or a hand-sewn technique. The Ivor Lewis approach is preferred for distal and mid-esophageal tumors because the intrathoracic anastomosis is at the level of or above the azygos vein.

McKeown (Three-Field) Esophagectomy

The McKeown approach adds a cervical phase to the Ivor Lewis operation — the esophagogastric anastomosis is performed in the neck rather than in the thorax. This requires three incisions (or equivalent minimally invasive access): abdominal (conduit creation), right thoracic (esophageal mobilization and mediastinal lymphadenectomy), and left cervical (esophagogastric anastomosis in the neck). The advantage of the cervical anastomosis is that it allows a wider proximal esophageal margin (relevant for proximal and mid-esophageal tumors) and, critically, an anastomotic leak in the neck is far more manageable than an intrathoracic leak — a cervical leak is controlled with local wound drainage, while an intrathoracic leak produces mediastinitis and empyema with high mortality. The disadvantage is a higher rate of anastomotic leak at the cervical site (10 to 25%) compared to the intrathoracic site (5 to 10%), likely because the conduit's blood supply is most tenuous at its most distal extent (the tip of the gastric tube in the neck), and a higher incidence of recurrent laryngeal nerve injury from the cervical dissection.

THE OPERATIVE DANGER ZONE ATLAS — Thoracic Duct Injury During Esophageal Mobilization

---

The Zone: The posterior mediastinum during esophageal mobilization — the plane between the esophagus and the thoracic spine, where the thoracic duct courses from the aortic hiatus to the junction of the left subclavian and internal jugular veins, crossing from right to left at approximately the T4–T5 level.

The Structure at Risk: Thoracic duct. The duct enters the posterior mediastinum through the aortic hiatus, courses between the aorta and the azygos vein posterior to the esophagus, and crosses from the right side to the left side of the mediastinum at the T4–T5 level. Multiple anatomical variants exist (duplicated ducts, variable crossover points), making identification difficult.

The Consequence: Thoracic duct injury produces chylothorax — accumulation of chyle (lymphatic fluid rich in triglycerides, fat-soluble vitamins, and lymphocytes) in the pleural space. A high-output chylothorax (greater than 1 liter per day) causes severe nutritional depletion, immunosuppression from lymphocyte loss, and dehydration. Uncontrolled chylothorax requires reoperation for thoracic duct ligation.

The Safe Maneuver: Ligate the thoracic duct en masse at the level of the diaphragmatic hiatus during esophagectomy — prophylactic ligation eliminates the risk of postoperative chylothorax and is standard practice in many centers. If chylothorax develops postoperatively, initial management is conservative (NPO with total parenteral nutrition or medium-chain triglyceride diet to reduce chyle production plus chest tube drainage); operative ligation is indicated if output exceeds 1 liter per day for more than 5 days or if the patient is clinically deteriorating.

Management of Esophageal Perforation

Etiology and Presentation

Esophageal perforation is a surgical emergency with mortality rates of 10 to 40% depending on the delay to treatment and the degree of mediastinal contamination. The most common cause is iatrogenic perforation during endoscopy (diagnostic or therapeutic), accounting for approximately 60% of cases. Boerhaave syndrome — spontaneous transmural perforation of the distal esophagus caused by forceful vomiting against a closed glottis — accounts for 15% of cases and classically produces a left posterolateral distal esophageal tear with contamination of the left pleural space. Other causes include foreign body impaction, caustic ingestion, trauma (penetrating or blunt), and intraoperative injury during thoracic, esophageal, or fundoplication surgery. The classic presentation of Boerhaave syndrome is Mackler triad — vomiting, chest pain, and subcutaneous emphysema — though all three elements are present in fewer than 50% of cases. CT with oral water-soluble contrast is the diagnostic study of choice, demonstrating extraluminal contrast extravasation, mediastinal air, pleural effusion, and pneumomediastinum.

Management Algorithm

Management of esophageal perforation is determined by four factors: the time from perforation to diagnosis, the location of the perforation, the degree of mediastinal contamination, and the condition of the underlying esophagus. Early perforations (diagnosed within 24 hours) with minimal contamination in a patient with a normal underlying esophagus are candidates for primary repair: the perforation is debrided, the mucosal defect is closed with interrupted absorbable sutures, the muscle layer is reapproximated over the mucosal closure, and the repair is reinforced with a vascularized tissue flap (intercostal muscle flap for thoracic perforations, sternocleidomastoid muscle flap for cervical perforations, or a fundoplication wrap for abdominal perforations). Late perforations (beyond 24 hours) with significant mediastinal contamination, sepsis, or a diseased underlying esophagus (cancer, end-stage achalasia, caustic stricture) may require esophageal diversion (cervical esophagostomy, distal esophageal staple closure, and feeding jejunostomy) with delayed reconstruction, or definitive esophagectomy if the patient's condition allows. Endoscopic management (endoscopic stent placement across the perforation, endoscopic vacuum therapy, or endoscopic clip closure) has emerged as a first-line option for contained perforations without sepsis, particularly iatrogenic perforations diagnosed immediately at the time of the causative endoscopy.

KEY POINT: The absence of a serosal layer on the esophagus is the fundamental reason that esophageal perforations are more dangerous than perforations elsewhere in the gastrointestinal tract. Without serosa, perforations rapidly contaminate the mediastinum and pleural spaces with saliva and gastric contents, producing fulminant mediastinitis — every hour of delay in diagnosis and treatment increases mortality.

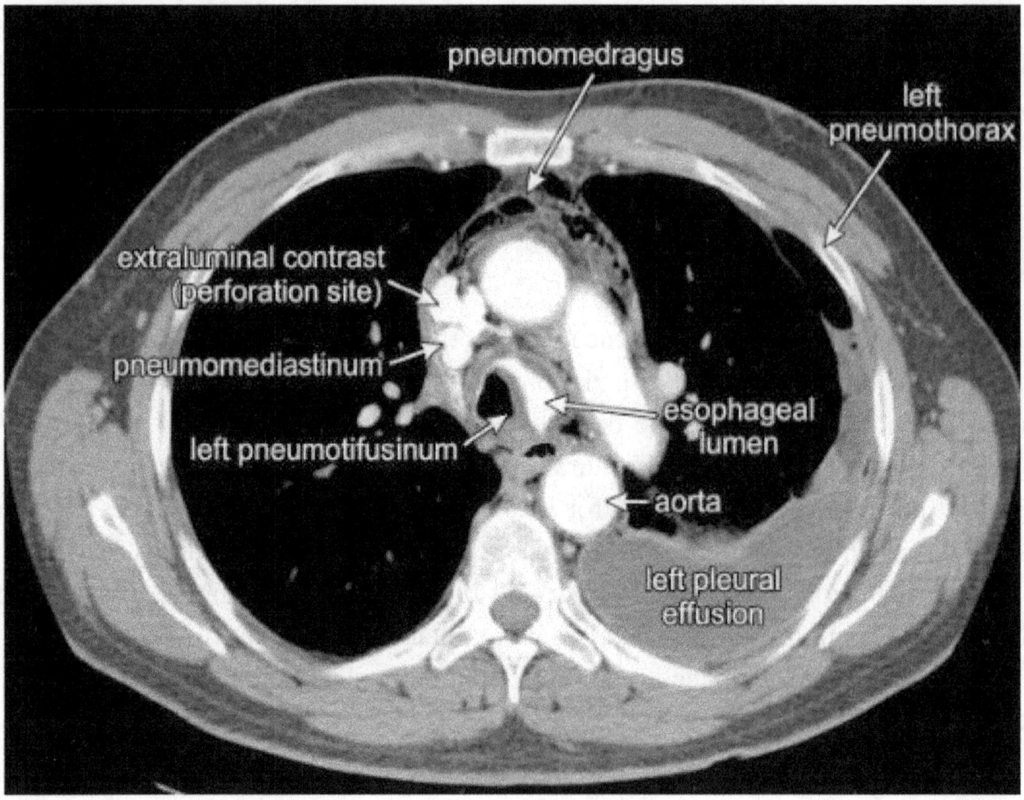

Clinical Case — Delayed Diagnosis of Boerhaave Syndrome

A 55-year-old man with a history of alcohol use disorder presents to the emergency department with 36 hours of left chest pain, fever, and progressive dyspnea following an episode of forceful vomiting after heavy alcohol consumption. He was initially evaluated at an outside facility where a chest radiograph showed a left pleural effusion, and he was discharged with oral antibiotics for presumed pneumonia. On arrival, he is febrile (39.2 degrees C), tachycardic, and hypotensive. Examination reveals subcutaneous crepitus in the left neck and chest wall. CT of the chest with oral water-soluble contrast demonstrates a distal esophageal perforation with extraluminal contrast in the left pleural space, pneumomediastinum, and a large left hydropneumothorax with complex fluid (suggesting empyema). Laboratory studies show leukocytosis and an elevated lactate.

The patient is resuscitated with intravenous fluids, broad-spectrum antibiotics are initiated, and a left chest tube is placed, draining 1.5 liters of turbid, foul-smelling pleural fluid. Given the delayed diagnosis (beyond 24 hours), the extent of mediastinal contamination, and the septic physiology, primary repair alone carries a high failure rate. The patient is taken to the operating room for left thoracotomy. The distal esophageal perforation is identified, the necrotic tissue edges are debrided, and the mucosal defect is closed with interrupted absorbable sutures. The muscle layer is reapproximated, and the repair is reinforced with an intercostal muscle flap pedicled on the intercostal vessels and sutured over the closure line. The pleural space and mediastinum are irrigated and debrided, and two chest tubes are left in place. A nasogastric tube is positioned proximal to the repair, and a feeding jejunostomy is placed during a subsequent brief abdominal exploration.

This case demonstrates why Boerhaave syndrome carries the highest mortality of all esophageal perforations — the combination of a full-thickness transmural tear (unlike an iatrogenic mucosal perforation, which may be contained), contamination of the mediastinum and pleural space with both saliva and gastric contents, and the frequent delay in diagnosis (because the presentation mimics pneumonia, myocardial infarction, or aortic dissection). Reinforcement of the primary repair with a vascularized tissue flap is essential for delayed perforations because the inflamed tissues hold sutures poorly and the flap provides an additional barrier and blood supply to the repair site.

THE OPERATIVE DANGER ZONE ATLAS — Esophageal Surgery Dangers

Vagal Trunk Injury During Esophageal Mobilization: The posterior vagal trunk lies on the posterior esophageal surface and is at risk during circumferential esophageal mobilization for fundoplication. Injury produces gastroparesis and post-vagotomy diarrhea. **Safe maneuver:** identify the posterior vagus before mobilization; use blunt dissection close to the esophageal wall; keep the vagus with the esophagus, not with the crura.

Esophageal Perforation During Paraesophageal Hernia Sac Dissection: The hernia sac is densely adherent to the esophageal adventitia at the gastroesophageal junction. Without serosa, the muscularis is the outermost layer and can be entered directly. **Safe maneuver:** dissect on the sac side; leave a cuff of sac on the esophagus if densely adherent; inspect the full circumference after sac excision.

Mucosal Perforation During Heller Myotomy: The submucosa is thinnest at the gastroesophageal junction where muscle fiber orientation changes. Mucosal perforation causes mediastinal contamination. **Safe maneuver:** divide muscle layers sequentially; use blunt spreading on circular fibers; test mucosal integrity with air insufflation under saline; repair immediately if found.

Thoracic Duct Injury During Esophageal Mobilization: The thoracic duct courses posterior to the esophagus in the posterior mediastinum and crosses from right to left at T4–T5. Injury produces high-output chylothorax with nutritional and immune depletion. **Safe maneuver:** prophylactically ligate the duct en masse at the diaphragmatic hiatus during esophagectomy; manage postoperative chylothorax conservatively initially, with operative ligation if output exceeds 1 L per day for more than 5 days.

Summary and Key Concepts

The esophagus lacks a serosal layer — anastomoses depend on the submucosa for holding strength and are inherently prone to leakage, and perforations rapidly contaminate the mediastinum because there is no serosal barrier to contain the spillage.

The antireflux barrier is a composite of the lower esophageal sphincter, crural diaphragm, phrenoesophageal membrane, angle of His, and gastric sling fibers — fundoplication restores this barrier by wrapping the gastric fundus around the distal esophagus to augment sphincter pressure.

Nissen (360-degree) fundoplication is standard for patients with normal esophageal peristalsis, while Toupet (270-degree posterior) fundoplication is preferred for impaired peristalsis and after Heller myotomy to reduce postoperative dysphagia.

Heller myotomy for achalasia must extend at least 6 cm proximal on the esophagus and 2 to 3 cm distal onto the gastric cardia to completely divide the lower esophageal sphincter, with a partial fundoplication added to prevent iatrogenic reflux.

The Ivor Lewis esophagectomy creates an intrathoracic anastomosis (lower leak rate, higher leak severity) while the McKeown approach creates a cervical anastomosis (higher leak rate, but cervical leaks are far more manageable than intrathoracic leaks).

Esophageal perforation management is determined by timing, location, contamination, and the condition of the underlying esophagus — early perforations with minimal contamination are repaired primarily with vascularized tissue flap reinforcement, while delayed perforations with sepsis may require diversion or esophagectomy.

CHAPTER 6: OPERATIONS OF THE STOMACH AND DUODENUM

Learning Objectives

1. Describe the surgical anatomy of the stomach and duodenum, including the blood supply from the celiac axis branches, the vagal innervation pattern, and the anatomical relationships of the duodenum to surrounding structures.
2. Differentiate truncal vagotomy from selective and highly selective vagotomy with respect to the extent of denervation, the need for a drainage procedure, and the incidence of post-vagotomy sequelae.
3. Perform the operative steps of subtotal and total gastrectomy, including construction of the Billroth I, Billroth II, and Roux-en-Y gastrojejunostomy reconstructions.
4. Describe pyloroplasty techniques and the indications for gastrojejunostomy as gastric drainage procedures.
5. Apply the operative decision algorithm for complicated peptic ulcer disease, including perforated, bleeding, and obstructing ulcers.
6. Describe the operative steps and anatomical danger zones of Roux-en-Y gastric bypass and sleeve gastrectomy for morbid obesity.

Surgical Anatomy of the Stomach and Duodenum

Gastric Blood Supply

The stomach has the richest blood supply of any organ in the gastrointestinal tract, receiving arterial flow from four major branches of the celiac axis that form two arterial arcades along the greater and lesser curvatures. The lesser curvature arcade is formed by the left gastric artery (arising directly from the celiac axis) and the right gastric artery (a branch of the common hepatic artery or, less commonly, the proper hepatic artery). The greater curvature arcade is formed by the left gastroepiploic artery (a terminal branch of the splenic artery) and the right gastroepiploic artery (a branch of the gastroduodenal artery). The fundus receives additional supply from the short gastric arteries (3 to 5 branches arising from the splenic artery or its terminal divisions). This abundant, redundant blood supply explains why the stomach tolerates extensive mobilization and devascularization during surgical procedures — a gastric conduit for esophageal replacement, for example, can survive on the right gastroepiploic artery alone after division of all other feeding vessels.

Vagal Innervation

The vagus nerves provide parasympathetic motor innervation to the stomach that controls acid secretion, gastric motility, and pyloric relaxation. The anterior vagal trunk (derived from the left vagus) descends on the anterior esophageal surface, gives off the hepatic branch (which courses in the gastrohepatic ligament to the liver and biliary tree), and continues as the anterior nerve of Latarjet along the lesser curvature, giving off branches to the anterior gastric wall before terminating in the crow's foot distribution at the antrum. The posterior vagal trunk (derived from the right vagus) descends on the posterior esophageal surface, gives off the celiac branch (which courses to the celiac plexus), and continues as the posterior nerve of Latarjet along the lesser curvature. The criminal nerve of Grassi — the highest branch of the posterior vagus to the fundus — is a frequent source of recurrent ulceration after incomplete vagotomy because it is easily missed during truncal vagotomy if the posterior vagus is not identified at or above the hiatus.

Duodenal Anatomy and Relationships

The duodenum is the C-shaped first portion of the small intestine, divided into four parts. The first part (D1, the duodenal bulb) is the most common site of duodenal ulcers, is partially retroperitoneal, and lies anterior to the common bile duct, portal vein, and gastroduodenal artery. The second part (D2, the descending duodenum) is entirely retroperitoneal, receives the common bile duct and the main pancreatic duct (of Wirsung) at the ampulla of Vater (major duodenal papilla), and is intimately attached to the head of the pancreas — this intimate relationship is why pancreaticoduodenectomy (Whipple procedure) requires en bloc resection of the duodenum with the pancreatic head. The third part (D3) crosses the midline anterior to the aorta and inferior vena cava and posterior to the superior mesenteric artery and vein. The fourth part (D4) ascends to the ligament of Treitz, where the duodenojejunal flexure marks the transition to the jejunum. The gastroduodenal artery — a branch of the common hepatic artery — courses posterior to the first part of the duodenum and is the most common source of massive hemorrhage from a posterior duodenal ulcer that erodes into this vessel.

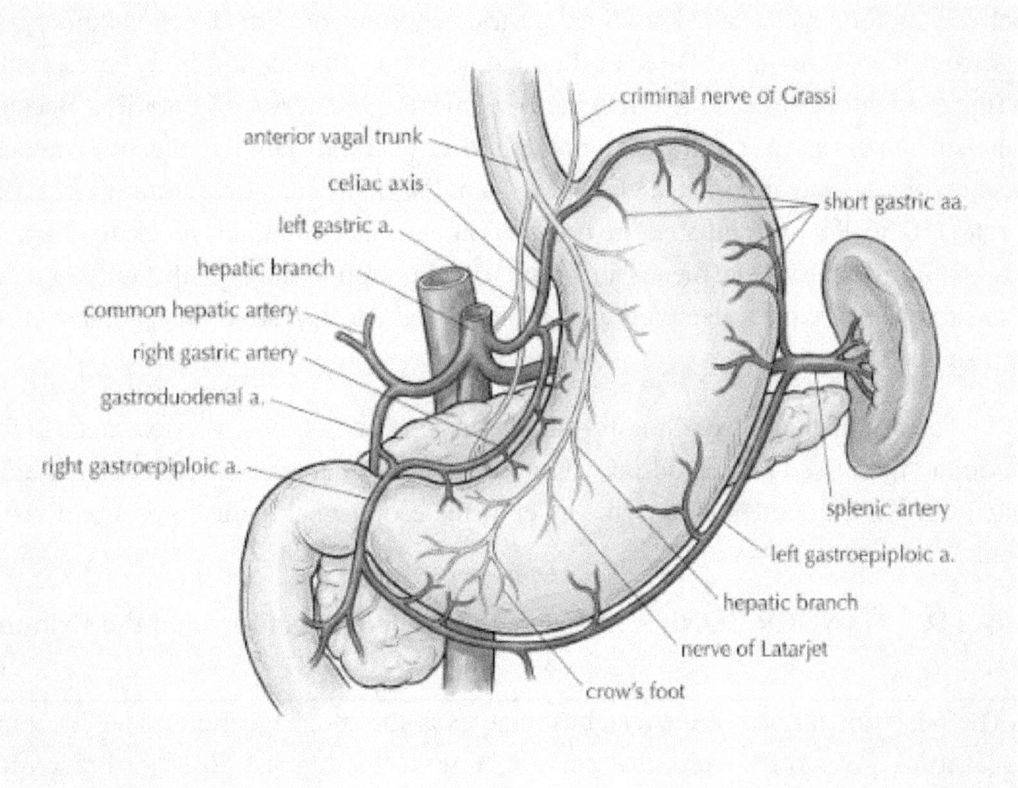

Truncal and Selective Vagotomy

Truncal Vagotomy

Truncal vagotomy divides both the anterior and posterior vagal trunks at the level of the distal esophagus, above all gastric branches. This eliminates vagal-mediated acid secretion (reducing basal acid output by approximately 80%) and was historically the standard anti-acid operation for peptic ulcer disease before the proton pump inhibitor era. Because truncal vagotomy also denervates the antral pump mechanism responsible for gastric emptying, a drainage procedure (pyloroplasty or gastrojejunostomy) is mandatory after truncal vagotomy to prevent gastric outlet obstruction from vagal-mediated pylorospasm and antral dysmotility. Truncal vagotomy also denervates the hepatic and celiac branches, producing post-vagotomy sequelae: post-vagotomy diarrhea (occurring in 5 to 10% of patients, caused by rapid intestinal transit from loss of vagal braking), dumping syndrome (early and late dumping from rapid gastric emptying of hyperosmolar contents into the jejunum), and bile reflux gastritis (from loss of pyloric control after the drainage procedure). These sequelae are the primary reason that selective and highly selective vagotomy were developed as alternatives.

Selective and Highly Selective Vagotomy

Selective vagotomy divides only the gastric branches of the anterior and posterior vagal trunks while preserving the hepatic branch (anterior) and the celiac branch (posterior), maintaining extragastric vagal innervation. This reduces (but does not eliminate) the incidence of post-vagotomy diarrhea. A drainage procedure is still required because the antral nerves of Latarjet are divided, impairing gastric emptying.

Highly selective vagotomy (also called proximal gastric vagotomy or parietal cell vagotomy) divides only the branches from the nerves of Latarjet to the acid-secreting fundus and body, preserving the antral innervation (thc crow's foot branches and the antral segment of the nerves of Latarjet). Because the antral pump mechanism is preserved, no drainage procedure is required. Highly selective vagotomy has the lowest incidence of post-vagotomy sequelae (less than 1% diarrhea, rare dumping) but a higher ulcer recurrence rate (10 to 15%) compared to truncal vagotomy with drainage (5 to 8%), because the preservation of antral innervation means incomplete acid suppression. In the current era, vagotomy procedures are rarely performed electively and are reserved for operative management of complicated peptic ulcer disease.

KEY POINT: The criminal nerve of Grassi — the highest branch of the posterior vagus to the fundus — is the most commonly missed branch during vagotomy and a frequent cause of recurrent ulceration. The posterior vagal trunk must be identified at the level of the esophageal hiatus to ensure division proximal to this branch.

THE OPERATIVE DANGER ZONE ATLAS — Incomplete Vagotomy and the Criminal Nerve of Grassi

The Zone: The posterior surface of the distal esophagus at the esophageal hiatus — the zone where the posterior vagal trunk gives off the criminal nerve of Grassi (the highest posterior branch to the gastric fundus) before descending as the posterior nerve of Latarjet.

The Structure at Risk: Criminal nerve of Grassi. This branch arises high on the posterior vagal trunk, often at or above the hiatus, and courses to the gastric fundus separately from the main trunk. It is easily missed during truncal vagotomy if the posterior vagus is divided too far distally.

The Consequence: An intact criminal nerve of Grassi maintains vagal-mediated acid secretion to the fundic parietal cells, producing an incomplete vagotomy. This results in persistent acid hypersecretion and recurrent peptic ulceration — the primary reason for vagotomy failure after technically planned truncal vagotomy.

The Safe Maneuver: Identify the posterior vagal trunk at the level of the esophageal hiatus — not on the stomach wall — and divide it at this proximal level to ensure the criminal nerve of Grassi is included in the specimen. Palpate the posterior esophageal surface for the cord-like posterior vagus, mobilize 5 cm of the distal esophagus, and divide the trunk with clamps or clips applied proximally and distally.

Gastric Resection (Subtotal and Total Gastrectomy)

Subtotal Gastrectomy — Operative Steps and Reconstruction

Subtotal (distal) gastrectomy removes the distal 60 to 80% of the stomach including the antrum and a portion of the body, along with the first part of the duodenum and the associated lymph node basins. The stomach is mobilized by dividing the gastrocolic ligament (entering the lesser sac), ligating the right and left gastroepiploic vessels, dividing the right gastric artery, and mobilizing the duodenum by performing a Kocher maneuver. The duodenum is divided distal to the pylorus with a linear stapler, and the stomach is divided at the level of the body using a linear stapler, creating the gastric remnant. The operative specimen includes the resected stomach, the proximal duodenum, the gastroduodenal and perigastric lymph nodes, and the greater and lesser omentum along the resected curvatures. For gastric cancer, a D2 lymphadenectomy (removal of perigastric nodes along the greater and lesser curvatures plus nodes along the left gastric, common hepatic, celiac, and splenic arteries) is the standard of care.

Reconstruction Options After Subtotal Gastrectomy

Three reconstruction options exist after subtotal gastrectomy. The Billroth I (gastroduodenostomy) creates an end-to-end or end-to-side anastomosis between the gastric remnant and the duodenal stump, restoring anatomic continuity through the duodenum — this is preferred when the duodenal stump is healthy and can be mobilized without tension, but it is limited by the reach of the duodenum and is rarely used for gastric cancer because the limited duodenal resection may compromise oncologic margins. The Billroth II (gastrojejunostomy) creates a loop gastrojejunostomy with an afferent limb (carrying bile and pancreatic secretions from the duodenal stump) and an efferent limb (carrying the food stream distally); the afferent limb should be short (less than 20 cm from the ligament of Treitz) to reduce the risk of afferent loop syndrome. The Roux-en-Y gastrojejunostomy is the preferred reconstruction for gastric cancer: the jejunum is divided 30 to 40 cm distal to the ligament of Treitz, the distal limb (Roux limb) is brought up and anastomosed to the gastric remnant, and the proximal jejunal limb is anastomosed to the Roux limb 40 to 60 cm distal to the gastrojejunostomy, creating a long jejunal limb that diverts bile away from the gastric remnant and prevents alkaline reflux gastritis.

Total Gastrectomy

Total gastrectomy removes the entire stomach from the gastroesophageal junction to the pylorus and is indicated for proximal gastric cancers, diffuse-type gastric cancer (linitis plastica), and hereditary diffuse gastric cancer (CDH1 mutation carriers). Reconstruction after total gastrectomy is exclusively Roux-en-Y esophagojejunostomy: the Roux limb is brought up to the distal esophagus, and a hand-sewn or circular-stapled esophagojejunal anastomosis is constructed. A jejunal pouch (J-pouch or Hunt-Lawrence pouch) may be created at the esophagojejunal anastomosis to increase the reservoir capacity and reduce the nutritional consequences of gastric loss, though evidence for functional benefit is mixed. D2 lymphadenectomy with omentectomy is standard. The spleen is preserved unless directly involved by tumor or required for adequate lymphadenectomy along the splenic hilum (station 10 nodes).

Postgastrectomy Syndromes

Several physiologic derangements follow gastric resection, regardless of the reconstruction type, because the stomach's reservoir, mixing, and controlled-emptying functions are lost. Dumping syndrome — the most common postgastrectomy syndrome — occurs in early and late forms. Early dumping (15 to 30 minutes after eating) results from rapid passage of hyperosmolar chyme into the jejunum, drawing fluid into the intestinal lumen and triggering a vasomotor response (tachycardia, diaphoresis, dizziness, cramping, diarrhea). Late dumping (1 to 3 hours after eating) results from reactive hypoglycemia: the rapid carbohydrate load triggers excessive insulin secretion, and the subsequent fall in blood glucose produces diaphoresis, tremor, and confusion. Dietary modification (small frequent meals, avoiding simple carbohydrates, separating liquids from solids) is the first-line treatment and is effective in 80% of patients. Alkaline reflux gastritis occurs after Billroth II reconstruction because bile refluxes freely through the gastrojejunostomy into the gastric remnant, producing chronic mucosal inflammation, epigastric pain, and bilious vomiting. Conversion to Roux-en-Y reconstruction diverts bile away from the gastric remnant and is the definitive treatment for medically refractory alkaline reflux gastritis.

Reconstruction	Anatomy	Advantages	Key Complications
Billroth I (gastroduodenostomy)	Gastric remnant to duodenal stump	Restores anatomic continuity; single anastomosis	Limited reach; risk of duodenal stump leak; limited oncologic application
Billroth II (gastrojejunostomy)	Loop gastrojejunostomy with afferent and efferent limbs	No duodenal stump tension; wider applicability	Afferent loop syndrome; bile reflux gastritis; internal hernia at the mesocolic defect
Roux-en-Y gastrojejunostomy	Roux limb to gastric remnant; jejunojejunostomy 40–60 cm distal	Eliminates bile reflux; preferred for cancer	Internal hernia at Petersen space and jejunojejunostomy mesenteric defect; Roux stasis syndrome

THE OPERATIVE DANGER ZONE ATLAS — Duodenal Stump Blowout After Subtotal Gastrectomy

---

The Zone: The duodenal stump — the stapled or sutured closure of the proximal duodenum after division distal to the pylorus during Billroth II or Roux-en-Y reconstruction.

The Structure at Risk: Duodenal stump closure. The stump contains the duodenal mucosa, submucosa, and muscularis without reinforcing serosa on its retroperitoneal surface. It receives bile and pancreatic secretions under positive pressure from the afferent limb.

The Consequence: Duodenal stump blowout (leak from the closed duodenal stump) produces uncontrolled leakage of bile and pancreatic secretions into the peritoneal cavity, causing bile peritonitis, sepsis, and multiorgan failure. This is one of the most feared complications after gastrectomy, with mortality rates of 10 to 30%.

The Safe Maneuver: Construct the duodenal stump closure with a secure staple line reinforced by oversewing with interrupted seromuscular sutures. Perform a Kocher maneuver to mobilize the duodenum and reduce tension on the stump. If the duodenal stump is edematous, inflamed, or friable (as in a scarred posterior duodenal ulcer), place a lateral duodenostomy tube (a catheter sewn into the stump that exits through the abdominal wall) for controlled decompression. If a stump blowout occurs postoperatively, manage with percutaneous drain placement, NPO status, parenteral nutrition, and octreotide — reoperation is reserved for diffuse peritonitis with source control failure.

Pyloroplasty and Gastrojejunostomy

Heineke-Mikulicz Pyloroplasty

The Heineke-Mikulicz pyloroplasty is the most common drainage procedure performed after truncal vagotomy. A longitudinal incision is made through the pylorus, extending 2 cm on the gastric side and 2 cm on the duodenal side of the pyloric sphincter. The pyloric muscle ring is divided, and the incision is closed transversely with interrupted full-thickness sutures, converting the longitudinal incision into a transverse closure that widens the pyloric channel. This eliminates the functional pyloric obstruction produced by vagal denervation. The Finney pyloroplasty creates a larger gastroduodenostomy by making a U-shaped incision extending farther along both the gastric and duodenal walls, producing a side-to-side gastroduodenostomy that provides a wider drainage channel. The Jaboulay pyloroplasty (gastroduodenostomy) bypasses the pylorus entirely by creating a side-to-side anastomosis between the gastric antrum and the duodenum without incising the pylorus — this is used when the pylorus is too scarred or inflamed for direct pyloroplasty.

Gastrojejunostomy as a Drainage Procedure

Gastrojejunostomy provides an alternative gastric drainage route when pyloroplasty is not feasible — typically in cases of duodenal scarring from chronic peptic ulcer disease that prevents safe pyloroplasty. A loop of jejunum is brought up to the posterior wall of the gastric antrum (retrocolic or antecolic), and a side-to-side gastrojejunostomy is constructed with a stapled or hand-sewn technique. The stoma should be placed on the dependent portion of the stomach to facilitate gravity-dependent emptying. A retrocolic gastrojejunostomy (the jejunal loop passes through an opening in the transverse mesocolon) provides a shorter, more dependent route but creates a mesocolic defect that must be closed to prevent internal hernia. Gastrojejunostomy is also used as a palliative bypass for unresectable gastric outlet obstruction from pancreatic or duodenal malignancy.

Operative Management of Peptic Ulcer Disease Complications

Perforated Duodenal Ulcer

Anterior duodenal ulcer perforation produces sudden-onset epigastric pain, free air on upright chest or CT imaging, and peritonitis. The standard operative approach is the Graham patch (omental patch) repair: through an upper midline laparotomy or laparoscopic approach, the perforation is identified on the anterior surface of the duodenal bulb, and a pedicled omental patch (a tongue of viable omentum on its vascular pedicle) is laid over the perforation and secured with three interrupted full-thickness sutures placed through the healthy duodenal wall on either side of the perforation, pulling the omentum into the defect. The sutures are tied over the omentum, not over the ulcer crater itself, so the repair relies on the omental plug rather than direct closure of friable ulcer edges. The peritoneal cavity is irrigated with warm saline, and the patient is placed on high-dose intravenous PPI therapy and tested for Helicobacter pylori. Definitive anti-ulcer surgery (vagotomy with drainage) is rarely added to the emergency perforation repair in the current era, because Helicobacter pylori eradication and PPI therapy are effective at preventing recurrence in the vast majority of patients.

Bleeding Duodenal Ulcer

A posterior duodenal ulcer that erodes into the gastroduodenal artery produces massive upper gastrointestinal hemorrhage. Endoscopic hemostasis (thermal coagulation, injection, hemoclips) is the first-line treatment and is successful in 80 to 90% of cases. Operative intervention is indicated for endoscopic failure, hemodynamic instability despite resuscitation, transfusion requirement exceeding 6 units of packed red blood cells within 24 hours, or rebleeding after two endoscopic attempts. The operative approach is a longitudinal pylorotomy (identical to the first step of a Heineke-Mikulicz pyloroplasty) that opens the pylorus and duodenal bulb to expose the bleeding posterior ulcer. The gastroduodenal artery is controlled with three-point suture ligation (the U-stitch technique): one suture is placed proximal to the bleeding point, one distal, and one medial (at the transverse pancreatic branch of the gastroduodenal artery), all placed deeply through the ulcer base to ligate the artery against the posterior duodenal wall and pancreatic head. After hemostasis, the pylorotomy is closed transversely as a Heineke-Mikulicz pyloroplasty. Truncal vagotomy is added only if the patient is hemodynamically stable and the ulcer history suggests Helicobacter pylori-negative, PPI-refractory disease.

THE OPERATIVE DANGER ZONE ATLAS — Gastroduodenal Artery Hemorrhage from Posterior Duodenal Ulcer

---

The Zone: The posterior wall of the first part of the duodenum (D1) — where a chronic posterior duodenal ulcer erodes through the duodenal wall into the gastroduodenal artery, which courses directly posterior to the duodenal bulb between the duodenum and the pancreatic head.

The Structure at Risk: Gastroduodenal artery (GDA). The GDA is a branch of the common hepatic artery that descends posterior to D1, gives off the right gastroepiploic artery and the superior pancreaticoduodenal artery, and lies directly against the posterior duodenal wall. Its transverse pancreatic branch crosses the ulcer base medially.

The Consequence: Erosion into the GDA produces life-threatening arterial hemorrhage presenting as hematemesis or melena with hemodynamic instability. The GDA is a large-caliber artery (3 to 5 mm diameter) under systemic arterial pressure, and bleeding is brisk, often exceeding the capacity of endoscopic hemostasis.

The Safe Maneuver: Control the GDA with three-point suture ligation through the ulcer base: one U-stitch proximal (toward the common hepatic artery), one distal (toward the right gastroepiploic), and one medial (across the transverse pancreatic branch). Place sutures deeply, incorporating the artery against the pancreatic head. Do not attempt to dissect the artery free from the ulcer crater — this risks uncontrolled hemorrhage. Close the pylorotomy as a Heineke-Mikulicz pyloroplasty.

Bariatric Procedures (Roux-en-Y Gastric Bypass and Sleeve Gastrectomy)

Roux-en-Y Gastric Bypass — Operative Steps

Roux-en-Y gastric bypass (RYGB) is performed laparoscopically. A small gastric pouch (approximately 30 mL volume) is created from the proximal stomach along the lesser curvature by dividing the stomach with sequential linear stapler firings, separating the pouch completely from the gastric remnant. The jejunum is divided 30 to 50 cm distal to the ligament of Treitz, and the distal (Roux) limb is brought up to the gastric pouch — the route may be antecolic antegastric (anterior to the transverse colon and gastric remnant) or retrocolic retrogastric (through the transverse mesocolon, posterior to the gastric remnant). A gastrojejunostomy is created between the pouch and the Roux limb, either with a linear stapler (with the common enterotomy closed with running suture) or a circular stapler. The biliopancreatic limb (the proximal jejunal segment carrying bile and pancreatic secretions) is anastomosed to the Roux limb 75 to 150 cm distal to the gastrojejunostomy, creating the jejunojejunostomy. The mesenteric defect at the jejunojejunostomy and the Petersen space (between the Roux limb mesentery and the transverse mesocolon) must be closed to prevent internal hernias.

Sleeve Gastrectomy

Laparoscopic sleeve gastrectomy (LSG) has become the most commonly performed bariatric procedure worldwide. The greater curvature vessels and short gastric arteries are divided from 4 to 6 cm proximal to the pylorus to the angle of His, completely mobilizing the greater curvature and fundus. A 36 to 40 French bougie dilator is positioned along the lesser curvature as a sizing guide, and the stomach is divided vertically with sequential linear stapler firings parallel to the bougie, excising approximately 75 to 80% of the stomach (the entire fundus, body, and greater curvature). The remaining stomach is a narrow, tubular sleeve along the lesser curvature. The staple line may be reinforced with buttress material or oversewing to reduce the risk of staple line bleeding and leak. The excised specimen is extracted, and the staple line is inspected for hemostasis and integrity using air insufflation under saline or methylene blue testing.

Complications After Bariatric Surgery

The most serious early complication of both RYGB and sleeve gastrectomy is anastomotic or staple line leak, which occurs in 1 to 5% of cases and presents with tachycardia (often the earliest sign), fever, abdominal pain, and leukocytosis typically between postoperative days 3 and 7. In RYGB, the gastrojejunostomy is the most common leak site; in sleeve gastrectomy, the proximal staple line at the angle of His is the most vulnerable location because of the thin gastric wall and high intraluminal pressure concentration at this point. Management ranges from conservative treatment (NPO, antibiotics, percutaneous drainage of fluid collections, endoscopic stent placement) for contained leaks to urgent operative re-exploration with washout, repair or revision, and wide drainage for free leaks with peritonitis. Marginal ulceration at the gastrojejunostomy after RYGB occurs in 5 to 15% of patients and is associated with smoking, NSAID use, and a large gastric pouch with residual parietal cells producing acid. Nutritional deficiencies after RYGB (iron, vitamin B12, calcium, fat-soluble vitamins) require lifelong supplementation and monitoring because the duodenum and proximal jejunum — the primary sites of absorption for these nutrients — are bypassed.

CLINICAL PEARL: The most common site of staple line leak after sleeve gastrectomy is at the angle of His — the most proximal aspect of the staple line where the gastric wall is thinnest and the blood supply is most tenuous. This is also the site of highest intraluminal pressure because the narrow lumen at the gastroesophageal junction concentrates pressure against the proximal staple line.

THE OPERATIVE DANGER ZONE ATLAS — Internal Hernia Through Petersen Space After Gastric Bypass

---

The Zone: Petersen space — the potential space between the mesentery of the Roux limb and the transverse mesocolon (in retrocolic Roux limb configuration) or between the Roux limb mesentery and the transverse colon mesentery (in antecolic configuration). This defect is created by the surgical rearrangement of bowel anatomy during gastric bypass.

The Structure at Risk: Small bowel mesentery and its contained superior mesenteric artery and vein branches. Bowel loops can herniate through Petersen space and become incarcerated, producing closed-loop small bowel obstruction with ischemia. The mesenteric vessels to the herniated loops are compressed at the hernia ring.

The Consequence: Internal hernia produces acute small bowel obstruction with a high risk of bowel ischemia and necrosis. The onset is often sudden (the hernia reduces and incarcerates intermittently, producing recurrent episodic abdominal pain before a definitive incarceration event). CT findings may be subtle — the swirl sign (mesenteric twist) and small bowel feces sign are characteristic. Delayed diagnosis leads to bowel necrosis, perforation, and peritonitis.

The Safe Maneuver: Close all mesenteric defects at the time of the index gastric bypass procedure. Close Petersen space with a running nonabsorbable suture. Close the mesenteric defect at the jejunojejunostomy with interrupted or running nonabsorbable suture. Defect closure reduces the incidence of internal hernia from 5 to 9% to less than 1%. If internal hernia is diagnosed postoperatively, emergent laparoscopic or open exploration with hernia reduction, bowel viability assessment, and defect closure is required.

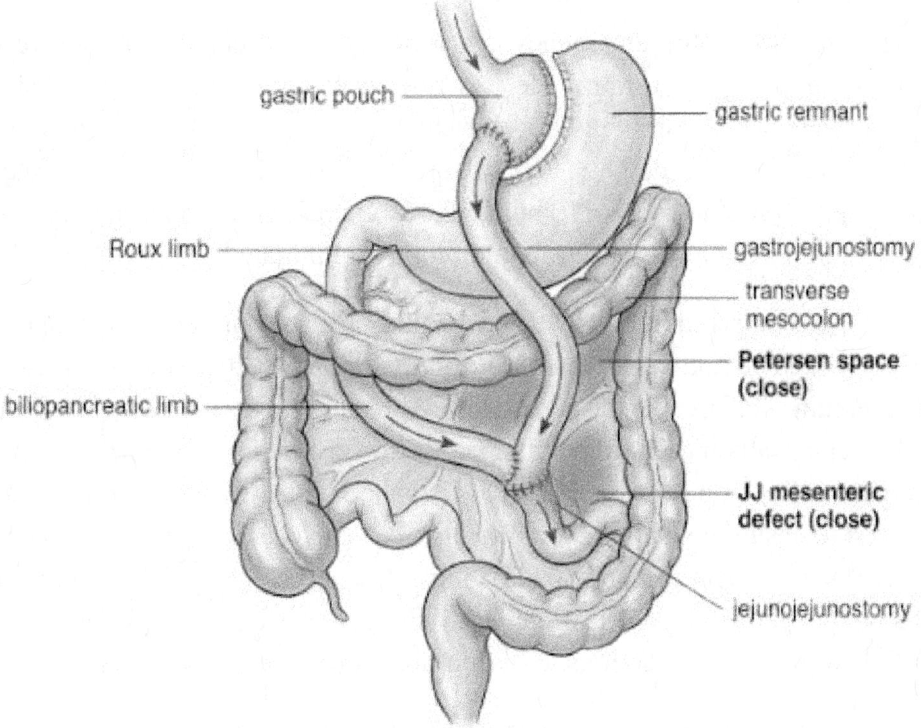
gastric pouch
gastric remnant
Roux limb
gastrojejunostomy
transverse
mesocolon
Petersen space
(close)
biliopancreatic limb
JJ mesenteric
defect (close)
jejunojejunostomy

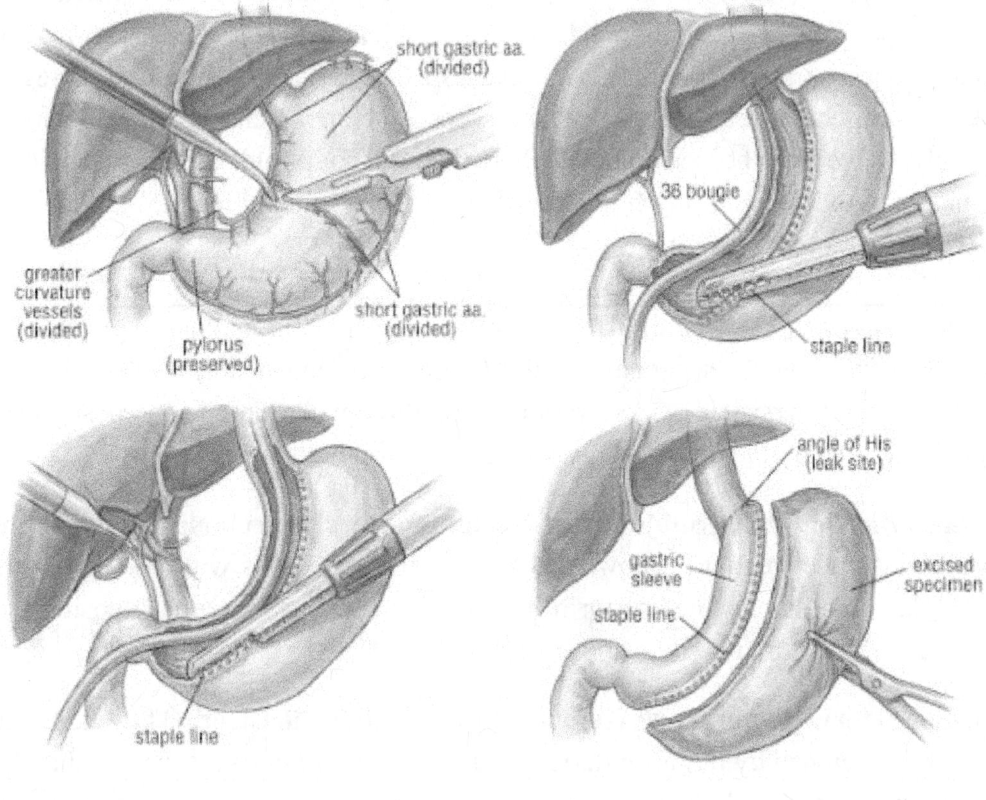
short gastric aa.
(divided)
greater
curvature
vessels
(divided)
pylorus
(preserved)
short gastric aa.
(divided)
36 bougie
staple line
staple line
angle of His
(leak site)
gastric
sleeve
excised
specimen
staple line

Clinical Case — Perforated Anterior Duodenal Ulcer With Peritonitis

A 42-year-old man presents to the emergency department with sudden-onset severe epigastric pain radiating to the right shoulder for 6 hours. He has a history of intermittent dyspepsia but has never undergone endoscopy. He takes ibuprofen daily for chronic knee pain. On examination, he has diffuse abdominal rigidity with rebound tenderness, and an upright chest radiograph demonstrates free air under the right hemidiaphragm. His heart rate is 110 bpm and blood pressure is 95/60 mmHg. He is resuscitated with intravenous crystalloid and broad-spectrum antibiotics are initiated.

At laparoscopy, a 5 mm perforation is identified on the anterior surface of the duodenal bulb with surrounding fibrinous exudate and bile-stained peritoneal fluid. A pedicled omental patch is mobilized from the greater omentum and laid over the perforation. Three interrupted seromuscular sutures are placed through healthy duodenal wall on each side of the perforation and tied over the omental patch, sealing the defect with the omental plug. The peritoneal cavity is irrigated with 3 liters of warm saline, and the upper abdomen is inspected to ensure no additional pathology. A closed suction drain is placed adjacent to the repair. Postoperatively, the patient is maintained on high-dose intravenous PPI therapy, and Helicobacter pylori testing by stool antigen returns positive. He is discharged on triple therapy for H. pylori eradication and long-term PPI therapy, with instructions to discontinue NSAID use.

This case illustrates the standard approach to perforated duodenal ulcer: the Graham omental patch repair seals the perforation without attempting to close the friable ulcer edges directly, which would risk suture cut-through and repair failure. Definitive anti-ulcer surgery is deferred to medical management in the majority of cases because H. pylori eradication and PPI therapy address the underlying cause in most NSAID-related and infection-related ulcers. The laparoscopic approach is preferred when the patient is hemodynamically stable and the perforation is less than 24 hours old, as laparoscopic repair reduces wound complications and hospital stay compared to open repair without increasing leak rates.

THE OPERATIVE DANGER ZONE ATLAS — Gastric and Duodenal Surgery Dangers

Incomplete Vagotomy and the Criminal Nerve of Grassi: The criminal nerve of Grassi arises high on the posterior vagus and courses separately to the fundus. Missing it during truncal vagotomy causes recurrent ulceration from persistent acid secretion. **Safe maneuver:** identify the posterior vagal trunk at the esophageal hiatus and divide it proximally above all gastric branches.

Duodenal Stump Blowout After Subtotal Gastrectomy: The closed duodenal stump receives bile and pancreatic secretions under pressure. Blowout produces bile peritonitis with 10 to 30% mortality. **Safe maneuver:** oversew the staple line; perform a Kocher maneuver to reduce tension; place a lateral duodenostomy tube if the stump is edematous or friable.

Gastroduodenal Artery Hemorrhage from Posterior Duodenal Ulcer: The GDA courses directly posterior to D1 and is eroded by posterior duodenal ulcers. **Safe maneuver:** three-point U-stitch ligation through the ulcer base (proximal, distal, and medial to the transverse pancreatic branch); do not attempt to dissect the artery free from the ulcer crater.

Internal Hernia Through Petersen Space After Gastric Bypass: Petersen space and the jejunojejunostomy mesenteric defect are created by the surgical rearrangement during RYGB. Small bowel can herniate and incarcerate, producing ischemia. **Safe maneuver:** close all mesenteric defects with nonabsorbable suture at the index procedure; defect closure reduces internal hernia incidence from 5 to 9% to less than 1%.

Summary and Key Concepts

The stomach receives arterial supply from four celiac axis branches forming two arcades (lesser and greater curvature), providing redundant blood supply that allows gastric conduit creation on the right gastroepiploic artery alone for esophageal replacement.

Truncal vagotomy denervates the entire stomach and requires a drainage procedure (pyloroplasty or gastrojejunostomy), while highly selective vagotomy preserves the antral crow's foot branches and the antral pump mechanism, eliminating the need for drainage but producing a higher recurrence rate.

The criminal nerve of Grassi is the most commonly missed vagal branch and the most frequent cause of recurrent ulceration after vagotomy — the posterior vagal trunk must be identified and divided at the esophageal hiatus to ensure complete denervation.

Roux-en-Y reconstruction is preferred after gastrectomy for cancer because it diverts bile away from the gastric remnant, preventing alkaline reflux gastritis, and all mesenteric defects (Petersen space and jejunojejunostomy defect) must be closed to prevent internal hernias.

The Graham omental patch repair for perforated duodenal ulcer seals the perforation with a viable omental plug without attempting to close the friable ulcer edges directly, and definitive anti-ulcer surgery is deferred to H. pylori eradication and PPI therapy in the vast majority of cases.

The most common staple line leak site after sleeve gastrectomy is at the angle of His, where the gastric wall is thinnest and intraluminal pressure is highest, making this the most vulnerable point on the proximal staple line.

CHAPTER 7: OPERATIONS OF THE GALLBLADDER AND BILIARY SYSTEM

Learning Objectives

1. Describe the surgical anatomy of the extrahepatic biliary tree, the hepatoduodenal ligament, and Calot triangle, including the most common anatomical variants that predispose to bile duct injury.
2. Achieve the critical view of safety during laparoscopic cholecystectomy and describe the specific criteria that define it.
3. Identify the indications for conversion from laparoscopic to open cholecystectomy and perform the key operative steps of open cholecystectomy.
4. Perform intraoperative cholangiography and interpret the findings to confirm biliary anatomy and exclude choledocholithiasis.
5. Describe the techniques of transcystic and choledochotomy common bile duct exploration for retained choledocholithiasis.
6. Classify bile duct injuries by the Strasberg system and select the appropriate repair strategy for each injury type.

Surgical Anatomy of the Biliary Tree and Calot's Triangle

Extrahepatic Biliary Anatomy

The extrahepatic biliary system consists of the right and left hepatic ducts, which emerge from the liver hilum and join to form the common hepatic duct (CHD). The cystic duct drains the gallbladder and joins the CHD to form the common bile duct (CBD), which descends in the hepatoduodenal ligament anterior to the portal vein and to the right of the hepatic artery, passes behind the first part of the duodenum and through the head of the pancreas, and enters the second part of the duodenum at the ampulla of Vater (major duodenal papilla). The CBD is approximately 6 to 8 cm long and 4 to 8 mm in diameter (greater than 8 mm is considered dilated when the gallbladder is in situ). The hepatoduodenal ligament — the free edge of the lesser omentum — contains the portal triad: the CBD (anterolateral and to the right), the proper hepatic artery (anterolateral and to the left), and the portal vein (posterior and between them). This arrangement is critical during the Pringle maneuver (temporary occlusion of the hepatoduodenal ligament to control hepatic inflow during liver surgery).

Calot Triangle and Its Significance

Calot triangle (the hepatocystic triangle) is defined by the cystic duct inferiorly, the common hepatic duct medially, and the inferior surface of the liver (specifically segment V) superiorly. This triangle contains the cystic artery (typically a branch of the right hepatic artery), the cystic lymph node (node of Lund), lymphatic channels, connective tissue, and, in anatomical variants, aberrant biliary or vascular structures. The entire rationale of the critical view of safety during laparoscopic cholecystectomy is to completely clear Calot triangle of all fat and fibrous tissue so that the two structures entering the gallbladder (the cystic duct and the cystic artery) are the only structures seen — confirming that neither is the common bile duct or the right hepatic artery.

Anatomical Variants Predisposing to Bile Duct Injury

Anatomical variants of the biliary tree and the hepatic artery are the single most important predisposing factor for bile duct injury during cholecystectomy. The most dangerous variant is a short cystic duct with a low junction to the CHD, because during upward retraction of the gallbladder infundibulum, the cystic duct and the CHD are aligned in parallel, creating the illusion that the CHD is the cystic duct — leading to inadvertent clip application and transection of the CHD (the classic mechanism of major bile duct injury). Other variants include a cystic duct that courses parallel to the CHD before joining it (a long cystic duct), an aberrant right hepatic duct draining directly into the cystic duct or into the CHD at the level of the cystic duct junction, a replaced or accessory right hepatic artery crossing posterior to the CHD (present in approximately 15 to 20% of patients), and a caterpillar hump of the right hepatic artery looping into Calot triangle where it can be mistaken for the cystic artery. Knowledge of these variants and meticulous adherence to the critical view of safety are the primary defenses against bile duct injury.

Epidemiology and Clinical Indications for Cholecystectomy

Gallstone disease affects approximately 10 to 15% of the adult population in Western countries, with higher prevalence in women, multiparous patients, patients with obesity, and those of Native American or Hispanic descent. Cholecystectomy is the most commonly performed elective abdominal operation, with approximately 1.2 million procedures performed annually in the United States. The most common indication is symptomatic cholelithiasis — recurrent episodes of biliary colic (postprandial right upper quadrant pain lasting 30 minutes to several hours, caused by transient cystic duct obstruction by a gallstone). Other indications include acute cholecystitis (sustained cystic duct obstruction with gallbladder inflammation and wall edema), gallstone pancreatitis (stones migrating through the cystic duct into the CBD and impacting at the ampulla, causing pancreatic duct obstruction), choledocholithiasis (stones within the CBD causing obstructive jaundice or cholangitis), gallbladder polyps greater than 10 mm (due to malignancy risk), and porcelain gallbladder (calcification of the gallbladder wall, historically associated with gallbladder carcinoma although the magnitude of cancer risk is debated in recent literature). Asymptomatic gallstones are generally not an indication for cholecystectomy except in specific populations — patients with sickle cell disease, patients undergoing bariatric surgery, and patients with congenital hemolytic anemias where the lifetime risk of symptomatic disease and pigment stone complications is high.

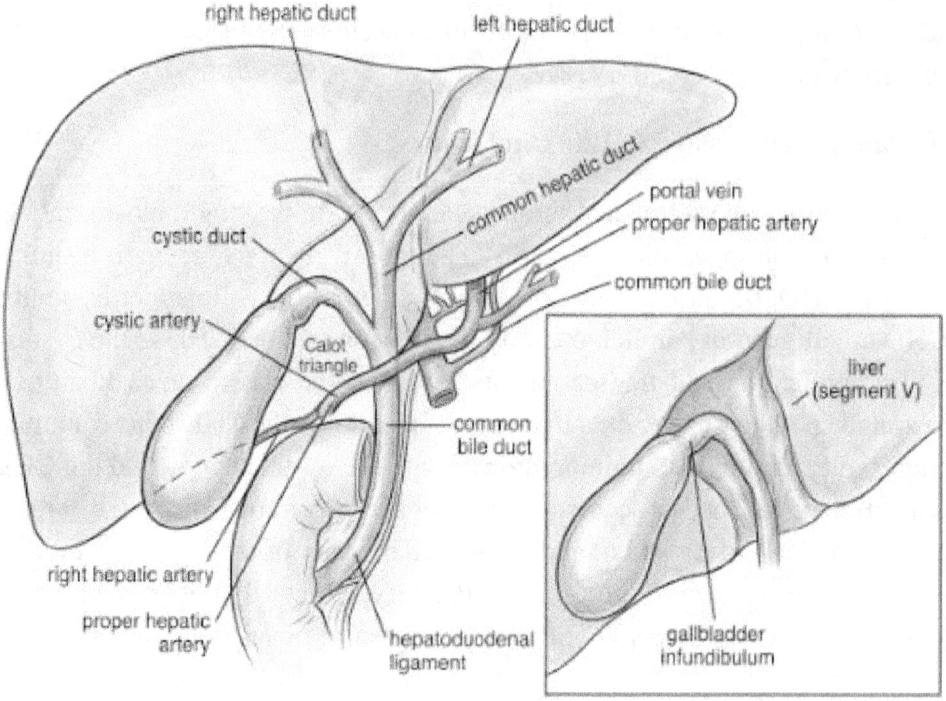

Laparoscopic Cholecystectomy (Critical View of Safety)

Operative Steps

Laparoscopic cholecystectomy is the most commonly performed abdominal operation worldwide. The patient is positioned supine in reverse Trendelenburg with left lateral tilt, and four trocars are placed (10 mm umbilical, 10 mm epigastric, and two 5 mm right subcostal). The gallbladder fundus is retracted cephalad toward the right shoulder to expose the infundibulum, and the infundibulum is retracted laterally and inferiorly to open Calot triangle. Dissection begins at the gallbladder infundibulum, not at the cystic duct — working from the gallbladder toward the bile duct, not from the bile duct toward the gallbladder. All peritoneum, fat, and fibrous tissue within Calot triangle are dissected off the gallbladder infundibulum until two and only two structures are seen entering the gallbladder: the cystic duct and the cystic artery. The inferior surface of the liver at the gallbladder bed (the hepatocystic plate of segment V) must be visible between and behind the two structures. This three-criteria endpoint is the critical view of safety (CVS): complete clearance of Calot triangle, two structures entering the gallbladder only, and visualization of the hepatocystic plate. Only after CVS is achieved are the cystic duct and cystic artery clipped and divided.

The Critical View of Safety — Definition and Rationale

The critical view of safety was described by Strasberg as the definitive method to prevent bile duct injury during laparoscopic cholecystectomy. It works because it establishes the identity of the cystic duct and cystic artery by proving that they are the only structures entering the gallbladder — no other structure can be inadvertently divided if only two structures connect the gallbladder to the rest of the anatomy. The most dangerous moment during laparoscopic cholecystectomy is when the surgeon misidentifies the CBD as the cystic duct. This misidentification most commonly occurs when inflammation, fibrosis, or aberrant anatomy in Calot triangle prevents complete visualization of the anatomy, and the surgeon clips and divides what appears to be the cystic duct without achieving the CVS. The infundibular technique (identifying the cystic duct by tracing it from the gallbladder infundibulum toward the CBD junction) is insufficient because it is precisely the technique that leads to injury when the cystic duct and CBD are aligned in parallel — the surgeon traces what they believe is the infundibulum-to-cystic duct junction but is actually the infundibulum-to-CBD junction.

KEY POINT: The critical view of safety requires three criteria simultaneously: (1) Calot triangle is cleared of all fat and fibrous tissue, (2) two and only two structures are seen entering the gallbladder (cystic duct and cystic artery), and (3) the hepatocystic plate (inferior liver surface at segment V) is visible between and behind the two structures. All three criteria must be met before any structure is clipped or divided. If the CVS cannot be achieved, the surgeon must convert to an alternative strategy (subtotal cholecystectomy, fundus-first technique, or open conversion).

THE OPERATIVE DANGER ZONE ATLAS — Common Bile Duct Misidentification and Transection

---

The Zone: Calot triangle during laparoscopic cholecystectomy — the zone where the cystic duct, common hepatic duct, common bile duct, cystic artery, and right hepatic artery converge in a small, often inflamed operative field with limited depth perception in two-dimensional laparoscopic imaging.

The Structure at Risk: Common bile duct and/or common hepatic duct. When upward traction on the gallbladder infundibulum aligns the cystic duct parallel to the CHD, the CHD can be mistaken for the cystic duct, clipped, and transected — the classic mechanism of major bile duct injury.

The Consequence: Major bile duct injury (Strasberg type D or E) produces bile leak, biliary peritonitis, or biliary obstruction depending on whether the duct was partially or completely transected. Delayed recognition worsens outcomes. Major bile duct injury requires hepaticojejunostomy (Roux-en-Y reconstruction) for definitive repair and is associated with significant long-term morbidity including biliary stricture, recurrent cholangitis, and secondary biliary cirrhosis.

The Safe Maneuver: Achieve the critical view of safety before clipping or dividing any structure. Never clip a structure that has not been definitively identified. If the anatomy cannot be clarified despite adequate dissection, use one of the rescue strategies: intraoperative cholangiography to delineate the biliary anatomy, subtotal (reconstituting or fenestrating) cholecystectomy that avoids dissection in Calot triangle entirely, fundus-first (top-down) dissection, or conversion to open cholecystectomy. The threshold for conversion should be low when inflammation or aberrant anatomy obscures the CVS.

Open Cholecystectomy

Indications and Operative Technique

Open cholecystectomy is performed when laparoscopic cholecystectomy cannot be completed safely — most commonly due to severe acute cholecystitis with a frozen Calot triangle (the gallbladder, cystic duct, and CBD are encased in a single inflammatory mass preventing identification of individual structures), Mirizzi syndrome (compression of the CHD by an impacted gallstone in the cystic duct or gallbladder neck), suspected gallbladder cancer (to allow en bloc resection and lymph node dissection), or uncontrolled bleeding or bile duct injury recognized intraoperatively during laparoscopic attempt. The open approach uses a right subcostal (Kocher) incision, identifies the cystic duct and cystic artery through retrograde (fundus-first) or antegrade dissection, and achieves the same critical view of safety as the laparoscopic approach. The advantage of the open approach in difficult cases is the availability of tactile feedback (palpation of the CBD to feel for stones, palpation of the hepatoduodenal ligament to identify the portal triad), direct three-dimensional visualization, and easier access for concomitant CBD exploration if needed.

Subtotal Cholecystectomy as a Bailout Strategy

When the critical view of safety cannot be achieved laparoscopically or at open surgery — because inflammation, fibrosis, or aberrant anatomy makes identification of the cystic duct and CBD impossible — subtotal cholecystectomy is the safest bailout strategy. The reconstituting subtotal cholecystectomy removes the anterior wall and most of the gallbladder body, leaving the posterior wall attached to the liver bed and oversewing or stapling the remaining gallbladder stump at the infundibulum, deliberately avoiding dissection into Calot triangle entirely. The fenestrating subtotal cholecystectomy leaves the posterior wall on the liver bed and opens the infundibulum to extract stones, then destroys the cystic duct orifice from within the opened stump using cautery — this avoids any external dissection of the cystic duct and prevents clip application near the CBD. Both techniques accept the trade-off of a higher rate of recurrent gallstone symptoms (from the retained stump) in exchange for eliminating the risk of bile duct injury.

Intraoperative Cholangiography

Technique and Interpretation

Intraoperative cholangiography (IOC) provides real-time fluoroscopic imaging of the biliary tree during cholecystectomy. After the cystic duct is partially dissected and clipped proximally (on the gallbladder side), a small incision is made in the cystic duct and a 4 or 5 French cholangiogram catheter is inserted into the cystic duct lumen and directed toward the CBD. Contrast agent (50% diluted iodinated contrast) is injected under fluoroscopy, and images are obtained to visualize the intrahepatic ducts, the common hepatic duct, the common bile duct, the cystic duct insertion point, and contrast flow into the duodenum through the ampulla of Vater. IOC serves two purposes: to confirm biliary anatomy (verifying that the structure clipped and about to be divided is in fact the cystic duct, not the CBD) and to detect choledocholithiasis (filling defects within the CBD that may require intraoperative bile duct exploration).

A normal cholangiogram shows free flow of contrast from the intrahepatic ducts through the CBD into the duodenum without filling defects, strictures, or extravasation. The CBD diameter on IOC is typically 4 to 8 mm — a duct measuring greater than 10 mm suggests distal obstruction.

Selective Versus Routine Cholangiography

Whether IOC should be performed routinely during every cholecystectomy or selectively in patients with elevated risk of choledocholithiasis remains debated. Advocates of routine IOC argue that it detects unexpected CBD stones in 3 to 5% of patients undergoing cholecystectomy for uncomplicated cholelithiasis and, more importantly, that it identifies aberrant biliary anatomy that predisposes to bile duct injury — providing an additional safeguard beyond the critical view of safety. Advocates of selective IOC argue that the low yield of routine IOC in low-risk patients (normal liver function tests, no biliary dilation on imaging, no history of pancreatitis) does not justify the additional operative time and radiation exposure, and that the critical view of safety is sufficient to prevent bile duct injury in experienced hands. Current practice guidelines support selective IOC based on risk stratification — IOC is strongly recommended when biliary anatomy is unclear, when the CVS cannot be confidently achieved, and when there is a moderate pretest probability of CBD stones.

Common Bile Duct Exploration (Transcystic and Choledochotomy)

Transcystic Common Bile Duct Exploration

Transcystic CBD exploration is performed when IOC demonstrates choledocholithiasis and the stones are amenable to extraction through the cystic duct. This approach avoids a choledochotomy and its associated morbidity. The cystic duct is dilated if necessary (using serial dilators or a balloon catheter), and a flexible choledochoscope or a wire basket is passed through the cystic duct into the CBD under fluoroscopic guidance. Small stones (less than 8 mm) can be retrieved with a wire basket or flushed into the duodenum with a saline flush after glucagon-induced sphincter relaxation. Transcystic exploration is limited by the diameter of the cystic duct (must accommodate the choledochoscope), the location of the stones (proximal intrahepatic stones are difficult to reach transcystically), and the number and size of stones (large or numerous stones are better managed by choledochotomy). If transcystic exploration fails or is not feasible, the options are choledochotomy for open CBD exploration or postoperative endoscopic retrograde cholangiopancreatography (ERCP) with sphincterotomy and stone extraction.

Choledochotomy for Common Bile Duct Exploration

Choledochotomy involves a longitudinal incision in the anterior wall of the supraduodenal CBD, typically 1 to 2 cm in length. The CBD is explored with forceps, balloon catheters, and a flexible choledochoscope passed both proximally (toward the hepatic ducts) and distally (toward the ampulla) to ensure complete stone clearance. After all stones are extracted and a completion cholangiogram or choledochoscopy confirms duct clearance, the choledochotomy is closed primarily over a T-tube (a latex or silicone T-shaped tube whose long limb exits through the abdominal wall and whose short crossbar sits within the CBD lumen). The T-tube decompresses the biliary system during healing, provides access for postoperative cholangiography to confirm complete stone clearance at 7 to 14 days, and creates a controlled fistula tract for tube removal at 4 to 6 weeks. Primary choledochotomy closure without a T-tube (using absorbable suture alone, with or without an internal biliary stent placed across the sphincter) has emerged as an alternative that eliminates the morbidity of T-tube management (bile leak at the insertion site, accidental dislodgement, retained tube tract stones).

THE OPERATIVE DANGER ZONE ATLAS — Right Hepatic Artery Injury in Calot Triangle

The Zone: Calot triangle — specifically the area posterior and medial to the cystic duct where the right hepatic artery crosses behind the common hepatic duct (in the standard anatomy) or, in the caterpillar hump variant, loops anteriorly into Calot triangle where it may be mistaken for the cystic artery.

The Structure at Risk: Right hepatic artery. In its standard course, the right hepatic artery passes behind the CHD and gives off the cystic artery within or near Calot triangle. In the caterpillar hump variant (approximately 10 to 15% of patients), the right hepatic artery loops cephalad into Calot triangle before giving off the cystic artery, creating a large tortuous vessel that can be mistaken for the cystic artery and clipped.

The Consequence: Ligation or transection of the right hepatic artery produces ischemia of the right liver lobe. While collateral arterial supply through the hepatic plexus may prevent frank infarction, right hepatic artery injury increases the risk of hepatic abscess, biliary stricture (from ischemia of the bile duct blood supply, which is predominantly arterial), and is a contributing factor in the severity of concomitant bile duct injuries.

The Safe Maneuver: The critical view of safety protects against right hepatic artery injury by requiring two and only two structures entering the gallbladder — the cystic duct and the cystic artery. A structure that does not enter the gallbladder cannot be the cystic artery and must not be divided. If a large or tortuous artery is encountered in Calot triangle, consider that it may be the right hepatic artery in a caterpillar hump configuration. IOC and intraoperative Doppler ultrasound can confirm the identity of vascular structures when in doubt.

Management and Repair of Bile Duct Injuries

Strasberg Classification of Bile Duct Injuries

The Strasberg classification is the standard system for categorizing bile duct injuries during cholecystectomy. Type A is a bile leak from a minor source — the cystic duct stump (from a dislodged clip or incomplete closure), a duct of Luschka (a small accessory duct draining directly from the liver bed into the gallbladder fossa), or a peripheral hepatic radical injured during liver bed dissection. Type B is occlusion (clip application without transection) of an aberrant right hepatic duct. Type C is transection (without ligation) of an aberrant right hepatic duct, producing a bile leak. Type D is a lateral injury to the CBD or CHD (partial wall laceration) without complete transection. Type E encompasses all injuries involving complete transection or excision of a segment of the main bile duct — subclassified by the Bismuth level (E1 through E5) based on the level of injury relative to the biliary confluence and whether the right and left hepatic ducts remain in communication.

Repair Strategies by Injury Type

Type A injuries (cystic duct stump leaks and duct of Luschka leaks) are managed by ERCP with sphincterotomy and temporary biliary stent placement — reducing the transpapillary pressure gradient diverts bile flow away from the leak site and allows spontaneous closure in the vast majority of cases. Type B and C injuries (aberrant duct injuries) are managed conservatively if the drained hepatic territory is small (less than one segment) or by hepaticojejunostomy if a major right sectoral duct is involved. Type D injuries (lateral CBD injuries) may be repaired primarily over a T-tube if recognized intraoperatively — the defect is closed with fine absorbable sutures and the T-tube is placed through a separate choledochotomy to decompress the repair. Type E injuries (complete transection or excision) require Roux-en-Y hepaticojejunostomy performed by a hepatobiliary specialist. The Roux limb is brought up to the proximal biliary stump, and a tension-free, mucosa-to-mucosa anastomosis is constructed with fine interrupted absorbable sutures. The level of the anastomosis determines long-term outcomes — higher injuries (E3–E5) have worse outcomes because the available proximal ductal tissue is smaller and the blood supply is more tenuous.

Timing of Definitive Repair

The timing of definitive bile duct repair is critical. If the injury is recognized intraoperatively by a surgeon experienced in biliary reconstruction, immediate repair is appropriate and achieves the best outcomes. If the injury is recognized postoperatively (the more common scenario — 70 to 80% of bile duct injuries are not recognized at the time of cholecystectomy), the initial management focuses on controlling sepsis and establishing biliary drainage: percutaneous drainage of bilomas, percutaneous transhepatic cholangiography to define the anatomy of the injury, and percutaneous or endoscopic biliary drainage. Definitive Roux-en-Y hepaticojejunostomy is then performed 6 to 12 weeks later, after the acute inflammation has resolved and the biliary anatomy has been fully delineated — delayed definitive repair at a specialized hepatobiliary center achieves the best long-term patency rates (85 to 90% at 10 years).

CAUTION: When a bile duct injury is recognized postoperatively and the operating surgeon is not experienced in hepatobiliary reconstruction, the patient should be transferred to a specialized hepatobiliary center for definitive repair. Attempted repair by a surgeon inexperienced in biliary reconstruction produces inferior outcomes and may convert a repairable injury into an unrepairable one.

Long-Term Outcomes After Bile Duct Repair

Long-term outcomes following bile duct repair are determined by the level of injury, the timing and setting of repair, and the experience of the surgeon performing the reconstruction. Roux-en-Y hepaticojejunostomy performed at a specialized hepatobiliary center achieves long-term patency rates of 85 to 90% at 10 years. However, 10 to 15% of patients develop anastomotic stricture, which typically presents with recurrent cholangitis, obstructive jaundice, or progressive secondary biliary cirrhosis months to years after the initial repair. Strictures can often be managed with percutaneous transhepatic balloon dilation or endoscopic dilation via the Roux limb, but a subset of patients require revision hepaticojejunostomy. The risk of stricture is highest in E3 to E5 injuries where the proximal ductal stump is small and the blood supply is compromised. Concomitant right hepatic artery injury — present in up to 30% of major bile duct injuries — further worsens outcomes because the arterial supply to the bile duct anastomosis is already tenuous, increasing the stricture rate to 50% or higher. Quality-of-life studies demonstrate that patients with major bile duct injury experience significantly worse physical and mental health scores compared to uncomplicated cholecystectomy patients, even after successful repair — reinforcing that prevention (the critical view of safety) is far superior to repair.

Special Populations — Cholecystectomy in Pregnancy and Cirrhosis

Cholecystectomy during pregnancy is indicated for recurrent biliary colic refractory to conservative management, acute cholecystitis, gallstone pancreatitis, and choledocholithiasis with cholangitis. The second trimester is the preferred operative window because organogenesis is complete, the uterus has not yet reached a size that limits laparoscopic working space, and the risk of preterm labor is lowest. Laparoscopic cholecystectomy is the preferred approach — the patient is positioned with left lateral tilt to avoid aortocaval compression by the gravid uterus, open (Hasson) technique is used for initial trocar placement to avoid uterine injury with a Veress needle, insufflation pressure is maintained at 12 to 15 mmHg, and intraoperative fetal heart rate monitoring is recommended. Cholecystectomy in patients with cirrhosis and portal hypertension carries significantly increased operative risk because of coagulopathy, thrombocytopenia, portosystemic venous collaterals in the gallbladder bed and hepatoduodenal ligament, and impaired hepatic regeneration. Child-Pugh class A cirrhosis is generally considered safe for laparoscopic cholecystectomy; class B cirrhosis carries intermediate risk and requires careful optimization; class C cirrhosis is a relative contraindication due to prohibitive operative mortality. In cirrhotic patients, meticulous hemostasis in the gallbladder bed is essential because portal hypertension engorges the small veins draining the gallbladder fossa into the liver, and subtotal cholecystectomy should be considered early if dissection of the gallbladder from the cirrhotic liver bed produces uncontrollable bleeding.

THE OPERATIVE DANGER ZONE ATLAS — Unrecognized Bile Duct Injury — Delayed Presentation

---

The Zone: The early postoperative period after laparoscopic cholecystectomy (postoperative days 1 to 7) — the critical window during which 70 to 80% of major bile duct injuries present with bile leak, biliary peritonitis, jaundice, or sepsis, but are often initially attributed to expected postoperative symptoms.

The Structure at Risk: Common hepatic duct or common bile duct — already injured during the cholecystectomy but not recognized intraoperatively. The injury may be a complete transection (Type E), a lateral laceration (Type D), or a clip-mediated obstruction without leak (Type B/E1), each presenting differently.

The Consequence: Delayed recognition of a bile duct injury allows ongoing bile leak to produce biliary peritonitis and sepsis (if the duct is transected or lacerated) or progressive obstructive jaundice, cholangitis, and secondary biliary cirrhosis (if the duct is clipped or strictured). Each day of delay in recognition worsens the prognosis — early recognition and referral to a hepatobiliary specialist are the most important determinants of long-term outcome.

The Safe Maneuver: Maintain a high index of suspicion for bile duct injury in any patient with unexplained postoperative symptoms after cholecystectomy. Persistent pain, nausea, fever, tachycardia, or elevated liver function tests in the first week after cholecystectomy should prompt urgent hepatobiliary imaging (CT abdomen with contrast, HIDA scan, or MRCP). If a bile duct injury is confirmed, control sepsis with percutaneous drainage and biliary decompression, fully delineate the anatomy with cholangiography, and refer to a hepatobiliary specialist for definitive Roux-en-Y hepaticojejunostomy at 6 to 12 weeks.

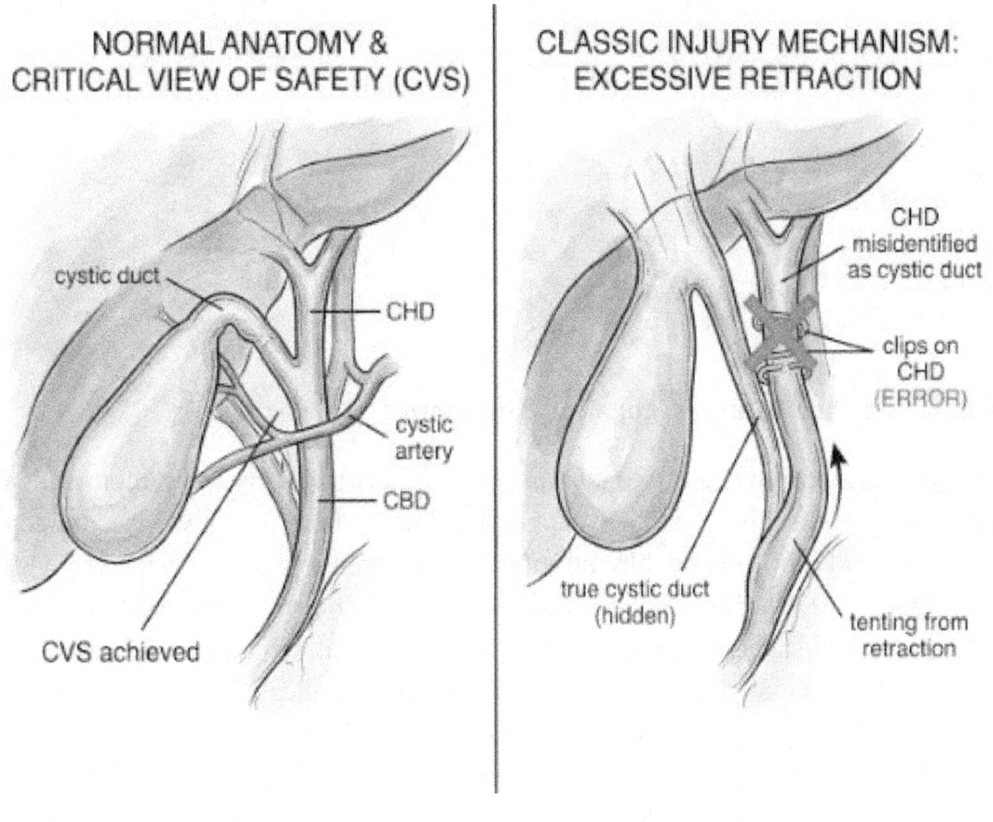

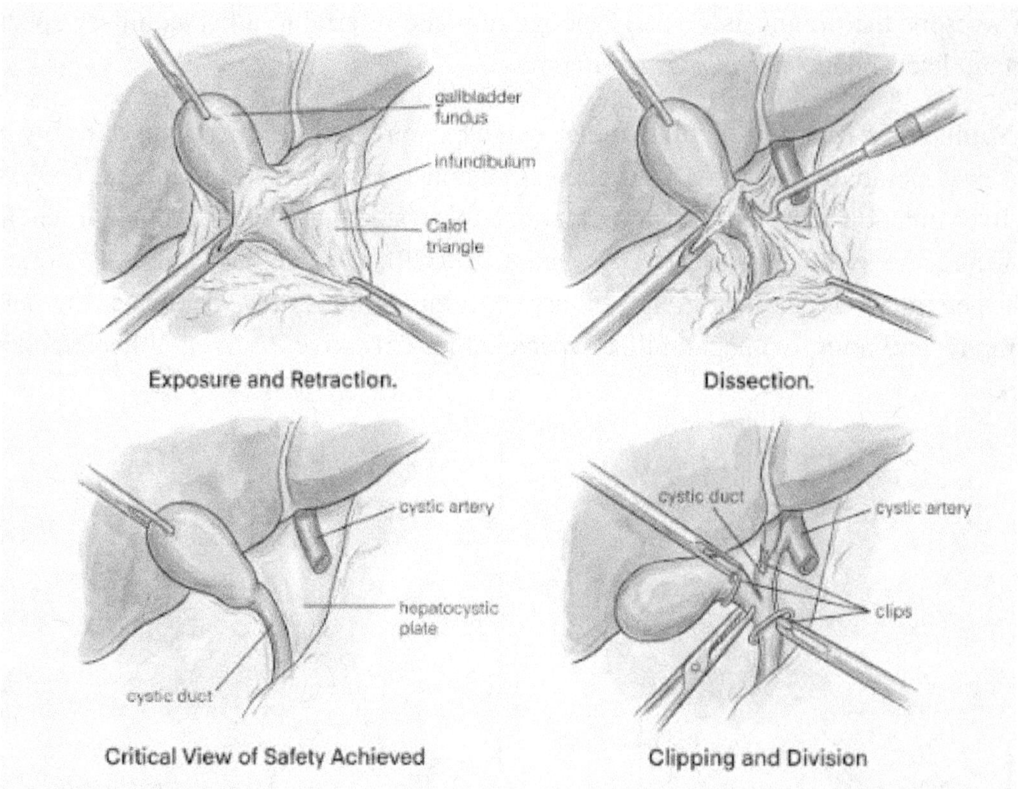

Clinical Case — Bile Duct Injury Recognized Postoperatively

A 48-year-old woman undergoes elective laparoscopic cholecystectomy for symptomatic cholelithiasis. The operation is described as difficult due to acute-on-chronic inflammation with a contracted gallbladder and dense adhesions in Calot triangle. No intraoperative cholangiogram is performed. On postoperative day 3, she develops fever (38.8 degrees C), right upper quadrant pain, and nausea. Laboratory studies reveal leukocytosis and elevated total bilirubin (4.2 mg/dL), alkaline phosphatase, and gamma-glutamyl transferase. CT of the abdomen demonstrates a 6 cm fluid collection in the gallbladder fossa and perihepatic free fluid. MRCP reveals a complete transection of the common hepatic duct at the level of the cystic duct takeoff (Strasberg E2 injury) with a proximal ductal segment ending blindly.

A percutaneous drain is placed into the perihepatic biloma, and a percutaneous transhepatic biliary drain is placed into the right intrahepatic duct for proximal biliary decompression. Broad-spectrum antibiotics are continued. After 8 weeks of drainage, during which the acute inflammation resolves and the patient recovers nutritionally, she undergoes definitive repair with Roux-en-Y hepaticojejunostomy at a hepatobiliary referral center. The proximal biliary stump is identified at the confluence of the right and left hepatic ducts, the scarred distal duct is excised, and a mucosa-to-mucosa anastomosis is constructed with interrupted 5-0 absorbable sutures over a transhepatic stent.

This case illustrates the consequences of failure to achieve the critical view of safety. In a difficult cholecystectomy with dense inflammation, the surgeon should have either performed an intraoperative cholangiogram to delineate the anatomy, converted to a subtotal cholecystectomy to avoid dissection in the dangerous area, or converted to open cholecystectomy for improved visualization and tactile feedback. The delayed presentation (postoperative day 3) is typical — bile duct injuries are frequently not recognized intraoperatively because the duct is divided under the misperception that it is the cystic duct. The principle of delayed definitive repair (6 to 12 weeks after initial drainage) at a specialized center achieves the best long-term outcomes because immediate reoperative repair in an acutely inflamed field carries a higher stricture rate.

THE OPERATIVE DANGER ZONE ATLAS — Biliary Surgery Dangers

Common Bile Duct Misidentification and Transection: Upward traction on the gallbladder infundibulum aligns the cystic duct parallel to the CHD, creating the illusion that the CHD is the cystic duct — the classic mechanism of major bile duct injury during laparoscopic cholecystectomy. **Safe maneuver:** achieve the critical view of safety (Calot triangle cleared, two structures only, hepatocystic plate visible) before clipping or dividing any structure.

Right Hepatic Artery Injury in Calot Triangle: The right hepatic artery crosses behind the CHD or, in caterpillar hump variants, loops into Calot triangle where it can be mistaken for the cystic artery. Ligation causes right hepatic ischemia, abscess, and biliary stricture. **Safe maneuver:** the CVS requires two structures only entering the gallbladder — any structure not entering the gallbladder is not the cystic artery and must not be divided.

Unrecognized Bile Duct Injury — Delayed Presentation: 70 to 80% of major bile duct injuries are not recognized intraoperatively and present postoperatively with bile leak, sepsis, or obstructive jaundice. Each day of delayed recognition worsens prognosis. **Safe maneuver:** maintain high index of suspicion for any unexplained postoperative symptoms after cholecystectomy; image promptly; control sepsis and refer to a hepatobiliary specialist for delayed definitive repair.

Bile Duct Repair by Inexperienced Surgeon: Attempted bile duct repair by a surgeon inexperienced in hepatobiliary reconstruction produces inferior outcomes and may convert a repairable injury into an unrepairable one. **Safe maneuver:** if a major bile duct injury is recognized intraoperatively or postoperatively and the surgeon is not experienced in biliary reconstruction, control the immediate problem (drain, decompress) and transfer to a hepatobiliary center for definitive repair.

Summary and Key Concepts

The critical view of safety during laparoscopic cholecystectomy requires three criteria: complete clearance of Calot triangle, visualization of two and only two structures entering the gallbladder, and visibility of the hepatocystic plate behind both structures — all three must be met before any structure is clipped or divided.

The classic mechanism of bile duct injury is misidentification of the common hepatic duct as the cystic duct when upward traction on the infundibulum aligns the two ducts in parallel, creating the visual illusion that the CHD is the cystic duct.

Subtotal cholecystectomy (reconstituting or fenestrating) is the safest bailout strategy when the critical view of safety cannot be achieved — it avoids dissection in Calot triangle entirely and eliminates the risk of bile duct injury at the cost of a higher rate of recurrent gallstone symptoms.

Bile duct injuries are classified by the Strasberg system — Type A (minor leaks from the cystic duct stump or duct of Luschka) are managed by ERCP with stenting, while Type E (complete transection) requires Roux-en-Y hepaticojejunostomy performed by a hepatobiliary specialist.

Definitive repair of a major bile duct injury is best performed 6 to 12 weeks after the initial injury, after acute inflammation has resolved and biliary anatomy has been fully delineated — immediate reoperation in an inflamed field carries a higher stricture rate.

Intraoperative cholangiography confirms biliary anatomy and detects choledocholithiasis, serving as an additional safeguard beyond the critical view of safety — it is strongly recommended when the anatomy is unclear or the CVS cannot be confidently achieved.

The right hepatic artery in the caterpillar hump variant loops into Calot triangle and can be mistaken for the cystic artery — the critical view of safety protects against this injury because a structure not entering the gallbladder cannot be the cystic artery.

CHAPTER 8: OPERATIONS OF THE LIVER

Learning Objectives

1. Describe the Couinaud segmental anatomy of the liver, including the eight functional segments, their portal pedicle supply, hepatic venous drainage, and the anatomical landmarks that define segment boundaries.
2. Differentiate anatomic from non-anatomic hepatic resections, state the indications for each, and describe the standardized Brisbane terminology for naming liver resections.
3. Explain the techniques of parenchymal transection (clamp-crush, CUSA, harmonic scalpel, stapler) and the methods of vascular control (Pringle maneuver, total vascular exclusion, selective hepatic vein control) used during hepatectomy.
4. Outline the operative management of pyogenic liver abscess, amebic liver abscess, and hepatic cystic disease (simple cysts, cystadenoma, and hydatid cysts).
5. Describe the operative approach to hepatic trauma, including damage-control strategies, perihepatic packing, the Pringle maneuver for hemorrhage control, and the indications for formal hepatic resection versus conservative operative management.

Surgical Anatomy of the Liver (Couinaud Segmental Anatomy)

Surface Anatomy and Peritoneal Attachments

The liver is the largest solid organ in the abdomen, weighing approximately 1,400 to 1,600 g in adults. It occupies the right upper quadrant and is suspended from the diaphragm and anterior abdominal wall by peritoneal reflections: the falciform ligament (containing the ligamentum teres, the obliterated umbilical vein) divides the liver surface into right and left lobes by surface anatomy (a distinction that does not correspond to functional anatomy); the coronary ligaments (anterior and posterior layers) create the bare area of the liver on the posterior surface, where the liver is in direct contact with the diaphragm without peritoneal covering; and the triangular ligaments (right and left) represent the lateral convergences of the coronary ligament layers. The lesser omentum attaches the liver to the lesser curvature of the stomach and the first part of the duodenum, containing the hepatoduodenal ligament with the portal triad (portal vein, hepatic artery, bile duct) at its free edge.

Couinaud Segmental Anatomy

The Couinaud classification divides the liver into eight functionally independent segments (segments I through VIII), each with its own portal pedicle (portal vein branch, hepatic artery branch, and bile duct branch) and hepatic venous drainage. This segmental anatomy is the foundation of modern hepatic surgery because it allows the surgeon to resect one or more segments while preserving the vascular inflow, outflow, and biliary drainage of the remaining liver — the basis of anatomic resection. The three major hepatic veins (right, middle, and left) run in the portal scissurae and divide the liver into four sectors. The right hepatic vein lies in the right portal scissura and divides the right liver into the right anterior sector (segments V and VIII) and the right posterior sector (segments VI and VII). The middle hepatic vein lies in the main portal scissura (Cantlie line) and divides the liver into the functional right and left hemilivers — this plane runs from the gallbladder fossa anteriorly to the left side of the inferior vena cava posteriorly, and it does NOT correspond to the falciform ligament. The left hepatic vein lies in the left portal scissura and divides the left liver into the left medial sector (segment IV, further subdivided into IVa and IVb) and the left lateral sector (segments II and III). Segment I (the caudate lobe) is anatomically unique because it receives portal inflow from both right and left portal pedicles and drains directly into the IVC through short hepatic veins (not through the three major hepatic veins), which explains why it is spared in Budd-Chiari syndrome when the major hepatic veins are occluded.

Hepatic Vascular Inflow and Outflow

The liver has a dual blood supply: the portal vein provides approximately 75% of hepatic blood flow (carrying nutrient-rich, partially deoxygenated blood from the splanchnic circulation), and the hepatic artery provides approximately 25% (carrying oxygenated blood from the celiac trunk). The proper hepatic artery arises from the common hepatic artery (a branch of the celiac trunk) and divides into right and left hepatic arteries at the hilum. Arterial anatomical variants are common and surgically important: a replaced right hepatic artery arising from the superior mesenteric artery (present in approximately 15 to 20% of patients, running posterior to the portal vein and the pancreatic head), a replaced left hepatic artery arising from the left gastric artery (approximately 10%), and accessory hepatic arteries (additional arteries that supplement rather than replace the standard arterial supply). The portal vein is formed by the confluence of the superior mesenteric vein and the splenic vein behind the neck of the pancreas, ascends in the hepatoduodenal ligament posterior to the bile duct and hepatic artery, and divides at the hilum into right and left portal vein branches. Hepatic venous outflow passes through the three major hepatic veins (right, middle, and left) and numerous short hepatic veins (draining the caudate lobe and the posterior aspect of the right lobe directly into the IVC).

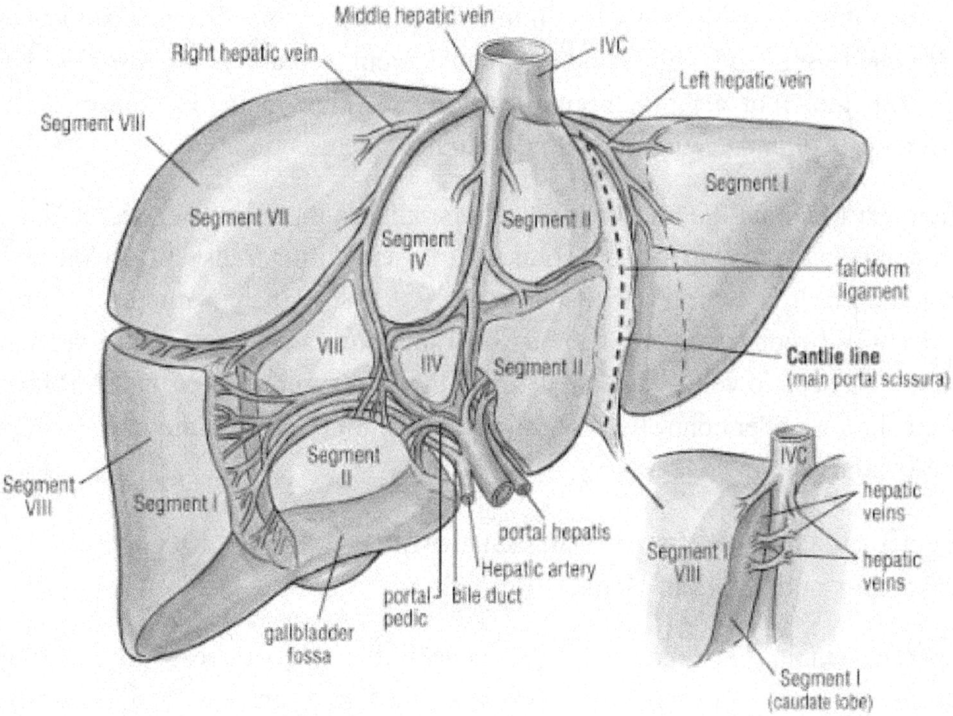

KEY POINT: The functional division of the liver into right and left hemilivers follows Cantlie line (the main portal scissura containing the middle hepatic vein), which runs from the gallbladder fossa to the left side of the IVC. This plane does NOT correspond to the falciform ligament, which divides the liver into surface right and left lobes. Understanding this distinction is essential for planning anatomic hepatic resections — a right hepatectomy removes segments V through VIII (everything to the right of Cantlie line), not everything to the right of the falciform ligament.

THE OPERATIVE DANGER ZONE ATLAS — Hepatic Vein Injury During Parenchymal Transection

The Zone: The plane of parenchymal transection during major hepatectomy — specifically the depth of the transection plane where the surgeon approaches the major hepatic veins running within the portal scissurae. The right hepatic vein is at greatest risk during right hepatectomy (it lies in the right portal scissura, directly in the transection plane for extended left hepatectomy), and the middle hepatic vein is at risk during both right and left hepatectomy (it lies in the main portal scissura at the center of the transection plane).

The Structure at Risk: Major hepatic veins (right, middle, or left) and the retrohepatic inferior vena cava. These thin-walled, high-flow vessels are fixed posteriorly where they enter the IVC and are easily torn by traction during parenchymal transection — particularly where short hepatic veins tether the liver to the IVC along the right posterior segment.

The Consequence: Hepatic vein laceration produces torrential hemorrhage (hepatic venous bleeding is under low pressure but high flow and is difficult to control because the torn vein retracts into the hepatic parenchyma). Air embolism is possible with large hepatic vein lacerations because the veins are in direct communication with the right atrium through a short, valveless path. Uncontrolled hepatic venous hemorrhage is the most common cause of death during hepatic resection.

The Safe Maneuver: Maintain the transection plane parallel to the major hepatic vein, not toward it — use intraoperative ultrasound to map the vein course before and during transection. Control hepatic venous pressure by maintaining low central venous pressure (CVP less than 5 mmHg) during parenchymal transection — low CVP reduces hepatic venous back-pressure and dramatically decreases blood loss during transection. If a hepatic vein is lacerated, apply direct pressure, lower the CVP further, and repair with fine vascular sutures under controlled conditions — do not blindly clamp into the depth of the liver, which risks further injury.

Hepatic Resection (Anatomic and Non-Anatomic)

Brisbane Terminology and Types of Hepatic Resection

The Brisbane 2000 terminology standardized the nomenclature for hepatic resections. A right hepatectomy (right hemihepatectomy) removes segments V, VI, VII, and VIII — the entire right hemiliver to the right of the main portal scissura (Cantlie line). A left hepatectomy (left hemihepatectomy) removes segments II, III, and IV — the entire left hemiliver to the left of the main portal scissura. An extended right hepatectomy (right trisectionectomy) removes the right hemiliver plus segment IV (segments IV, V, VI, VII, VIII), leaving only segments II and III (the left lateral section). An extended left hepatectomy (left trisectionectomy) removes the left hemiliver plus the right anterior section (segments II, III, IV, V, VIII), leaving only segments VI and VII (the right posterior section). A left lateral sectionectomy removes segments II and III only. A right posterior sectionectomy removes segments VI and VII. Segmentectomy refers to the removal of an individual Couinaud segment. Each resection follows the portal scissurae and preserves the vascular pedicles and venous drainage of the remaining segments — the definition of an anatomic resection.

Non-Anatomic Resection and Indications

Non-anatomic (or atypical) resection removes a portion of the liver parenchyma without following the segmental boundaries defined by the portal scissurae. The resection margin is determined by the tumor margin rather than by anatomical planes — the surgeon transects liver parenchyma at a specified distance (typically 1 cm or greater) from the tumor edge regardless of whether the resection plane crosses segment boundaries or portal pedicles. Non-anatomic resection is preferred when a small peripheral tumor can be removed with adequate margins while preserving more functional liver volume than a formal anatomic resection would, when the tumor lies at the junction of multiple segments (making formal segmentectomy impractical), or when the background liver has limited regenerative capacity (cirrhosis, steatohepatitis, prior chemotherapy) and every centimeter of preserved parenchyma reduces the risk of postoperative liver failure. In patients with hepatocellular carcinoma on cirrhosis, preserving functional liver volume is often the primary constraint on resection extent — the Child-Pugh score, the indocyanine green retention rate at 15 minutes (ICG-R15), and volumetric CT assessment of the future liver remnant (FLR) guide the decision between anatomic and non-anatomic resection.

Future Liver Remnant and Preoperative Assessment

The future liver remnant (FLR) is the volume of functional liver that will remain after the planned resection. Adequate FLR is the single most important determinant of whether a patient will survive hepatectomy without liver failure. In patients with normal liver parenchyma, the minimum safe FLR is 20 to 25% of the total liver volume. In patients with significant steatosis or post-chemotherapy hepatic injury, the minimum is 30%. In patients with cirrhosis, the minimum is 40%. If the planned resection will leave an FLR below the safe threshold, portal vein embolization (PVE) of the segments to be resected is performed 4 to 6 weeks before hepatectomy — PVE redirects portal blood flow to the FLR segments, inducing compensatory hypertrophy that can increase FLR volume by 10 to 40%. Associating liver partition and portal vein ligation for staged hepatectomy (ALPPS) is a more aggressive two-stage approach that produces faster and greater FLR hypertrophy but carries higher morbidity.

Resection Type	Segments Removed	Minimum FLR (Normal Liver)	Key Vascular Structure Divided
Right hepatectomy	V, VI, VII, VIII	30–40% (left lobe remains)	Right portal pedicle, right hepatic vein
Left hepatectomy	II, III, IV	60–70% (right lobe remains)	Left portal pedicle, left and middle hepatic veins
Extended right hepatectomy	IV, V, VI, VII, VIII	20–25% (segments II–III remain)	Right portal pedicle, right and middle hepatic veins, segment IV pedicle
Extended left hepatectomy	II, III, IV, V, VIII	25–30% (segments VI–VII remain)	Left portal pedicle, left and middle hepatic veins, right anterior pedicle
Left lateral sectionectomy	II, III	75–80%	Left lateral portal pedicle, left hepatic vein
Right posterior sectionectomy	VI, VII	60–70%	Right posterior portal pedicle

Techniques of Parenchymal Transection and Vascular Control

Parenchymal Transection Methods

The goal of parenchymal transection is to divide the liver tissue along the planned resection plane while identifying, isolating, and controlling the intrahepatic vascular and biliary structures that cross the plane — dividing those that belong to the resected portion and preserving those that supply the FLR. The clamp-crush (Kelly clamp fracture) technique is the oldest and most widely used method: the liver parenchyma is crushed between the jaws of a Kelly clamp, which fractures the soft hepatocytes and exposes the tougher vascular and biliary pedicles running through the parenchyma. These pedicles are then individually ligated, clipped, or cauterized and divided. The technique is inexpensive, universally available, and has been shown in randomized trials to produce transection times and blood loss comparable to more expensive technologies. The Cavitron Ultrasonic Surgical Aspirator (CUSA) uses ultrasonic energy to fragment and aspirate hepatocytes while sparing the fibrous walls of vascular and biliary structures, producing a skeletonized operative field with excellent visualization of individual pedicles. The harmonic scalpel and bipolar sealing devices (LigaSure, Enseal) coagulate and divide small vessels and parenchyma simultaneously. Stapler hepatectomy uses vascular staplers (Endo GIA with vascular loads) to fire through the entire thickness of the liver parenchyma in sequential firings — this technique is fastest but provides the least selective control of individual intrahepatic structures.

Vascular Control — The Pringle Maneuver and Total Vascular Exclusion

The Pringle maneuver is the temporary occlusion of the hepatoduodenal ligament (portal triad) using a vascular clamp or a Rumel tourniquet, which interrupts all hepatic arterial and portal venous inflow to the liver. By eliminating inflow, the Pringle maneuver reduces bleeding during parenchymal transection and is the most commonly used method of vascular control during hepatectomy. The normal liver tolerates continuous Pringle clamping for up to 60 minutes and intermittent clamping (15 minutes on, 5 minutes off) for a total ischemia time of 90 to 120 minutes — intermittent clamping is preferred because it allows reperfusion and reduces the cumulative ischemic injury to the FLR. In cirrhotic livers, ischemic tolerance is reduced and the total safe clamping time is shorter (30 to 40 minutes continuous). The Pringle maneuver controls inflow bleeding but does NOT control outflow (hepatic venous) bleeding — backflow from the hepatic veins and the IVC continues despite Pringle clamping. Total hepatic vascular exclusion (THVE) adds clamping of the suprahepatic and infrahepatic IVC to the Pringle maneuver, completely isolating the liver from the circulation — this eliminates both inflow and outflow bleeding and is reserved for resections involving the major hepatic veins or the retrohepatic IVC (such as extended hepatectomy for tumors invading the hepatocaval confluence). THVE produces significant hemodynamic instability (decreased venous return, decreased cardiac output, hypotension) and requires close anesthetic coordination with volume loading and vasopressor support.

CLINICAL PEARL: Low central venous pressure (CVP less than 5 mmHg) anesthesia during hepatectomy reduces hepatic venous back-pressure and decreases blood loss during parenchymal transection by 40 to 50% compared to standard CVP management. The anesthesiologist restricts intravenous fluids, uses vasodilators if needed, and positions the patient in slight Trendelenburg. Low

CVP is the single most effective strategy for reducing transfusion requirements during liver surgery — it is used in combination with, not instead of, the Pringle maneuver.

THE OPERATIVE DANGER ZONE ATLAS — Portal Pedicle Injury During Hilar Dissection

The Zone: The hepatic hilum (porta hepatis) during hilar dissection for anatomic hepatectomy — the zone where the surgeon isolates and divides the portal pedicle (portal vein branch, hepatic artery branch, bile duct branch) supplying the segments to be resected. The hilum is a congested space where the right and left portal pedicles, the hepatic arterial branches, and the biliary confluence are separated by only millimeters.

The Structure at Risk: Contralateral portal pedicle — the portal vein branch, hepatic artery branch, or bile duct branch supplying the future liver remnant. During right hepatectomy, the left portal pedicle is at risk (it lies immediately to the left of the right portal pedicle at the hilum); during left hepatectomy, the right portal pedicle and especially the right posterior sectoral duct (which has a short extrahepatic course and joins the confluence close to the left hepatic duct) are at risk.

The Consequence: Inadvertent ligation, clip application, or transection of the contralateral portal pedicle devascularizes or obstructs the future liver remnant — precisely the portion of liver the surgeon intended to preserve. If the portal vein branch is injured, the FLR loses portal inflow and the patient develops acute liver failure. If the bile duct branch is injured, the FLR develops biliary obstruction, cholangitis, and biliary cirrhosis. The outcome is often fatal because the resected segments are already removed and the remaining liver cannot function.

The Safe Maneuver: Perform intraoperative ultrasound to map the portal pedicle anatomy and the planned transection plane before dividing any hilar structures. Use the intrahepatic Glissonian approach (pedicle ligation within the liver parenchyma) rather than extrahepatic hilar dissection when hilar anatomy is distorted by tumor, prior surgery, or portal lymphadenopathy — this avoids the hilum entirely and secures the pedicle where it enters the resected segment. Before dividing any pedicle, perform a test clamp and confirm by demarcation (ischemic color change) on the liver surface that the clamped pedicle supplies ONLY the segments to be resected. Never divide a hilar structure that has not been definitively identified.

Surgical Management of Liver Abscess and Cystic Disease

Pyogenic Liver Abscess — Etiology and Operative Management

Pyogenic liver abscess arises from biliary infection (ascending cholangitis from choledocholithiasis or malignant biliary obstruction), portal pyemia (from intra-abdominal sepsis — appendicitis, diverticulitis, inflammatory bowel disease), hepatic artery bacteremia, direct extension from adjacent infection, or cryptogenic (no identifiable source, in up to 40% of cases). The most common causative organisms are Escherichia coli, Klebsiella pneumoniae, and streptococcal species; in East and Southeast Asian populations, K. pneumoniae is the predominant pathogen, often associated with gas-forming abscess and a characteristic clinical syndrome (K. pneumoniae liver abscess syndrome) that carries a risk of metastatic endophthalmitis and central nervous system infection. Initial management is intravenous antibiotics and percutaneous catheter drainage (for abscesses greater than 3 cm) — this is curative in 80 to 90% of cases. Operative drainage is reserved for abscesses that fail to resolve with percutaneous drainage (persistent fever and leukocytosis after 72 hours of adequate drainage), multiloculated abscesses with thick septations that prevent effective percutaneous drainage, and abscesses associated with a biliary etiology that requires simultaneous surgical correction (choledocholithiasis, biliary stricture). Operative drainage involves laparotomy, abscess unroofing, debridement of necrotic material, irrigation, and placement of a large-bore closed-suction drain. Formal hepatic resection is rarely required for pyogenic abscess unless the abscess has destroyed an entire segment or lobe and the necrotic parenchyma is a persistent source of sepsis.

Amebic Liver Abscess

Amebic liver abscess is caused by Entamoeba histolytica, which reaches the liver via the portal vein from the colon. The abscess is typically solitary, large, located in the right lobe (because portal flow from the superior mesenteric vein preferentially distributes to the right liver), and filled with sterile, dark-brown (anchovy paste) material that represents liquefied hepatocytes. Treatment is metronidazole (the drug of choice, which kills trophozoites in the abscess and in the intestinal wall), followed by a luminal agent (paromomycin or diloxanide furoate) to eliminate cysts in the colon. Percutaneous aspiration is indicated for large abscesses (greater than 5 to 10 cm) at risk of rupture, left-lobe abscesses that may rupture into the pericardium, and abscesses that fail to respond clinically to metronidazole within 72 hours. Operative intervention is rarely needed — indications include rupture into the peritoneum or pericardium (requiring operative lavage and drainage) and failure of repeated percutaneous drainage.

Hepatic Cystic Disease — Simple Cysts and Hydatid Cysts

Simple hepatic cysts are common incidental findings on imaging, present in approximately 5% of the population. They are lined by biliary-type cuboidal epithelium, filled with serous fluid, and are virtually never malignant. The vast majority are asymptomatic and require no treatment. Symptomatic simple cysts (causing right upper quadrant pain or early satiety from mass effect) are treated by laparoscopic cyst unroofing (fenestration or deroofing): the cyst is decompressed, the dome is excised broadly back to the liver surface, and the base is inspected for bile leaks or suspicious nodularity. Aspiration alone is not curative (the cyst recurs in virtually all cases). Hepatic cystadenoma (now reclassified as mucinous cystic neoplasm of the liver) is a premalignant lesion that occurs predominantly in women and requires complete enucleation or formal hepatic resection — fenestration is inadequate because it does not remove the neoplastic epithelium and leaves the patient at risk for recurrence and malignant transformation. Hydatid cysts (Echinococcus granulosus) require operative treatment when large, symptomatic, or at risk of rupture. The operative technique centers on killing the protoscolices before opening the cyst (to prevent peritoneal dissemination): hypertonic saline (20%) or cetrimide is injected into the cyst as a scolicidal agent, the cyst is then aspirated and opened, the endocyst (germinal layer) and daughter cysts are removed, and the pericyst (the host-derived fibrous capsule) is left in place. The residual cavity is managed by omentoplasty (packing with omentum) or by capitonnage (suture obliteration of the cavity). Formal pericystectomy (complete excision of the cyst including the pericyst) or hepatic resection is performed for thick-walled, calcified, or multiple cysts.

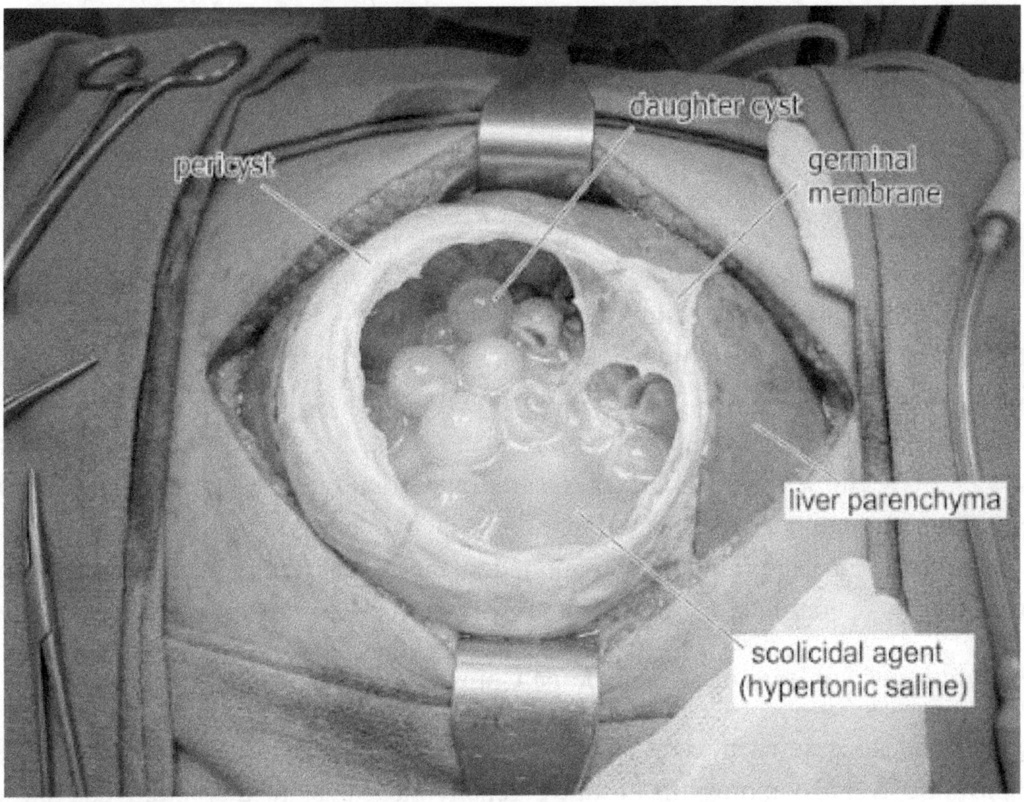

THE OPERATIVE DANGER ZONE ATLAS — Inadvertent Rupture of Hydatid Cyst Contents

The Zone: The operative field during surgical management of a hepatic hydatid cyst — specifically the moment of cyst puncture and the initial aspiration phase, before scolicidal treatment has been completed.

The Structure at Risk: The peritoneal cavity and the systemic circulation. Hydatid cyst fluid contains millions of viable protoscolices (the infective larval forms of Echinococcus granulosus). Each protoscolex can develop into a new hydatid cyst wherever it implants.

The Consequence: Spillage of hydatid cyst contents into the peritoneal cavity causes disseminated peritoneal hydatidosis — hundreds of secondary cysts developing across the peritoneal surfaces, mesentery, and omentum over months to years, requiring multiple operations and prolonged albendazole therapy with poor eradication rates. Spillage into the systemic circulation (through an open hepatic vein within the cyst wall) can cause anaphylaxis — the hydatid fluid contains highly antigenic proteins that trigger IgE-mediated systemic anaphylactic reactions, which can be fatal.

The Safe Maneuver: Before puncturing any hydatid cyst, pack the operative field around the cyst with scolicidal-soaked gauze pads to contain any spillage. Puncture the cyst with a large-bore trocar connected to suction, aspirate a portion of the cyst fluid (send for microscopy to confirm protoscolices), and instill hypertonic saline (20%) or cetrimide into the cyst for a minimum of 15 minutes as a scolicidal agent before opening the cyst. Only after scolicidal treatment is the cyst opened widely for evacuation of daughter cysts and the germinal membrane. Pre-operative albendazole (for 1 to 3 months before surgery) reduces cyst viability and the risk of intraperitoneal dissemination from inadvertent spillage.

Operative Management of Hepatic Trauma

AAST Grading of Liver Injuries and Initial Assessment

Hepatic injuries are graded by the American Association for the Surgery of Trauma (AAST) scale from grade I (subcapsular hematoma less than 10% of liver surface area, capsular tear less than 1 cm in parenchymal depth) to grade VI (hepatic avulsion — the liver is completely separated from its vascular attachments). Grades I through III are managed non-operatively in hemodynamically stable patients with serial clinical examinations, hemoglobin monitoring, and repeat imaging if clinically indicated — non-operative management is successful in 80 to 90% of blunt liver injuries. Operative management is indicated for hemodynamic instability (systolic blood pressure less than 90 mmHg despite resuscitation), peritonitis, ongoing transfusion requirement (more than 4 units of packed red blood cells in the first 4 hours), grade IV or V injuries with active contrast extravasation on CT, and associated intra-abdominal injuries requiring laparotomy. The operative approach to hepatic trauma follows damage-control principles: control hemorrhage, control contamination, and close temporarily — definitive repair is deferred to the second operation after physiologic resuscitation in the intensive care unit.

Operative Techniques for Hepatic Hemorrhage Control

At laparotomy for hepatic trauma, the first maneuver is perihepatic packing — laparotomy pads are packed above and below the liver to compress the hepatic parenchyma against the diaphragm and retroperitoneum, tamponading parenchymal and venous bleeding. Perihepatic packing alone controls hemorrhage in approximately 50 to 60% of operative hepatic trauma cases and is the definitive damage-control maneuver — the packs are left in place, the abdomen is closed temporarily, and the patient is transferred to the ICU for resuscitation (correction of hypothermia, acidosis, and coagulopathy — the lethal triad). Packs are removed at planned re-laparotomy 24 to 72 hours later. If packing alone fails to control hemorrhage, the Pringle maneuver is applied. If bleeding stops with the Pringle (suggesting hepatic arterial or portal venous bleeding), the surgeon identifies the bleeding vessel within the hepatic parenchyma, ligates or sutures it, and repairs the laceration. If bleeding continues despite the Pringle (suggesting hepatic venous or retrohepatic IVC injury), the injury involves the major hepatic veins or the retrohepatic IVC — the most lethal hepatic injuries. Options include selective hepatic vein repair (direct suture repair with vascular clamps), hepatic vein ligation (the liver can tolerate ligation of one major hepatic vein if the other two are patent), or total hepatic vascular exclusion to isolate the liver completely while the venous injury is repaired. Liver resection (formal hepatectomy or non-anatomic resection) is performed only when a lobe or segment is devascularized or destroyed by the injury and cannot be salvaged — resectional debridement removes only the non-viable tissue.

THE OPERATIVE DANGER ZONE ATLAS — Retrohepatic Inferior Vena Cava Injury

The Zone: The retrohepatic space — the 6 to 10 cm segment of the inferior vena cava that lies posterior to the liver, receiving the short hepatic veins and the three major hepatic veins. This segment of the IVC is partially or completely surrounded by liver parenchyma and is inaccessible without mobilizing or resecting liver tissue.

The Structure at Risk: The retrohepatic inferior vena cava and the hepatic vein-IVC junctions. The retrohepatic IVC is a large, thin-walled, low-pressure vessel carrying the entire venous return from the lower body. The short hepatic veins are small, fragile vessels draining directly from the posterior liver surface into the IVC that are easily torn during liver mobilization.

The Consequence: Retrohepatic IVC injury produces massive, exsanguinating hemorrhage that is extremely difficult to control because the injury is in an anatomically inaccessible location (posterior to the liver), the vein is large and thin-walled (direct suture repair is difficult under pressure), and standard vascular clamp placement is hazardous (clamping the suprahepatic IVC eliminates venous return and produces cardiac arrest). Retrohepatic IVC injuries carry an operative mortality exceeding 50 to 80%, even in experienced trauma centers.

The Safe Maneuver: When retrohepatic IVC injury is suspected (persistent venous hemorrhage despite Pringle clamping, hemorrhage from behind the liver), the first maneuver is aggressive perihepatic packing — direct tamponade of the retrohepatic space may control the bleeding sufficiently for damage-control closure and ICU resuscitation. If packing fails, total hepatic vascular exclusion (clamping the suprahepatic IVC, infrahepatic IVC, and the porta hepatis simultaneously) isolates the retrohepatic IVC and allows direct repair — but this requires rapid volume resuscitation and causes severe hemodynamic compromise. An atriocaval shunt (Schrock shunt — a large-bore chest tube inserted through the right atrial appendage, passed through the suprahepatic IVC, and positioned with its tip in the infrahepatic IVC, with a side hole at the level of the renal veins) diverts venous return around the injured retrohepatic IVC, allowing repair under controlled conditions — but the technique is rarely used and carries high mortality.

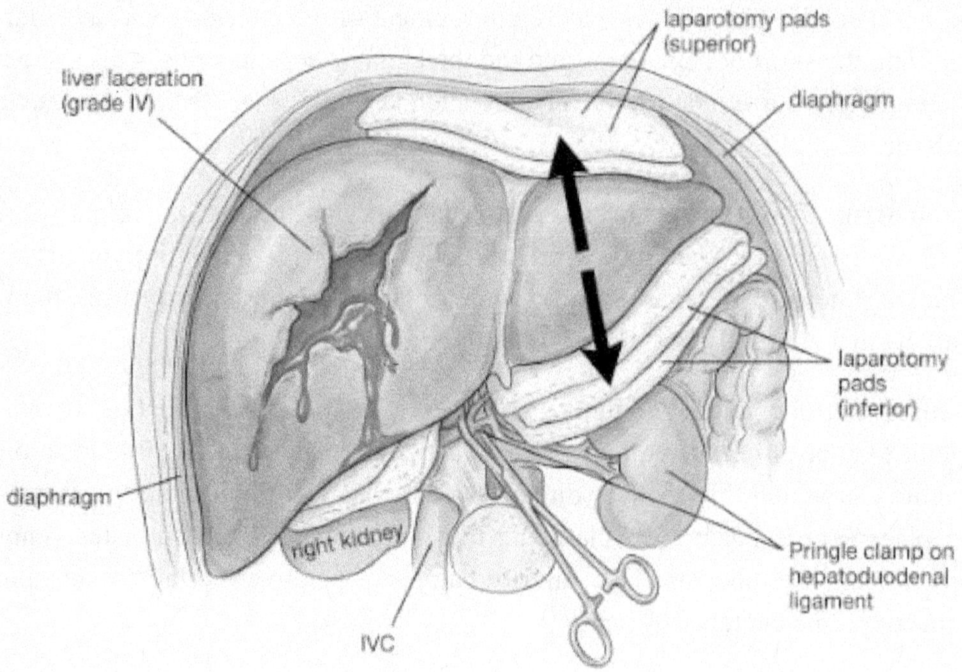

Clinical Case — Damage-Control Hepatectomy for Grade V Liver Injury

A 32-year-old man presents after a high-speed motor vehicle collision with hemodynamic instability (blood pressure 72/40 mmHg, heart rate 128 bpm) despite 2 liters of crystalloid and 2 units of packed red blood cells in the emergency department. A focused assessment with sonography for trauma (FAST) examination demonstrates free fluid in the right upper quadrant and the pelvis. The patient is taken directly to the operating room without CT imaging.

At laparotomy, 2 liters of hemoperitoneum are evacuated. A grade V stellate laceration is identified through the right lobe of the liver involving segments V, VI, VII, and VIII, with active arterial hemorrhage from a transected right hepatic artery branch within the parenchyma and venous bleeding from the right hepatic vein. Perihepatic packing is applied immediately, and the Pringle maneuver is performed. Arterial hemorrhage is controlled, but venous bleeding continues (indicating hepatic vein injury). The devitalized right lobe is resected using clamp-crush technique as a non-anatomic resectional debridement, the right hepatic vein stump is suture-ligated, and the raw transection surface is packed. The abdomen is closed temporarily with a negative-pressure dressing. The patient receives massive transfusion protocol (12 units of packed red blood cells, 8 units of fresh frozen plasma, 2 units of platelets, and 2 units of cryoprecipitate) and is transferred to the ICU for correction of hypothermia, acidosis, and coagulopathy. At planned re-laparotomy 48 hours later, the packs are removed, hemostasis is confirmed, the abdomen is irrigated, and the fascia is closed primarily.

This case demonstrates the damage-control sequence for high-grade hepatic trauma: hemorrhage control (packing plus Pringle), resection of devitalized tissue only, damage-control closure, ICU resuscitation to correct the lethal triad, and planned re-laparotomy. The decision to resect the right lobe was driven by the extent of devitalization (the right hepatic artery and right hepatic vein were both disrupted, rendering segments V through VIII non-viable), not by elective oncologic principles. In trauma, the goal is to stop the bleeding and remove only what is already dead — not to perform a formal anatomic hepatectomy.

CAUTION: Formal anatomic hepatic resection should NOT be the primary approach to hepatic trauma. The vast majority of operative liver injuries are managed by packing, direct suture repair, and selective vessel ligation. Formal hepatectomy carries high mortality in the trauma setting (30 to 50%) and is reserved for devitalized lobes or segments where the major vascular inflow and outflow are irreversibly disrupted — resectional debridement of non-viable tissue, not planned oncologic resection.

THE OPERATIVE DANGER ZONE ATLAS — Hepatic Surgery Dangers

Hepatic Vein Injury During Parenchymal Transection: The major hepatic veins run within the portal scissurae directly in the transection plane during hepatectomy. Laceration produces torrential venous hemorrhage and risk of air embolism. **Safe maneuver:** maintain the transection plane parallel to the vein using intraoperative ultrasound guidance, operate under low CVP anesthesia (less than 5 mmHg), and control bleeding with direct pressure and fine suture repair — never blindly clamp into the liver depth.

Portal Pedicle Injury During Hilar Dissection: At the hepatic hilum, the right and left portal pedicles are separated by only millimeters. Inadvertent ligation of the contralateral pedicle devascularizes the future liver remnant. **Safe maneuver:** map pedicle anatomy with intraoperative ultrasound, use intrahepatic Glissonian approach when hilar anatomy is distorted, and perform a test clamp with demarcation confirmation before dividing any pedicle.

Inadvertent Rupture of Hydatid Cyst Contents: Spillage of hydatid cyst fluid causes disseminated peritoneal hydatidosis (secondary cysts throughout the peritoneum) and can trigger fatal anaphylaxis. **Safe maneuver:** pack the operative field with scolicidal-soaked gauze, aspirate before opening, instill hypertonic saline for 15 minutes minimum, and only then open the cyst widely for evacuation.

Retrohepatic Inferior Vena Cava Injury: The retrohepatic IVC is inaccessible, thin-walled, and carries the entire lower body venous return — injury produces exsanguinating hemorrhage with operative mortality exceeding 50 to 80%. **Safe maneuver:** aggressive perihepatic packing as first-line tamponade; if packing fails, total hepatic vascular exclusion for direct repair under rapid volume resuscitation.

Summary and Key Concepts

The Couinaud classification divides the liver into eight functionally independent segments defined by their portal pedicles and hepatic venous drainage — each segment can be resected while preserving the vascular supply and biliary drainage of the remaining segments.

The functional division of the liver into right and left hemilivers follows Cantlie line (the main portal scissura, containing the middle hepatic vein), running from the gallbladder fossa to the IVC — not the falciform ligament.

The future liver remnant (FLR) must exceed 20 to 25% in normal livers, 30% in steatotic livers, and 40% in cirrhotic livers to prevent post-hepatectomy liver failure — portal vein embolization can increase FLR volume by 10 to 40% over 4 to 6 weeks.

Low CVP anesthesia (less than 5 mmHg) during hepatectomy reduces hepatic venous back-pressure and decreases blood loss by 40 to 50% — it is the single most effective strategy for reducing transfusion requirements during liver surgery.

The Pringle maneuver controls hepatic inflow bleeding but not hepatic venous bleeding — the normal liver tolerates up to 60 minutes of continuous clamping and 90 to 120 minutes of intermittent clamping.

Perihepatic packing controls hemorrhage in 50 to 60% of operative hepatic trauma cases and is the definitive damage-control maneuver — packs are removed at planned re-laparotomy 24 to 72 hours later after correction of hypothermia, acidosis, and coagulopathy.

Retrohepatic IVC injuries carry operative mortality exceeding 50 to 80% even in experienced trauma centers — perihepatic packing (direct tamponade) is the first-line maneuver before escalating to total hepatic vascular exclusion or atriocaval shunt placement.

CHAPTER 9: OPERATIONS OF THE PANCREAS

Learning Objectives

1. Describe the surgical anatomy of the pancreas, its arterial supply from the celiac and superior mesenteric systems, its venous drainage through the portal-splenic-mesenteric confluence, and the intimate anatomical relationships that make pancreatic surgery technically demanding.
2. Outline the indications, critical operative steps, and reconstructive phase of pancreaticoduodenectomy (Whipple procedure), including the management of the superior mesenteric vein during uncinate dissection.
3. Describe the technique of distal pancreatectomy with and without splenectomy, including the indications for spleen-preserving distal pancreatectomy (Kimura and Warshaw techniques).
4. Explain the operative management of infected pancreatic necrosis, including the step-up approach and open necrosectomy.
5. Compare the techniques of internal drainage for pancreatic pseudocysts (cystogastrostomy versus cystojejunostomy) and state the criteria for operative drainage.
6. Describe the indications for and technique of lateral pancreaticojejunostomy (Puestow procedure) in chronic pancreatitis with a dilated pancreatic duct.

Surgical Anatomy of the Pancreas and Peripancreatic Vasculature

Anatomical Relationships of the Pancreas

The pancreas is a retroperitoneal organ extending from the C-loop of the duodenum to the splenic hilum. It is divided into five anatomical regions: the head (which includes the uncinate process), the neck, the body, the tail, and the uncinate process (which hooks posteriorly and medially behind the superior mesenteric vessels). The head of the pancreas is intimately adherent to the medial wall of the duodenum — the two organs share a common blood supply through the pancreaticoduodenal arcades, which is why the head of the pancreas and the duodenum must be resected together (the Whipple procedure). The neck of the pancreas overlies the confluence of the superior mesenteric vein (SMV) and the splenic vein, which join to form the portal vein directly posterior to the pancreatic neck — this relationship is the basis for the critical step of creating a tunnel behind the pancreatic neck during pancreaticoduodenectomy. The body and tail extend to the left, crossing anterior to the aorta, the left kidney, and the left adrenal gland. The tail of the pancreas enters the splenorenal ligament and lies in close proximity to the splenic hilum — this intimate relationship explains why splenectomy is frequently performed together with distal pancreatectomy.

Arterial Supply and Venous Drainage

The arterial supply of the pancreas derives from both the celiac trunk and the superior mesenteric artery (SMA), creating a watershed anastomosis between the two systems. The head and uncinate process are supplied by the anterior and posterior pancreaticoduodenal arcades, each formed by a superior branch (from the gastroduodenal artery, a branch of the celiac trunk via the common hepatic artery) and an inferior branch (from the SMA). The body and tail are supplied by branches of the splenic artery (dorsal pancreatic artery, great pancreatic artery of von Haller, and transverse pancreatic artery) and by the inferior pancreatic artery from the SMA. The venous drainage mirrors the arterial supply and flows into the portal venous system: the head drains through the pancreaticoduodenal veins into the SMV and the portal vein; the body and tail drain through small pancreatic veins directly into the splenic vein along its posterior surface. The splenic vein runs along the posterior surface of the pancreatic body and tail, receiving multiple small, fragile pancreatic branches — these short pancreatic veins are easily torn during mobilization of the pancreatic body from the splenic vein, and their avulsion is a common source of operative hemorrhage during distal pancreatectomy.

The Pancreatic Duct System

The main pancreatic duct (duct of Wirsung) runs the entire length of the gland from the tail to the head, where it joins the common bile duct at the ampulla of Vater and opens into the second part of the duodenum through the major duodenal papilla. The accessory pancreatic duct (duct of Santorini) drains the superior portion of the head and opens through the minor duodenal papilla, approximately 2 cm proximal to the major papilla. In approximately 10% of the population, the main and accessory ducts do not communicate (pancreas divisum — the dorsal and ventral pancreatic anlage fail to fuse during embryological development), so the majority of pancreatic secretion drains through the minor papilla. The normal main pancreatic duct diameter is 2 to 3 mm in the body and tail; a duct diameter exceeding 7 mm in the body suggests obstruction or chronic pancreatitis. In chronic pancreatitis, the duct may dilate to 10 to 15 mm or more, with interspersed strictures and calculi — this chain-of-lakes pattern is the indication for lateral pancreaticojejunostomy (Puestow procedure).

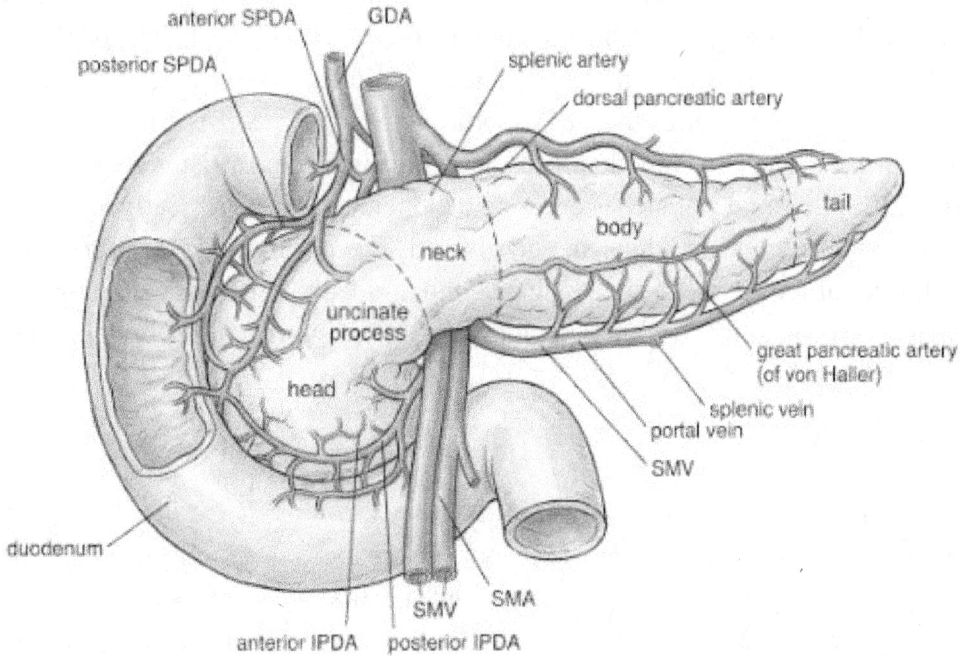

Pancreaticoduodenectomy (Whipple Procedure)

Indications and Resectability Assessment

Pancreaticoduodenectomy is the standard curative-intent operation for malignant and premalignant tumors of the pancreatic head, uncinate process, distal common bile duct, ampulla of Vater, and duodenum. Resectability depends on the relationship of the tumor to the major mesenteric vessels — the SMV-portal vein confluence, the SMA, and the celiac trunk. By the National Comprehensive Cancer Network (NCCN) criteria, a pancreatic head tumor is resectable when there is no tumor contact with the SMV-portal vein or SMA (or contact is less than 180 degrees with no vein contour deformity), borderline resectable when there is tumor contact with the SMV-portal vein of 180 degrees or greater or contact with the SMA of less than 180 degrees, and locally advanced (unresectable) when there is encasement (greater than 180 degrees contact) of the SMA or celiac trunk. Borderline resectable tumors may undergo neoadjuvant chemotherapy (with or without radiation) to downstage the tumor before resection. Benign indications for pancreaticoduodenectomy include chronic pancreatitis with an inflammatory head mass causing intractable pain, duodenal obstruction, or biliary obstruction unresponsive to endoscopic management.

Critical Operative Steps — Resection Phase

The resection phase of pancreaticoduodenectomy removes the head of the pancreas, the duodenum, the distal stomach (in the classic Whipple) or preserves the stomach and proximal duodenum (in the pylorus-preserving modification), the distal common bile duct, the gallbladder, and the proximal jejunum. The critical operative step is the creation of a tunnel behind the neck of the pancreas, anterior to the SMV-portal vein confluence. This tunnel is created by carefully dissecting the loose areolar tissue between the posterior surface of the pancreatic neck and the anterior surface of the SMV-portal vein, passing a Penrose drain or an umbilical tape through the tunnel to encircle the pancreatic neck. The pancreas is then divided at the neck, typically with a scalpel, exposing the anterior surface of the SMV. The uncinate process is dissected off the right lateral wall of the SMV-portal vein and the SMA using a combination of sharp dissection and bipolar cautery — this uncinate dissection is the most dangerous step of the operation because the small, fragile venous branches draining the uncinate process directly into the SMV and portal vein must be individually identified, ligated, and divided. The gastroduodenal artery (GDA) is identified at the superior border of the pancreatic head, ligated and divided (after a test clamp to confirm that proper hepatic artery flow is maintained, excluding celiac artery stenosis), and the common bile duct is divided above the pancreatic head.

Reconstruction Phase

After en bloc resection of the specimen, three anastomoses are constructed to restore gastrointestinal and biliary continuity — the pancreaticojejunostomy (or pancreaticogastrostomy), the hepaticojejunostomy, and the gastrojejunostomy (or duodenojejunostomy in the pylorus-preserving modification). The pancreaticojejunostomy is the most critical anastomosis because it is the most prone to leakage — the pancreatic anastomotic leak (postoperative pancreatic fistula, POPF) is the most common and most dangerous complication of pancreaticoduodenectomy, occurring in 10 to 25% of cases. The anastomosis is constructed either as a duct-to-mucosa anastomosis (the pancreatic duct is sutured directly to a small enterotomy in the jejunal wall with fine interrupted sutures, and the seromuscular layer of the jejunum is sutured to the pancreatic capsule as an outer layer) or as an invagination (dunking) anastomosis (the pancreatic stump is telescoped into the jejunal lumen). A pancreatic duct stent (internal or external) is often placed to decompress the duct and protect the anastomosis during healing. The hepaticojejunostomy is constructed 10 to 15 cm distal to the pancreaticojejunostomy on the same jejunal limb, and the gastrojejunostomy is constructed an additional 40 to 50 cm distally.

Postoperative Complications of Pancreaticoduodenectomy

Pancreaticoduodenectomy carries a perioperative mortality of 2 to 5% at high-volume centers and a morbidity rate of 30 to 50%. The most important complication is postoperative pancreatic fistula (POPF), defined by the International Study Group of Pancreatic Surgery (ISGPS) as drain output of any measurable volume of fluid with an amylase content greater than 3 times the upper limit of normal serum amylase. POPF is graded as biochemical leak (no clinical impact), grade B (requiring maintenance of drains beyond 3 weeks, percutaneous drainage, or interventional radiology procedures), or grade C (requiring reoperation, organ failure, or causing death). The risk of clinically relevant POPF (grade B or C) is highest in patients with a soft, non-fibrotic pancreatic remnant and a small pancreatic duct (less than 3 mm) — these features predict poor healing at the pancreaticojejunal anastomosis. Other major complications include delayed gastric emptying (15 to 25%, managed conservatively with nasogastric decompression and prokinetics), postpancreatectomy hemorrhage (5 to 10%, classified as early intraluminal or delayed extraluminal — delayed hemorrhage is often caused by erosion of the GDA stump pseudoaneurysm into the intestinal lumen and requires angiographic embolization), and bile leak from the hepaticojejunostomy (3 to 5%). The Fistula Risk Score (FRS) — based on gland texture, pathology, duct diameter, and intraoperative blood loss — stratifies patients into negligible, low, moderate, and high POPF risk categories and guides postoperative drain management (early drain removal in low-risk patients reduces infectious complications).

THE OPERATIVE DANGER ZONE ATLAS — SMV-Portal Vein Hemorrhage During Uncinate Dissection

The Zone: The uncinate process of the pancreas during the dissection of the uncinate from the right lateral wall of the SMV-portal vein confluence — the most technically demanding step of pancreaticoduodenectomy.

The Structure at Risk: Superior mesenteric vein and portal vein. The uncinate process is attached to the right lateral wall of the SMV-portal vein by multiple small, fragile venous branches (3 to 6 tributaries, including the first jejunal branch of the SMV) that drain the uncinate directly into the SMV-portal vein. These branches are short (often only 2 to 5 mm long), thin-walled, and surrounded by pancreatic parenchyma that obscures them until they are encountered during dissection.

The Consequence: Avulsion of an uncinate venous branch from the SMV produces a side-wall venous tear with rapid hemorrhage that obscures the operative field, risks air embolism, and requires immediate vascular repair. Uncontrolled SMV hemorrhage during the Whipple procedure is the most common reason for intraoperative death or conversion to an incomplete resection.

The Safe Maneuver: Divide uncinate venous branches individually between suture ligatures or clips — never by electrocautery or blunt avulsion. Maintain complete visualization of the SMV-portal vein surface throughout uncinate dissection by proceeding from superior to inferior along the right lateral wall. If a venous branch avulses, apply direct pressure with a sponge stick, control inflow with the Pringle maneuver, and repair the SMV with a fine running vascular suture (5-0 Prolene). Have vascular sutures, sponge sticks, and Satinsky clamps on the operative field at all times during uncinate dissection.

Distal Pancreatectomy With and Without Splenectomy

Standard Distal Pancreatectomy With Splenectomy

Distal pancreatectomy removes the body and tail of the pancreas (and, variably, the neck) to the left of the SMV-portal vein confluence. The most common indications are pancreatic ductal adenocarcinoma of the body or tail, neuroendocrine tumors of the distal pancreas, mucinous cystic neoplasms, and symptomatic chronic pancreatitis localized to the distal gland. In the standard operation for malignancy, the spleen is removed en bloc with the distal pancreas because the splenic artery and vein are intimately adherent to the posterior surface of the pancreatic body and tail, and en bloc splenectomy ensures adequate lymph node harvest (station 10 and 11 nodes) and an adequate margin of clearance around the tumor. The operation begins with mobilization of the splenic flexure of the colon, entry into the lesser sac, and identification of the inferior border of the pancreas. The pancreas is mobilized from left (tail) to right (neck) in a lateral-to-medial approach, dividing the splenocolic, splenorenal, and splenophrenic ligaments, and taking the splenic artery and vein at the left lateral aspect of the dissection. The pancreatic neck is divided at the chosen transection line, and the stump is managed with a fish-mouth closure (suture closure of the transected pancreatic duct and oversewing of the parenchymal surface) or a stapled closure with or without a reinforced bioabsorbable buttress.

Spleen-Preserving Distal Pancreatectomy

Spleen preservation is indicated for benign and low-grade neoplastic indications (mucinous cystic neoplasm, intraductal papillary mucinous neoplasm with low-grade dysplasia, serous cystadenoma, small neuroendocrine tumors) where lymph node dissection is not oncologically required and the splenic vessels can be separated from the pancreas. Two techniques exist. The Kimura technique preserves the splenic artery and vein by meticulously dissecting the pancreas off the anterior and posterior surfaces of the splenic vessels, individually ligating and dividing each small pancreatic branch entering the vessels — this technique preserves normal splenic perfusion but is time-consuming and technically demanding. The Warshaw technique ligates the splenic artery and vein at the level of the pancreatic transection and distally at the splenic hilum, removing the vessels en bloc with the distal pancreas — the spleen survives on collateral blood flow through the short gastric arteries and the left gastroepiploic artery via the gastrosplenic ligament. The Warshaw technique is faster but carries a 2 to 5% risk of splenic infarction (requiring delayed splenectomy) and a higher rate of perigastric varices because the splenic venous drainage is rerouted through the short gastric veins.

THE OPERATIVE DANGER ZONE ATLAS — Splenic Vein Avulsion During Distal Pancreatectomy

The Zone: The posterior surface of the pancreatic body and tail during distal pancreatectomy — specifically the plane between the posterior pancreatic parenchyma and the anterior wall of the splenic vein, where multiple short, fragile pancreatic venous tributaries (3 to 8 branches) drain directly into the splenic vein.

The Structure at Risk: Splenic vein and its direct pancreatic tributaries. These short veins (2 to 5 mm long) are tethered between the pancreatic parenchyma and the splenic vein wall — traction during mobilization of the pancreas avulses them from the splenic vein, creating side-wall tears.

The Consequence: Avulsion of a pancreatic tributary produces a side-wall tear in the splenic vein with rapid venous hemorrhage. If the tear extends or involves the splenic vein-SMV confluence, repair becomes complex and may require segmental vein resection with reconstruction. Uncontrolled splenic vein hemorrhage during distal pancreatectomy is the most common reason for conversion from laparoscopic to open approach and may necessitate portal vein repair.

The Safe Maneuver: Dissect the pancreas off the splenic vein from left to right (tail to neck), maintaining the dissection directly on the posterior pancreatic capsule (not on the vein wall). Identify, clip, and divide each pancreatic tributary before it comes under tension — never avulse a tributary by pulling the pancreas away from the vein. If a tributary avulses, apply direct pressure, obtain proximal and distal vascular control of the splenic vein, and repair with a fine running vascular suture. In cases where the splenic vein is densely adherent to the pancreas (tumor invasion, chronic pancreatitis), abandon splenic vein preservation early and perform en bloc splenectomy rather than risking a major venous injury.

Surgical Management of Acute Pancreatitis Complications (Necrosectomy and Drainage)

The Step-Up Approach to Infected Pancreatic Necrosis

Approximately 20% of patients with acute pancreatitis develop pancreatic and peripancreatic necrosis, and approximately one-third of those patients develop secondary infection of the necrotic tissue (infected pancreatic necrosis, IPN) — the primary indication for operative intervention in acute pancreatitis. The step-up approach (validated by the PANTER and TENSION trials) is now the standard of care. Step 1 is percutaneous or endoscopic transgastric catheter drainage of the infected collection, performed as the initial intervention. If the patient does not improve clinically (persistent fever, leukocytosis, organ failure) after 72 hours of adequate drainage, Step 2 is minimally invasive necrosectomy — either video-assisted retroperitoneal debridement (VARD) through a left flank incision using the drain tract as a guide, or endoscopic transgastric necrosectomy through a cystogastrostomy created by interventional endoscopy. Step 3 is open necrosectomy, reserved for patients who fail minimally invasive approaches. Operative intervention is delayed as long as possible (ideally 4 weeks or more from disease onset) to allow the necrotic tissue to demarcate and encapsulate (walled-off necrosis), which facilitates debridement and reduces the complication rate.

Open Necrosectomy Technique

When open necrosectomy is required, the retroperitoneum is accessed through the gastrocolic ligament (entering the lesser sac) or through a left flank incision (retroperitoneal approach). The necrotic pancreatic and peripancreatic tissue is debrided by blunt finger dissection and gentle irrigation — the necrotic material separates from the viable tissue along a natural cleavage plane in walled-off necrosis. Aggressive sharp debridement is avoided because the necrotic cavity walls are in intimate contact with the splenic vein, SMV, portal vein, SMA, and transverse mesocolon — sharp instruments in these areas risk catastrophic vascular injury. After debridement, the cavity is managed by closed continuous lavage (large-bore drains with continuous saline irrigation at 1 to 2 liters per hour for 7 to 14 days) or by open packing with planned re-laparotomy every 48 to 72 hours until the cavity is clean. The mortality of infected pancreatic necrosis managed by the step-up approach is approximately 15 to 20%, compared to 30 to 40% with primary open necrosectomy — the step-up approach reduces organ failure, new-onset diabetes, and incisional hernia.

Vascular Complications of Necrotizing Pancreatitis

Necrotizing pancreatitis produces vascular complications through enzymatic digestion and inflammation of the peripancreatic vessels. Splenic vein thrombosis (from direct contact with the inflamed pancreatic body and tail) occurs in 10 to 20% of cases, causing sinistral (left-sided) portal hypertension with gastric varices that may bleed — the treatment is splenectomy if variceal hemorrhage occurs. Pseudoaneurysm formation affects the splenic artery, gastroduodenal artery, or pancreaticoduodenal arteries in 5 to 10% of patients with necrotizing pancreatitis — the enzymatic erosion weakens the arterial wall, producing a contained pseudoaneurysm that can rupture into the necrotic cavity, the peritoneum, or the gastrointestinal tract (hemosuccus pancreaticus — bleeding through the pancreatic duct into the duodenum). Pseudoaneurysm rupture is a surgical emergency with high mortality. The first-line treatment for pseudoaneurysm is angiographic embolization (coil embolization of the feeding artery) — operative ligation is reserved for failed embolization or hemodynamic instability precluding angiography. During open necrosectomy, the surgeon must be aware that the necrotic cavity walls may contain a pseudoaneurysm — any pulsatile structure within the cavity should not be debrided.

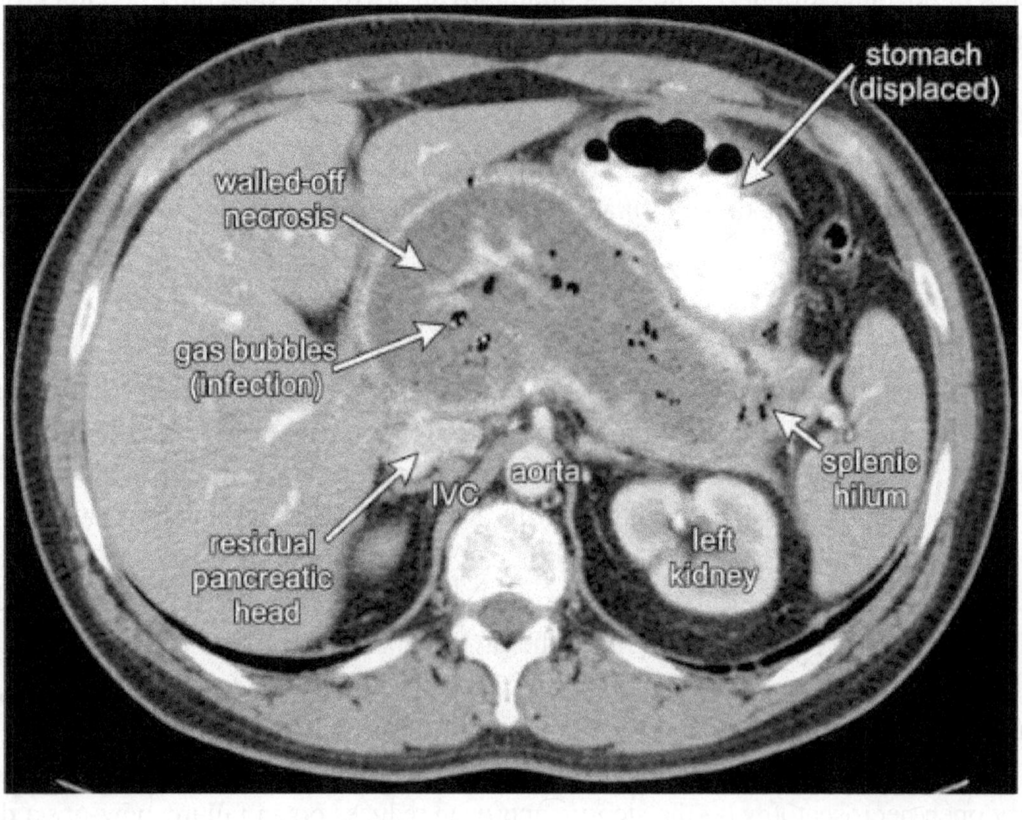

Pancreatic Pseudocyst Drainage (Cystogastrostomy and Cystojejunostomy)

Indications for Operative Drainage

A pancreatic pseudocyst is an encapsulated collection of pancreatic fluid surrounded by a fibrous wall (lacking an epithelial lining — distinguishing it from a true cyst), arising from pancreatic ductal disruption during acute or chronic pancreatitis. Most pseudocysts resolve spontaneously within 6 weeks. Intervention is indicated for pseudocysts that are symptomatic (abdominal pain, gastric outlet obstruction, biliary obstruction, early satiety), enlarging on serial imaging, greater than 6 cm and persisting beyond 6 weeks, or complicated (infected pseudocyst, pseudocyst hemorrhage into the cyst cavity, or pseudocyst rupture). Before any drainage procedure, the cyst must be evaluated for neoplastic features — a cystic neoplasm (mucinous cystic neoplasm, intraductal papillary mucinous neoplasm) masquerading as a pseudocyst requires resection, not drainage. Features suggesting neoplasm include the absence of a pancreatitis history, an epithelial lining on imaging, septations, mural nodules, and elevated cyst fluid CEA.

Cystogastrostomy and Cystojejunostomy Techniques

Internal drainage creates a communication between the pseudocyst and the gastrointestinal tract, allowing the cyst contents to drain internally and the cyst cavity to collapse. Cystogastrostomy (cyst-to-stomach drainage) is performed when the pseudocyst is adherent to the posterior wall of the stomach — the posterior gastric wall and the anterior cyst wall are opened through a common gastrotomy, creating a large stoma (at least 3 to 4 cm) between the cyst cavity and the gastric lumen. The cyst wall is biopsied to exclude neoplasm, and the stoma edges are sutured with absorbable suture for hemostasis and to prevent premature closure. Cystogastrostomy can be performed laparoscopically or endoscopically (endoscopic ultrasound-guided cystogastrostomy with lumen-apposing metal stent placement is now the preferred first-line approach for pseudocysts accessible from the stomach). Cystojejunostomy (cyst-to-jejunum drainage) is performed when the pseudocyst is not adherent to the stomach — a Roux-en-Y jejunal limb is brought up to the pseudocyst, and a wide anastomosis (at least 3 to 4 cm) is created between the cyst wall and the jejunal wall. Cystojejunostomy is preferred for pseudocysts in the pancreatic tail, pseudocysts extending into the mesentery, and pseudocysts associated with a pancreatic duct stricture that requires simultaneous pancreatic duct drainage (a combined Puestow-cystojejunostomy).

CLINICAL PEARL: Before draining any pancreatic cystic lesion presumed to be a pseudocyst, confirm that the patient has a documented history of pancreatitis and that the cyst lacks epithelial features (no septations, no mural nodules, no solid component). A cystic neoplasm (MCN, IPMN, SCA) masquerading as a pseudocyst requires resection — internal drainage of a cystic neoplasm delays definitive treatment and may seed the peritoneum if the lesion is malignant.

Lateral Pancreaticojejunostomy (Puestow Procedure)

Indications and Patient Selection

Lateral pancreaticojejunostomy (the modified Puestow procedure, also called the Partington-Rochelle modification) is the standard operation for chronic pancreatitis with a dilated main pancreatic duct (greater than 7 mm in the body) and intractable abdominal pain. The procedure decompresses the obstructed pancreatic duct along its entire length by creating a side-to-side anastomosis between the opened duct and a Roux-en-Y jejunal limb — the ductal pressure drops, the inflammatory cascade driven by ductal hypertension diminishes, and the pain improves or resolves in 70 to 80% of patients. The primary indication is the chain-of-lakes pattern seen on cross-sectional imaging or MRCP: alternating strictures and dilations of the main pancreatic duct, often with intraductal calculi. The procedure is not appropriate for small-duct chronic pancreatitis (duct less than 5 mm) because there is insufficient duct caliber to create a reliable anastomosis — these patients are managed with total pancreatectomy with islet autotransplantation (TPIAT) or the Frey or Beger procedures (which combine limited pancreatic head resection with lateral pancreaticojejunostomy).

Operative Technique

The anterior surface of the pancreas is exposed by opening the gastrocolic ligament and entering the lesser sac. The main pancreatic duct is identified by palpation (feeling the dilated, often calcified duct through the anterior pancreatic capsule) or by intraoperative ultrasound. A longitudinal incision is made in the anterior pancreatic capsule and parenchyma directly over the duct, extending from the tail to within 1 cm of the duodenal wall (do not extend the ductal opening into the pancreatic head within 1 cm of the duodenal wall — this risks injury to the intrapancreatic CBD). The duct is opened along its full length (typically 8 to 12 cm), and all intraductal calculi are extracted. A Roux-en-Y jejunal limb (60 cm in length, constructed with a stapled or sutured jejunojejunostomy) is brought up through a defect in the transverse mesocolon or in a retrocolic fashion. The opened jejunal lumen is anastomosed side-to-side to the opened pancreatic duct using a single layer of interrupted absorbable sutures (3-0 or 4-0 PDS or Vicryl), creating a wide, tension-free pancreaticojejunostomy that drains the entire length of the decompressed duct into the jejunum.

THE OPERATIVE DANGER ZONE ATLAS — Intrapancreatic Common Bile Duct Injury During Puestow Procedure

---

The Zone: The head of the pancreas during lateral pancreaticojejunostomy — specifically the area where the main pancreatic duct approaches the intrapancreatic segment of the common bile duct within the pancreatic head, typically within 1 cm of the duodenal wall.

The Structure at Risk: Intrapancreatic common bile duct. The CBD passes through the posterior aspect of the pancreatic head before entering the ampulla of Vater. In chronic pancreatitis with extensive fibrosis and calcification of the head, the CBD may be displaced, compressed, or encased in calcified tissue, making it difficult to distinguish from the pancreatic duct during ductal opening.

The Consequence: Incision into or transection of the intrapancreatic CBD during opening of the pancreatic duct produces bile leak, biliary peritonitis, and biliary obstruction. If unrecognized, the CBD injury leads to biliary stricture and cholangitis. Repair of the intrapancreatic CBD injury in a field of chronic pancreatitis fibrosis and calcification is technically extremely difficult.

The Safe Maneuver: Stop the ductal opening 1 cm before reaching the duodenal wall — do not extend the pancreatic ductotomy into the pancreatic head. If the head is the primary site of disease (inflammatory mass, dominant head stricture), perform a Frey procedure (coring out the pancreatic head parenchyma while preserving a thin rim of posterior pancreatic tissue overlying the CBD and the posterior pancreaticoduodenal arcade) rather than a simple lateral pancreaticojejunostomy. Palpate or use intraoperative ultrasound to identify the CBD within the head before extending the ductotomy medially. Place a biliary stent endoscopically before the operation to make the CBD palpable (the stent is easily felt through the pancreatic head tissue).

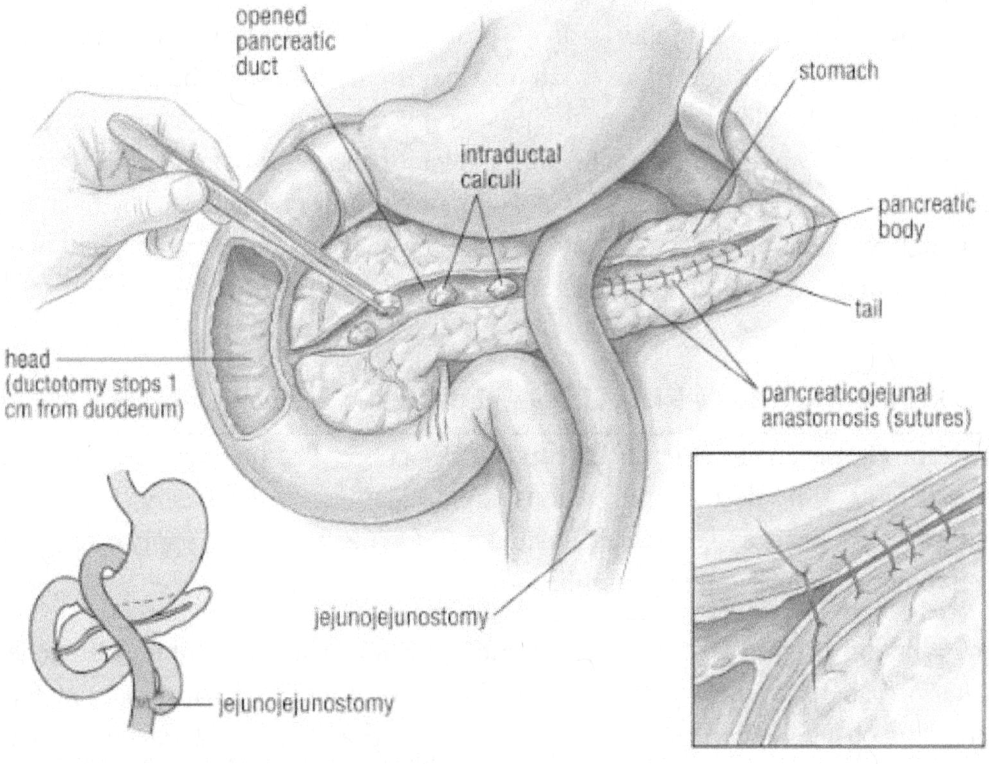

Clinical Case — Pancreaticoduodenectomy for Periampullary Carcinoma

A 67-year-old man presents with painless obstructive jaundice (total bilirubin 14.2 mg/dL), pruritus, dark urine, and 10 kg unintentional weight loss over 3 months. CT of the abdomen reveals a 2.8 cm hypodense mass in the head of the pancreas with abrupt cutoff of the pancreatic duct and common bile duct (double-duct sign), no evidence of vascular involvement (the SMV-portal vein confluence and SMA have clear fat planes), and no distant metastases. Endoscopic ultrasound with fine-needle biopsy confirms adenocarcinoma. A plastic biliary stent is placed during ERCP for preoperative biliary decompression, and the patient is nutritionally optimized over 2 weeks.

At operation, the abdomen is explored and no peritoneal metastases are found. Intraoperative ultrasound confirms no liver metastases. The tumor is confirmed to be limited to the pancreatic head with no vascular involvement. A standard pancreaticoduodenectomy (pylorus-preserving modification) is performed. During uncinate dissection, three small venous branches draining into the SMV are individually ligated with 4-0 silk ties and divided. The pancreatic duct diameter at the transection margin is 4 mm (not dilated — a soft gland, which carries a higher risk of postoperative pancreatic fistula). A duct-to-mucosa pancreaticojejunostomy is constructed over an internal stent, followed by hepaticojejunostomy and duodenojejunostomy. Two closed-suction drains are placed near the pancreaticojejunostomy. The postoperative course is complicated by a clinically relevant pancreatic fistula (ISGPS grade B) managed by maintaining the surgical drains for 3 weeks. The patient is discharged on postoperative day 14 and started on adjuvant gemcitabine-based chemotherapy at 6 weeks postoperatively. Final pathology reveals a T2N1 pancreatic ductal adenocarcinoma with negative margins (R0 resection) and 3 of 18 lymph nodes positive.

THE OPERATIVE DANGER ZONE ATLAS — Pancreatic Surgery Dangers

SMV-Portal Vein Hemorrhage During Uncinate Dissection: The uncinate process is tethered to the SMV-portal vein by 3 to 6 short, fragile venous tributaries that avulse easily during dissection. **Safe maneuver:** individually ligate and divide each tributary; if avulsion occurs, apply direct pressure, Pringle maneuver, and repair with fine running vascular suture.

Splenic Vein Avulsion During Distal Pancreatectomy: Short pancreatic venous branches (2 to 5 mm) along the posterior pancreatic body drain into the splenic vein and tear with traction. **Safe maneuver:** dissect left to right on the posterior pancreatic capsule, clip and divide each tributary before tension develops.

Intrapancreatic CBD Injury During Puestow Procedure: The intrapancreatic CBD lies within 1 cm of the duodenal wall in the pancreatic head, near the termination of the opened pancreatic duct. **Safe maneuver:** stop the ductotomy 1 cm from the duodenal wall, palpate or ultrasound the CBD, and use a Frey procedure for head-dominant disease.

Vascular Injury During Open Necrosectomy: The walls of the necrotic cavity in acute pancreatitis are in intimate contact with the splenic vein, SMV, portal vein, and SMA. Sharp debridement risks catastrophic vascular injury. **Safe maneuver:** debride by blunt finger dissection only, following the natural cleavage plane of walled-off necrosis.

Summary and Key Concepts

The uncinate process hooks behind the SMV-portal vein confluence, and its small, fragile venous branches draining directly into the SMV are the most dangerous structures encountered during pancreaticoduodenectomy — each must be individually ligated and divided.

The critical view in pancreaticoduodenectomy is the tunnel behind the pancreatic neck anterior to the SMV-portal vein confluence — creating this tunnel confirms that the tumor has not invaded the portal venous system and defines the transection line.

Postoperative pancreatic fistula (POPF) is the most common and most dangerous complication of pancreaticoduodenectomy, occurring in 10 to 25% of cases — the risk is highest with a soft pancreatic remnant and a small (non-dilated) pancreatic duct.

The step-up approach to infected pancreatic necrosis (percutaneous drainage, then minimally invasive necrosectomy if needed, then open necrosectomy as a last resort) reduces organ failure and mortality compared to primary open necrosectomy.

Internal drainage of pancreatic pseudocysts by cystogastrostomy or cystojejunostomy requires confirmation that the lesion is a true pseudocyst (documented pancreatitis history, no epithelial features) and not a cystic neoplasm that requires resection.

Lateral pancreaticojejunostomy (Puestow) decompresses the dilated main pancreatic duct along its full length — the ductotomy must stop 1 cm from the duodenal wall to avoid injury to the intrapancreatic common bile duct.

The splenic vein runs along the posterior surface of the pancreatic body and tail, receiving multiple short pancreatic tributaries — avulsion of these tributaries during distal pancreatectomy is the most common source of operative hemorrhage.

CHAPTER 10: OPERATIONS OF THE SMALL INTESTINE

Learning Objectives

1. Describe the surgical anatomy of the small intestine — the duodenum, jejunum, and ileum — including the mesenteric vascular arcades, the vasa recta, and the anatomical features that distinguish jejunum from ileum.
2. Perform a small bowel resection with primary anastomosis using both handsewn and stapled techniques, and explain the principles of adequate blood supply, tension-free approximation, and mucosal apposition.
3. Describe the indications for and techniques of strictureplasty in Crohn disease, including the Heineke-Mikulicz and Finney techniques, and state when strictureplasty is contraindicated.
4. Outline the operative management of small bowel obstruction, including adhesiolysis, assessment of bowel viability, and the decision to resect versus preserve borderline-viable bowel.
5. Describe Meckel diverticulum, its embryological basis, clinical presentations, and the technique of Meckel diverticulectomy versus segmental ileal resection.
6. Describe the techniques of loop and end ileostomy creation and ileostomy closure, including parastomal considerations and common complications.

Surgical Anatomy of the Small Bowel and Mesentery

Anatomical Divisions and Distinguishing Features

The small intestine extends from the pylorus to the ileocecal valve and is divided into three segments: the duodenum (approximately 25 cm, largely retroperitoneal), the jejunum (approximately 100 to 110 cm of the remaining intraperitoneal small bowel), and the ileum (approximately 150 to 160 cm). The jejunum and ileum are suspended from the posterior abdominal wall by the mesentery, whose root runs obliquely from the ligament of Treitz (the duodenojejunal flexure, at the level of L2 on the left) to the ileocecal junction (at the right iliac fossa). Surgically important features distinguish jejunum from ileum: the jejunum has a thicker wall, a larger lumen, more prominent circular folds (plicae circulares or valvulae conniventes), fewer and larger mesenteric vascular arcades with long vasa recta, and a mesentery with less fat (making the vascular arcades visible through translucent windows in the mesentery). The ileum has a thinner wall, a smaller lumen, fewer circular folds, more numerous and smaller vascular arcades with shorter vasa recta, and a mesentery with more fat (obscuring the vascular arcades). These differences are clinically important: the thicker jejunal wall holds sutures better and heals more reliably, making jejunal anastomoses generally more secure than ileal anastomoses — and the jejunal arcade pattern (fewer, larger arcades with long vasa recta) allows the surgeon to divide fewer arcade vessels when mobilizing a jejunal loop for reconstruction.

Mesenteric Vascular Anatomy

The superior mesenteric artery (SMA) supplies the entire jejunum, ileum, and proximal colon. It arises from the anterior aorta at the level of L1, passes behind the neck of the pancreas and the splenic vein, crosses anterior to the third part of the duodenum and the uncinate process, and enters the mesenteric root. From its left side, it gives off 12 to 18 jejunal and ileal branches that course within the mesentery, forming a series of vascular arcades — loops of interconnecting arteries that run parallel to the intestinal wall. From the most peripheral arcade, the vasa recta (straight arteries) pass directly to the mesenteric border of the intestinal wall, where they penetrate the muscularis to supply the intestinal wall. The vasa recta are end arteries — each supplies a segment of bowel wall approximately 1 to 2 cm wide, and division of a vas rectum produces ischemia in that segment. This is why the mesenteric division during small bowel resection must be performed by dividing the mesentery in a V-shaped pattern (preserving the proximal arcades while dividing only the vasa recta at the resection margin), and why the anastomosis must be located at a point where intact vasa recta supply both cut ends.

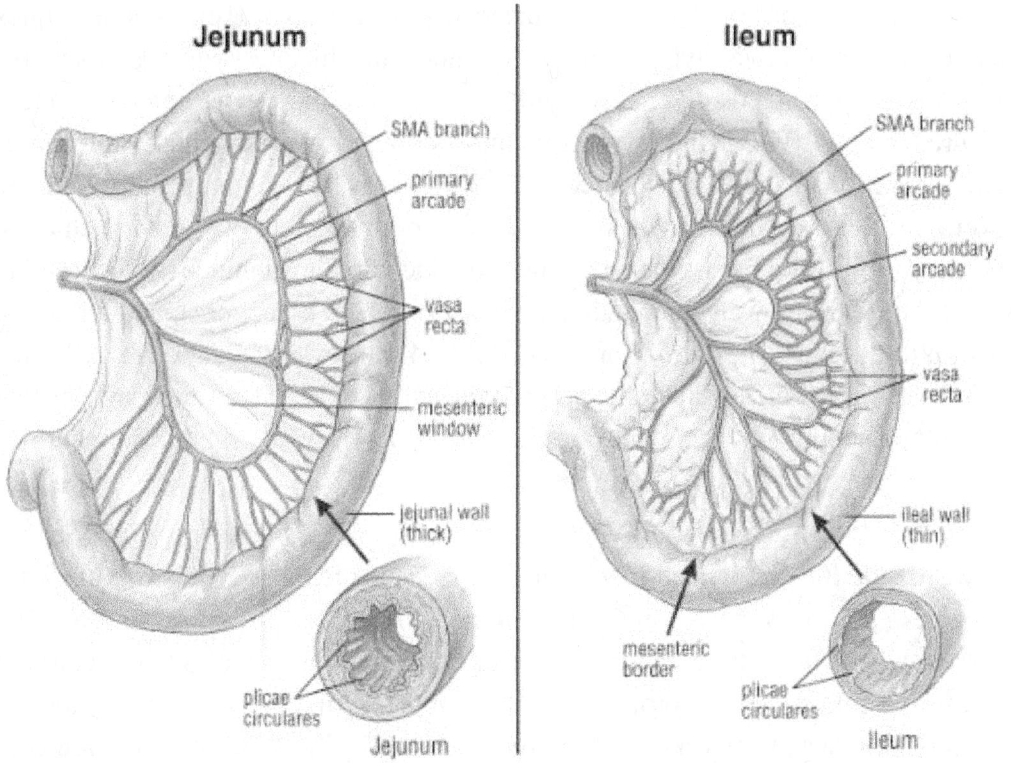

Small Bowel Resection and Anastomosis

Principles of Small Bowel Anastomosis

The fundamental principles of a safe intestinal anastomosis are adequate blood supply at both cut ends (confirmed by visible bleeding from the cut mesenteric edge and the presence of pulsatile vasa recta), a tension-free approximation (the two ends of the bowel come together without traction — tension on the anastomosis is the most common technical cause of leak), accurate mucosal apposition (the mucosal surfaces of both bowel ends are in contact, which promotes primary healing), and the absence of distal obstruction (an anastomosis proximal to an untreated obstruction will break down because of intraluminal pressure). The anastomosis may be constructed as end-to-end (the standard configuration for small bowel resection), side-to-side (functional end-to-end, the standard stapled configuration), or end-to-side (used when there is a significant size discrepancy between the two limbs or for specific reconstructions).

Handsewn Anastomosis Technique

The handsewn end-to-end anastomosis is constructed in a single layer (full-thickness bites through all layers of the bowel wall) or a two-layer technique (an inner full-thickness running absorbable suture and an outer seromuscular interrupted silk or absorbable suture). The single-layer interrupted technique using absorbable suture (3-0 or 4-0 PDS or Vicryl) is the most commonly used handsewn technique in current practice — it is faster than the two-layer technique, produces less luminal narrowing (the two-layer technique inverts more tissue and reduces the lumen by approximately 30%), and achieves comparable leak rates. The key technical point is that each bite must include the submucosa — the submucosa is the strength layer of the intestinal wall (it contains the densest collagen network), and a bite that misses the submucosa will pull through. The sutures are placed 3 to 4 mm from the cut edge and 3 to 4 mm apart. The mesenteric border is the most vulnerable point of the anastomosis (it has the least peritoneal coverage and the poorest blood supply), and care must be taken to achieve a watertight closure at this point.

Stapled Anastomosis Technique

The stapled side-to-side (functional end-to-end) anastomosis is the most widely used technique for small bowel anastomosis. The two bowel ends are aligned side by side in an antimesenteric fashion, enterotomies are made on the antimesenteric border of each end, one arm of a linear cutting stapler (GIA 60 or 80) is inserted into each enterotomy, and the stapler is fired — creating a side-to-side stapled anastomosis with simultaneous cutting of the intervening wall. The resulting common enterotomy (the defect at the apex where the stapler arms were inserted) is closed with a second firing of a linear stapler (TA 60) or with handsewn sutures. The stapled technique is faster, more reproducible (less operator-dependent), and produces a wider lumen than an end-to-end handsewn anastomosis, making it the preferred technique in most clinical settings including emergency surgery and anastomoses in irradiated or edematous bowel.

KEY POINT: The submucosa is the strength layer of the intestinal wall. Every suture bite during a handsewn anastomosis must include the submucosa — a bite that captures only the mucosa or only the serosa will pull through under tension, leading to dehiscence. The mesenteric border is the weakest point of any anastomosis because it has the least serosal coverage and the entry point of the vasa recta creates a gap — ensure a meticulous, watertight closure at this point.

Complications of Small Bowel Resection — Short Bowel Syndrome

Short bowel syndrome (SBS) results when the residual functional small bowel length is insufficient to maintain adequate nutrient, fluid, and electrolyte absorption without parenteral supplementation. The critical threshold depends on the segment remaining and the presence or absence of the colon in continuity: patients with an end-jejunostomy (no colon) require at least 100 to 150 cm of jejunum to maintain enteral autonomy; patients with a jejunocolonic anastomosis (colon in continuity) may achieve enteral autonomy with as little as 60 to 80 cm of small bowel because the colon absorbs water, electrolytes, and short-chain fatty acids produced by bacterial fermentation of malabsorbed carbohydrates. The ileum is more important to preserve than the jejunum because the ileum contains specialized absorptive functions that the jejunum cannot replace: vitamin B12 absorption (intrinsic factor-B12 complex receptor in the terminal ileum), bile salt reabsorption (the enterohepatic circulation of bile salts depends on the ileal bile salt transporter), and the ileocecal valve (which slows intestinal transit and prevents colonic bacterial reflux into the small bowel). Loss of the terminal ileum produces bile salt malabsorption (cholerheic diarrhea, bile salt depletion, fat malabsorption, fat-soluble vitamin deficiency) and B12 deficiency (megaloblastic anemia, neuropathy). Management of SBS involves dietary optimization (small frequent meals, complex carbohydrates, medium-chain triglycerides), pharmacotherapy (loperamide, codeine, proton pump inhibitors to reduce gastric hypersecretion, cholestyramine for bile salt diarrhea), parenteral nutrition for patients who cannot achieve enteral autonomy, and glucagon-like peptide 2 (GLP-2) analogues (teduglutide, which stimulates intestinal adaptation and villous growth, reducing parenteral nutrition dependency). Intestinal transplantation is reserved for patients with irreversible intestinal failure and life-threatening complications of parenteral nutrition.

Special Populations — Small Bowel Surgery in Crohn Disease

Operative decision-making in Crohn disease is fundamentally different from other surgical indications because Crohn disease cannot be cured by surgery — the disease recurs after resection in 50 to 70% of patients by 5 years (endoscopic recurrence at the anastomotic site), and each recurrence may require additional surgery. Every operative decision must therefore minimize the amount of bowel resected while achieving the immediate operative goal. The principle of limited resection (resecting only macroscopically diseased bowel with grossly clear margins of 2 cm, without attempting to achieve microscopically negative margins) has been validated by prospective studies showing that the recurrence rate is independent of microscopic margin status. Strictureplasty preserves bowel length at stricture sites. When resection is unavoidable, a stapled side-to-side (functional end-to-end) anastomosis is preferred over handsewn end-to-end because it produces a wider lumen (reducing the risk of anastomotic stricture, the most common site of Crohn recurrence). Medical prophylaxis against postoperative recurrence (mesalamine, thiopurines, anti-TNF agents, or vedolizumab) is started within 4 weeks of surgery in patients at high risk of recurrence.

THE OPERATIVE DANGER ZONE ATLAS — Mesenteric Vascular Injury During Adhesiolysis

The Zone: The mesentery of the small bowel during adhesiolysis for small bowel obstruction — the zone where dense inflammatory or postoperative adhesions tether loops of small bowel to the abdominal wall, to other loops, or to the mesentery itself. Traction on these adhesions to separate the bowel loops places the mesenteric vascular arcades and the vasa recta under tension.

The Structure at Risk: Mesenteric vascular arcades and vasa recta. These thin-walled arteries and veins run within the mesentery and are easily torn when adhesions involving the mesentery are divided sharply or avulsed by traction. The SMA branches and the SMV tributaries at the mesenteric root are at risk during deep adhesiolysis near the retroperitoneum.

The Consequence: Avulsion of a mesenteric vascular arcade produces hemorrhage within the mesentery (mesenteric hematoma) that can compress or thrombose adjacent vasa recta, causing segmental ischemia of the bowel wall supplied by the affected vessels. Division of multiple vasa recta at the mesenteric border devascularizes a segment of bowel wall, leading to delayed ischemic perforation at the devascularized segment — a complication that may not be apparent at the time of adhesiolysis but presents 3 to 7 days postoperatively with peritonitis.

The Safe Maneuver: Divide adhesions sharply with scissors directly on the bowel wall (not in the mesentery), staying in the avascular plane between the adhesion and the bowel serosa. Never use electrocautery to divide adhesions adherent to the mesenteric border — thermal spread damages the vasa recta. When adhesions involve the mesentery itself, divide them close to the adhesion point (not in the mid-mesentery where the arcades run). After completing adhesiolysis, inspect the entire mesenteric border of the freed bowel loops for mesenteric hematoma or serosal tears — any segment with compromised mesenteric vascularity should be resected.

Strictureplasty for Crohn Disease

Indications and Contraindications

Strictureplasty is a bowel-preserving operation for fibrous strictures in Crohn disease that widens the intestinal lumen at the stricture site without resecting bowel. The fundamental rationale is conservation of intestinal length — Crohn disease is a lifelong relapsing condition that produces multiple strictures over decades, and repeated resections progressively shorten the small bowel, ultimately producing short bowel syndrome (a functional small bowel length less than 200 cm). Strictureplasty is indicated for short fibrotic strictures (less than 10 cm for Heineke-Mikulicz, up to 20 cm for Finney), multiple strictures in a short segment of bowel (where resection would sacrifice too much length), recurrent strictures at or near prior anastomotic sites, and patients with previous extensive small bowel resection who cannot afford to lose more length. Contraindications to strictureplasty include active sepsis at the stricture site (abscess, fistula, phlegmon), strictures with dysplasia or carcinoma on preoperative biopsy, free perforation at the stricture, severe malnutrition with albumin less than 2.0 g/dL (impaired healing makes strictureplasty unsafe), and colonic strictures (which are better treated by resection because of the higher malignancy risk in colonic Crohn disease).

Heineke-Mikulicz and Finney Strictureplasty Techniques

The Heineke-Mikulicz strictureplasty is used for short strictures (less than 10 cm). A longitudinal enterotomy is made along the antimesenteric border of the stricture, extending 1 cm beyond the stricture into normal bowel at each end. The enterotomy is then closed transversely with a single layer of interrupted full-thickness absorbable sutures (3-0 Vicryl or PDS), widening the lumen at the stricture site — the same principle as the pyloroplasty. The Finney strictureplasty is used for longer strictures (10 to 20 cm). The strictured segment is folded on itself in a U-shape, the antimesenteric borders of the two arms are sutured together as a posterior outer layer, a longitudinal enterotomy is made through both walls of the folded segment, and the enterotomy is closed as a side-to-side anastomosis (inner full-thickness running suture, outer seromuscular interrupted suture) — creating a wide side-to-side channel that bypasses the stricture. For very long strictures (greater than 20 cm), the Michelassi strictureplasty (side-to-side isoperistaltic strictureplasty) divides the strictured segment in the middle, overlaps the two halves side by side, and creates a long side-to-side anastomosis — preserving the entire length of bowel while creating a wide channel.

Management of Small Bowel Obstruction (Adhesiolysis and Bowel Viability Assessment)

Operative Decision-Making

Small bowel obstruction (SBO) is caused by postoperative adhesions in approximately 60 to 75% of cases, followed by hernias (15 to 20%), malignancy (5 to 10%), and Crohn disease (5%). Initial management of adhesive SBO is non-operative — nasogastric decompression, intravenous fluid resuscitation, and serial clinical assessments — which resolves the obstruction in approximately 65 to 80% of cases. Operative intervention is indicated for complete SBO that fails to resolve after 48 to 72 hours of non-operative management (some guidelines use water-soluble contrast studies — if contrast does not reach the colon within 24 hours, operative intervention is recommended), suspected closed-loop obstruction on CT (a segment of bowel obstructed at two points, creating a closed loop that cannot decompress — closed-loop obstruction carries a high risk of ischemia and perforation), signs of strangulation (continuous rather than colicky pain, fever, tachycardia, leukocytosis, elevated lactate, peritoneal signs), and irreducible or incarcerated hernias with signs of ischemia.

Adhesiolysis Technique and Bowel Viability Assessment

At laparotomy, the entire small bowel is run from the ligament of Treitz to the ileocecal valve, identifying and dividing all adhesive bands causing obstruction. The transition point (where dilated proximal bowel transitions to decompressed distal bowel) is identified and the obstructing adhesion is divided. After relieving the obstruction, the viability of any compromised bowel segment must be assessed. Clinical signs of viability include the return of normal pink color after release of the obstruction, the return of peristalsis (spontaneous contractile activity of the bowel wall), the presence of mesenteric arterial pulsations at the mesenteric border, and bleeding from the cut mesenteric edge (if a test incision is made). Bowel that is frankly necrotic (black, non-bleeding, non-peristaltic, no mesenteric pulsations) must be resected. The difficult decision is the borderline-viable segment — dusky (dark purple) bowel that may or may not recover after release of the obstruction. For borderline-viable bowel, the surgeon wraps the segment in warm saline-soaked laparotomy pads and reassesses after 15 to 20 minutes. If color and peristalsis return, the bowel is viable and is preserved. If the segment remains dusky and non-peristaltic after the observation period, resection is indicated. Intravenous fluorescein with Wood lamp examination or indocyanine green (ICG) fluorescence angiography may be used as adjuncts to confirm perfusion in equivocal cases.

THE OPERATIVE DANGER ZONE ATLAS — Enterotomy During Adhesiolysis

---

The Zone: The interface between dense postoperative adhesions and the small bowel serosa — particularly where adhesion bands are broad, vascularized, and fused to the bowel wall, making the plane between adhesion and serosa indistinguishable.

The Structure at Risk: The small bowel wall itself. In dense adhesions, the serosal surface is obscured, and the dissection plane passes through the muscularis or mucosa rather than between the adhesion and the serosa — producing a full-thickness enterotomy (inadvertent perforation) or a seromuscular injury that weakens the wall and leads to delayed perforation.

The Consequence: An unrecognized enterotomy during adhesiolysis produces postoperative peritonitis (typically presenting on postoperative day 3 to 5), which carries significant morbidity and mortality — especially in the debilitated patient with small bowel obstruction. Multiple serosal injuries weaken the bowel wall and produce delayed perforations even if each individual injury appears superficial at the time of operation.

The Safe Maneuver: Divide adhesions sharply with scissors, not electrocautery — electrocautery causes thermal injury to the bowel wall that is wider and deeper than the visible burn mark. Stay on the bowel wall surface (the plane of safety is between the adhesion and the serosa, not through the adhesion). When the plane between adhesion and bowel wall is obliterated, divide the adhesion on the abdominal wall side (leave a patch of adhesion on the bowel serosa) rather than risking an enterotomy by dissecting into the bowel wall. After completing adhesiolysis, inspect the ENTIRE length of the freed bowel — both the mesenteric and antimesenteric borders — for enterotomies and serosal injuries. Repair all serosal injuries with seromuscular sutures (3-0 Vicryl or silk, interrupted Lembert), and oversew or resect any full-thickness enterotomies.

Meckel Diverticulectomy

Embryology and the Rule of Twos

Meckel diverticulum is a true diverticulum (containing all layers of the intestinal wall — mucosa, submucosa, muscularis, serosa) that arises from incomplete obliteration of the omphalomesenteric (vitelline) duct during embryological development. It is the most common congenital anomaly of the gastrointestinal tract, present in approximately 2% of the population. It is located on the antimesenteric border of the ileum, typically within 60 to 100 cm (approximately 2 feet) of the ileocecal valve. It contains heterotopic mucosa in approximately 50% of symptomatic cases — most commonly gastric mucosa (which secretes acid, causing peptic ulceration of the adjacent ileal mucosa) and less commonly pancreatic tissue. The majority of Meckel diverticula are asymptomatic and discovered incidentally. Symptomatic presentations include painless lower gastrointestinal bleeding (most common in children — from acid-induced ulceration of the ileal mucosa adjacent to heterotopic gastric mucosa), intestinal obstruction (from intussusception with the diverticulum as the lead point, or from a Meckel band tethering the diverticulum to the umbilicus), and diverticulitis (inflammation of the diverticulum mimicking appendicitis but located more proximally in the ileum).

Operative Management

The two operative options are simple diverticulectomy and segmental ileal resection. Simple diverticulectomy is performed by applying a linear stapler (GIA or TA) across the base of the diverticulum, perpendicular to the long axis of the ileum, excising the diverticulum and oversewing the staple line. This technique is appropriate when the diverticulum has a narrow base, when the pathology is confined to the diverticulum itself (diverticulitis without surrounding ileal disease), and when the clinical presentation is obstruction or incidental discovery. Segmental ileal resection (removing the diverticulum along with a short segment of adjacent ileum and performing a primary anastomosis) is indicated when the presentation is gastrointestinal bleeding (because the ulceration is in the adjacent ileal mucosa, not in the diverticulum — simple diverticulectomy may not remove the bleeding ulcer), when the diverticulum has a wide base (risk of narrowing the ileal lumen with a transverse staple line), or when the adjacent ileum is inflamed or necrotic. The incidental Meckel diverticulum (discovered during laparotomy or laparoscopy for another indication) is resected if the patient is young (less than 50 years), if the diverticulum is palpably thickened (suggesting heterotopic mucosa), or if a Meckel band is present. Incidental diverticulectomy is generally not recommended in elderly patients or when the diverticulum appears normal and thin-walled, because the lifetime risk of complications is low (approximately 4%) and the added procedure carries its own morbidity.

Enterostomy Creation and Closure

Loop Ileostomy Creation

A diverting loop ileostomy is created to protect a distal anastomosis (most commonly a low anterior rectal anastomosis or an ileal pouch-anal anastomosis) by diverting the fecal stream away from the anastomosis during healing. The terminal ileum is identified and a point approximately 20 to 30 cm proximal to the ileocecal valve is selected. A 2.5 to 3 cm circular disc of skin and subcutaneous tissue is excised at the pre-marked stoma site (typically in the right lower quadrant, through the rectus abdominis muscle), a cruciate incision is made in the anterior rectus sheath, the rectus muscle fibers are split (not divided), and a cruciate incision is made in the posterior rectus sheath and peritoneum. The loop of ileum is delivered through the abdominal wall defect — the opening must accommodate two fingers alongside the bowel (too tight causes venous congestion and ischemia; too loose predisposes to parastomal hernia). A rod or bridge is placed beneath the loop to prevent retraction during the first 5 to 7 postoperative days. The loop is opened on the distal (efferent) limb, and the proximal (afferent) limb is everted and sutured to the skin edge to create a spouted stoma (the Brooke ileostomy) — the spout protrudes 2 to 3 cm above the skin surface, which directs the corrosive ileal effluent into the appliance and away from the peristomal skin.

End Ileostomy and Ileostomy Closure

An end (Brooke) ileostomy is created after total proctocolectomy, when there is no downstream bowel for restoration of continuity. The terminal ileum is divided, the cut end is delivered through the abdominal wall, and the stoma is matured with eversion (the bowel is folded back on itself and sutured to the skin) to create the characteristic protruding spout. Ileostomy closure (reversal of a diverting loop ileostomy) is typically performed 8 to 12 weeks after the primary operation, after confirming the integrity of the distal anastomosis with a water-soluble contrast enema or flexible endoscopy. The stoma is mobilized circumferentially by incising the mucocutaneous junction and dissecting the bowel free from the abdominal wall fascia. For loop ileostomy closure, the two limbs are identified, the stoma is excised, and the bowel is anastomosed using a handsewn or stapled technique — the closure may be performed as a resection with a new anastomosis or as a simple closure of the enterotomy if the bowel is healthy. The fascia is closed primarily and the skin may be closed primarily or left partially open (to reduce the wound infection rate, which is 5 to 15% for stoma closure).

THE OPERATIVE DANGER ZONE ATLAS — Parastomal Vascular Compromise During Ileostomy Maturation

---

The Zone: The abdominal wall defect through which the ileum is delivered during ileostomy creation — specifically the fascial aperture and the mesenteric passage through the abdominal wall.

The Structure at Risk: The mesenteric vessels supplying the delivered ileal loop. As the ileum passes through the abdominal wall fascial opening, the mesentery is compressed between the fascial edges and the bowel wall. If the fascial aperture is too tight, the mesenteric veins are compressed (while the higher-pressure arteries remain patent), producing venous congestion, edema, and ultimately ischemic necrosis of the stoma.

The Consequence: Stomal ischemia from mesenteric venous compression produces a dusky, edematous, and ultimately necrotic stoma. Superficial mucosal necrosis (limited to the everted portion above the fascial level) may be managed conservatively — the mucosa sloughs and re-epithelializes. Necrosis extending below the fascial level indicates that the ischemia involves the bowel within the abdominal cavity and requires urgent revision to prevent perforation and peritonitis.

The Safe Maneuver: Size the fascial aperture to admit two fingers alongside the delivered bowel loop — this ensures that the mesentery is not compressed by the fascial edges. Avoid excessive tension on the mesentery (shorten the mesenteric root mobilization if needed so the ileum reaches the skin without traction). After maturation, inspect the stoma for color (healthy stoma is beefy red), capillary refill, and mucosal bleeding when gently rubbed — a dusky or cyanotic stoma within the first 24 hours requires immediate assessment of the fascial aperture and consideration of revision.

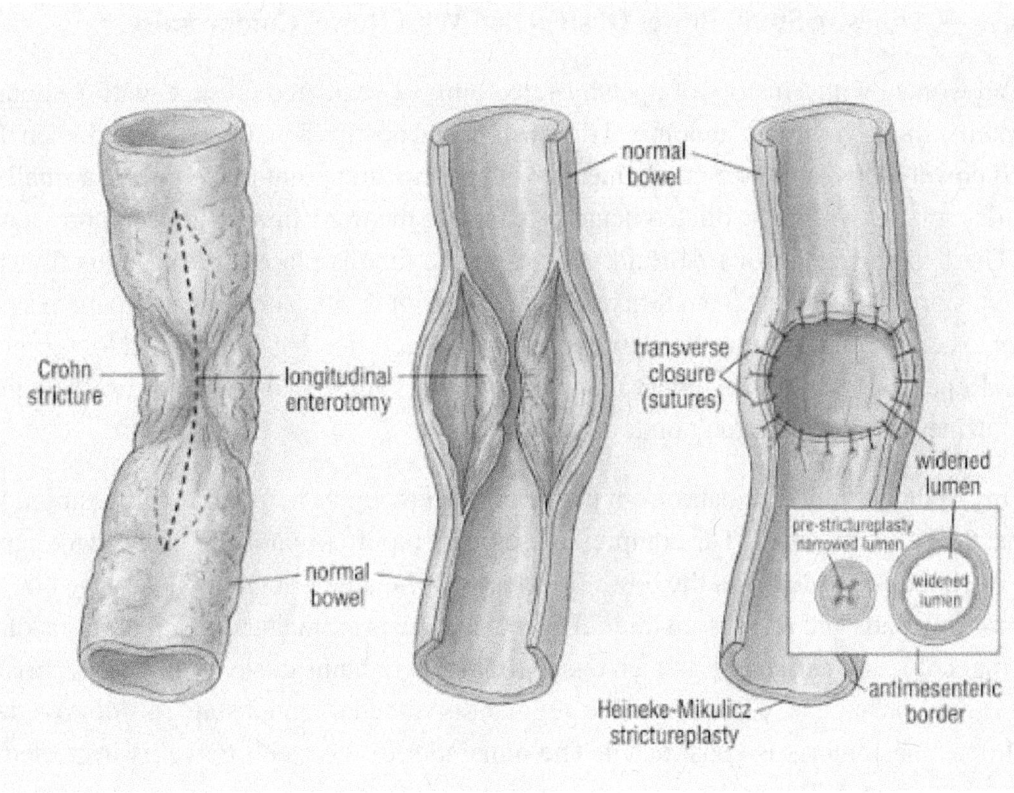
Crohn stricture
longitudinal enterotomy
normal bowel
normal bowel
transverse closure (sutures)
widened lumen
pre-strictureplasty narrowed lumen
widened lumen
antimesenteric border
Heineke-Mikulicz strictureplasty

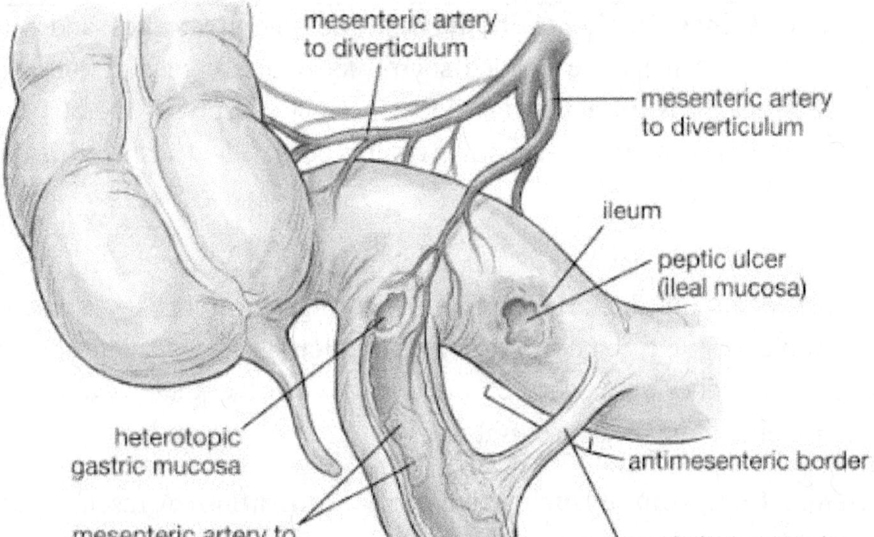
mesenteric artery to diverticulum
mesenteric artery to diverticulum
ileum
peptic ulcer (ileal mucosa)
heterotopic gastric mucosa
antimesenteric border
mesenteric artery to diverticulum
omphalomesenteric band

Clinical Case — Adhesive Small Bowel Obstruction With Bowel Compromise

A 58-year-old woman with a history of open hysterectomy 12 years ago presents with 36 hours of crampy abdominal pain, bilious vomiting, abdominal distension, and obstipation. CT of the abdomen demonstrates dilated small bowel loops (up to 4.5 cm diameter) with a transition point in the pelvis, a small-bowel feces sign (particulate matter within the dilated ileum proximal to the transition), and decompressed distal ileum and colon. There is no free air or free fluid. A nasogastric tube is placed, intravenous fluids are started, and electrolytes are corrected. After 48 hours of non-operative management, the patient's pain changes from colicky to continuous, and she develops tachycardia (heart rate 108 bpm) and a low-grade fever (38.1 degrees C). Repeat CT shows an interval increase in the volume of small bowel dilation and new mesenteric haziness at the transition point.

At laparotomy, a dense adhesive band from the prior hysterectomy is found compressing a loop of mid-ileum against the pelvic sidewall. The compressed segment (approximately 15 cm) is dark purple and non-peristaltic. The band is divided, and the bowel is released. The dusky segment is wrapped in warm saline-soaked laparotomy pads and reassessed after 20 minutes. The proximal and distal portions of the segment recover normal color and peristalsis, but a 6 cm central zone remains dusky with absent peristalsis and no mesenteric arterial pulsations. The non-viable segment is resected, and a stapled side-to-side (functional end-to-end) ileal anastomosis is constructed. The remainder of the small bowel is inspected — no other adhesive bands are found. The patient recovers uneventfully and is discharged on postoperative day 5.

THE OPERATIVE DANGER ZONE ATLAS — Small Bowel Surgery Dangers

Mesenteric Vascular Injury During Adhesiolysis: Mesenteric arcades and vasa recta tear when adhesions involving the mesentery are divided sharply or avulsed, causing mesenteric hematoma and segmental bowel ischemia. **Safe maneuver:** divide adhesions sharply on the bowel wall surface (not in the mesentery), avoid electrocautery near the mesenteric border, and inspect for mesenteric hematoma after adhesiolysis.

Enterotomy During Adhesiolysis: Dense adhesions fused to the bowel serosa obscure the dissection plane, leading to inadvertent full-thickness perforation during adhesiolysis — unrecognized enterotomies present as postoperative peritonitis on day 3 to 5. **Safe maneuver:** divide adhesions sharply with scissors on the bowel wall, leave adhesion patches on the serosa when the plane is obliterated, and inspect the entire freed bowel for enterotomies and serosal injuries.

Parastomal Vascular Compromise During Ileostomy Maturation: A fascial aperture that is too tight compresses the mesenteric veins of the delivered ileal loop, producing venous congestion and stomal ischemia — necrosis below the fascial level requires urgent revision. **Safe maneuver:** size the aperture to admit two fingers alongside the bowel, avoid mesenteric tension, and assess stomal color and perfusion within 24 hours.

Vasa Recta Injury During Mesenteric Division: The vasa recta are end arteries — division of multiple vasa recta at the mesenteric border devascularizes the corresponding segment of bowel wall, causing delayed ischemic perforation. **Safe maneuver:** divide the mesentery in a V-shaped pattern preserving proximal arcades, confirm pulsatile vasa recta at both cut ends, and ensure the anastomosis is located where intact vasa recta supply the bowel.

Summary and Key Concepts

The jejunum has thicker walls, larger vascular arcades, longer vasa recta, and less mesenteric fat than the ileum — jejunal anastomoses are generally more secure than ileal anastomoses because the thicker wall holds sutures better.

The submucosa is the strength layer of the intestinal wall — every suture bite during a handsewn anastomosis must include the submucosa, and the mesenteric border (the weakest point) requires meticulous closure.

Strictureplasty conserves bowel length in Crohn disease by widening strictured segments without resection — the Heineke-Mikulicz technique (longitudinal enterotomy closed transversely) is used for strictures less than 10 cm.

Borderline-viable bowel after release of strangulated obstruction is reassessed after wrapping in warm saline pads for 15 to 20 minutes — if color and peristalsis do not return, the segment is resected.

Meckel diverticulum bleeding originates from acid-induced ulceration of the adjacent ileal mucosa (not the diverticulum itself), so segmental ileal resection rather than simple diverticulectomy is indicated for bleeding presentations.

The fascial aperture for ileostomy creation must admit two fingers alongside the delivered bowel to prevent mesenteric venous compression — stomal necrosis extending below the fascial level requires urgent revision.

Dense adhesions obliterating the plane between the adhesion and the bowel serosa should be divided on the abdominal wall side (leaving adhesion on the bowel) rather than dissecting into the bowel wall and risking enterotomy.

CHAPTER 11: APPENDECTOMY

Learning Objectives

1. Describe the surgical anatomy of the appendix, including its arterial supply, positional variants, and the surface landmarks used to locate it intraoperatively.
2. Perform a laparoscopic appendectomy using the three-trocar technique, including identification and division of the mesoappendix and the appendiceal base.
3. Perform an open appendectomy through a McBurney (muscle-splitting) incision, including the retrograde technique for a retrocecal appendix.
4. Manage the difficult appendix — retrocecal appendicitis, perforated appendicitis with abscess, and the appendiceal mass (phlegmon) — using both operative and non-operative strategies.
5. Explain the rationale, timing, and technique of interval appendectomy after initial non-operative management of a periappendiceal abscess.

Surgical Anatomy of the Appendix and Its Variants

Anatomy and Embryology

The vermiform appendix is a blind-ending tubular diverticulum arising from the posteromedial aspect of the cecum, approximately 2 to 3 cm below the ileocecal valve. It arises at the convergence of the three taeniae coli on the cecal surface — the taeniae coli can be traced distally from the ascending colon to their convergence at the base of the appendix, providing a reliable intraoperative landmark when the appendix is not immediately visible. The appendix averages 6 to 9 cm in length (range 2 to 20 cm) and has a complete peritoneal covering with its own mesentery (the mesoappendix), which extends from the lower leaf of the mesentery of the terminal ileum and contains the appendicular artery — a terminal branch of the ileocolic artery. Because the appendicular artery is an end artery with no collateral supply, thrombosis (from inflammation and infection) produces transmural gangrene and perforation — the pathophysiology that makes perforated appendicitis a surgical emergency.

Positional Variants

The position of the appendix relative to the cecum is variable and directly affects both clinical presentation and operative difficulty. The retrocecal position (behind the cecum, either intraperitoneal or retroperitoneal) is the most common variant, present in approximately 65% of the population — retrocecal appendicitis produces posterior or flank pain rather than classic McBurney point tenderness, may present with psoas sign (pain on hip extension) rather than peritoneal signs, and is more difficult to access laparoscopically because the appendix is hidden behind the cecum. The pelvic position (descending into the pelvis) is present in approximately 30% and may produce suprapubic pain, dysuria, rectal tenesmus, or diarrhea — mimicking urinary tract infection, pelvic inflammatory disease, or gynecological pathology. The preileal position (anterior to the terminal ileum), the postileal position (posterior to the terminal ileum), and the subhepatic position (in patients with incomplete intestinal rotation where the cecum lies in the right upper quadrant) are less common but produce atypical clinical presentations that delay diagnosis.

Epidemiology and Pathophysiology of Acute Appendicitis

Acute appendicitis is the most common surgical emergency worldwide, with a lifetime risk of approximately 7 to 8%. Peak incidence occurs between ages 10 and 30 years. The pathophysiology begins with luminal obstruction — most commonly by a fecalith (hardened stool pellet), lymphoid hyperplasia (particularly in children and young adults), or, less commonly, a tumor (carcinoid, adenocarcinoma, mucocele), parasitic infection, or foreign body. Obstruction leads to continued mucosal secretion into a closed space, rising intraluminal pressure, venous congestion, arterial ischemia, transmural gangrene, and finally perforation. The time from symptom onset to perforation is typically 36 to 72 hours, although the progression is variable and is influenced by the patient's age (elderly patients perforate earlier and present with fewer classic signs) and immune status. The diagnosis is clinical (periumbilical pain migrating to the right lower quadrant, anorexia, nausea, fever, leukocytosis) supplemented by CT imaging (sensitivity and specificity both exceeding 95%) in equivocal cases. The Alvarado score (MANTRELS criteria) risk-stratifies patients to guide the need for imaging versus proceeding directly to surgery.

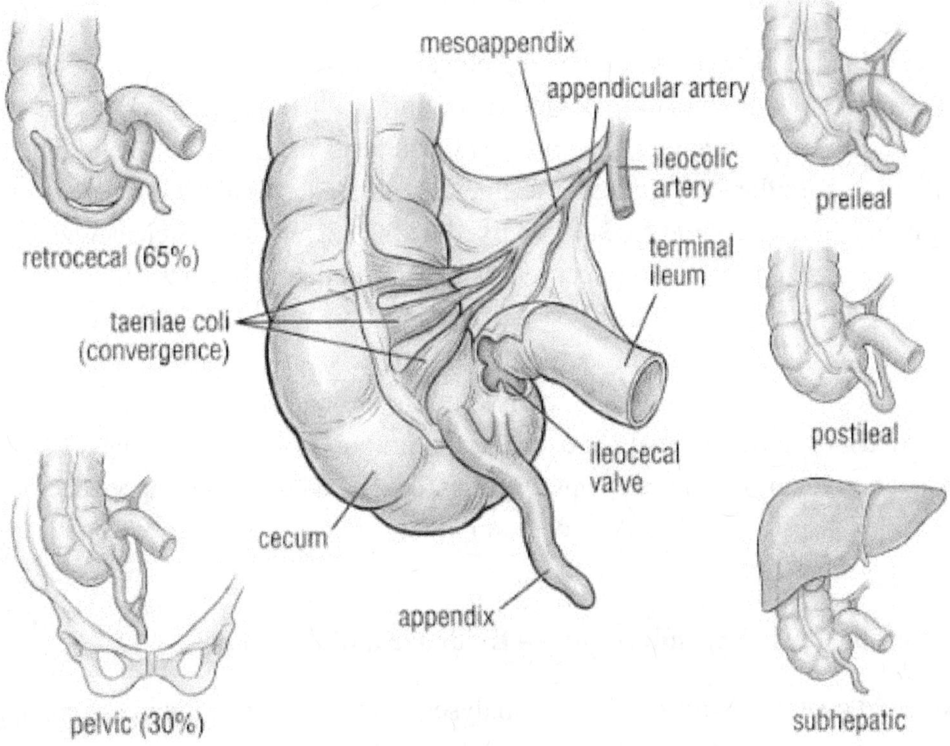

KEY POINT: The three taeniae coli converge at the base of the appendix on the cecal surface. When the appendix is retrocecal, adhesed, or buried in an inflammatory mass and cannot be immediately identified, tracing the anterior taenia coli distally from the ascending colon to its convergence on the cecum will reliably lead to the appendiceal base — this is the most dependable intraoperative landmark for locating a difficult appendix.

Laparoscopic Appendectomy

Patient Positioning and Trocar Placement

Laparoscopic appendectomy is the standard operative approach for acute appendicitis in most clinical settings. The patient is positioned supine with the left arm tucked, and the surgeon stands on the patient's left side (operating across the abdomen). Pneumoperitoneum is established and a three-trocar technique is used: a 10 or 12 mm umbilical trocar (camera), a 5 mm left lower quadrant trocar (working port for the surgeon's left hand), and a 5 or 12 mm suprapubic trocar (working port for the surgeon's right hand). The patient is placed in Trendelenburg position with left lateral tilt to allow the small bowel to fall away from the right lower quadrant and expose the cecum and appendix. The cecum is identified, and the appendix is located by following the taeniae coli to their convergence.

Operative Steps — Mesoappendix Division and Appendiceal Base Management

The appendix is grasped at its tip or mid-body and elevated to create a window in the mesoappendix. The mesoappendix is divided with an energy device (harmonic scalpel, bipolar vessel sealer, or monopolar electrocautery with clip application to the appendicular artery) from the tip of the appendix toward its base. Alternatively, a vascular-load endoscopic linear stapler can divide the mesoappendix in a single firing. After complete division of the mesoappendix, the appendiceal base is clearly visible at its junction with the cecum. The appendiceal base is secured using one of three methods: endoscopic loop ligatures (two pre-tied Endoloop sutures placed at the base of the appendix and a third placed 1 cm distal to the first two — the appendix is divided between the ligatures with scissors), endoscopic linear stapler (a single firing across the appendiceal base using a blue or white tissue-load stapler — this is the fastest and most reproducible method), or intracorporeal handsewn ligation (a 0-Vicryl or chromic suture tied at the base — used when neither Endoloops nor a stapler are available). The divided appendix is retrieved in an endoscopic specimen bag to avoid wound contamination, and the right lower quadrant is irrigated if purulent fluid is present.

Laparoscopic Versus Open Appendectomy — Evidence and Outcomes

Multiple randomized controlled trials and meta-analyses have established laparoscopic appendectomy as the preferred approach for acute appendicitis in adults, demonstrating lower wound infection rates (approximately 3% versus 8% for open surgery), shorter hospital stays (by 0.5 to 1 day), reduced postoperative pain scores, and faster return to normal activity. The advantages are particularly pronounced in obese patients — where the open McBurney incision must be enlarged significantly to provide adequate exposure, increasing wound morbidity — and in women of reproductive age, where diagnostic laparoscopy simultaneously evaluates gynecological pathology that may mimic appendicitis (ovarian cyst torsion, ruptured ectopic pregnancy, tubo-ovarian abscess). The principal disadvantage of laparoscopic appendectomy is a slightly higher rate of intra-abdominal abscess formation compared to the open technique (approximately 2 to 3% versus 1%), which may reflect the increased pneumoperitoneum-driven dispersion of infected peritoneal fluid and the reduced capacity for effective tactile irrigation compared with open lavage. In complicated appendicitis with perforation and diffuse peritonitis, the evidence supports either approach — meta-analyses show comparable outcomes, although operative times are longer for the laparoscopic approach in complicated cases, and conversion rates to open surgery increase to 10 to 20%.

The decision to convert from laparoscopic to open surgery should be made when the anatomy cannot be clearly identified, when dense adhesions prevent safe dissection, when the appendiceal base is too necrotic to manage laparoscopically, or when bleeding cannot be controlled endoscopically. Conversion is a judgment of surgical wisdom, not a complication — it should be made early when difficulty is encountered rather than persisting with an unsafe laparoscopic dissection. In pediatric practice, laparoscopic appendectomy has become the standard approach in most centers, with the technique modified to use smaller trocars (3 to 5 mm) and instruments. Single-incision laparoscopic appendectomy (through a single umbilical incision using a multi-channel port) has been described as a cosmetic alternative but has not demonstrated clinical superiority over conventional three-trocar laparoscopy and is associated with longer operative times and increased port-site hernia risk.

Management of the Inflamed or Friable Appendiceal Base

When the appendiceal base is necrotic, gangrenous, or too friable to hold a ligature or staple line (which occurs in advanced perforated appendicitis), simple ligation or stapling is unsafe because the suture or staples will cut through the compromised tissue. In this situation, partial cecectomy is required — a segment of the cecal wall surrounding the appendiceal base is resected using an endoscopic stapler, excising the necrotic appendiceal base with a rim of healthy cecal wall. The stapler is applied across viable cecal tissue, not across necrotic tissue, and the specimen (appendix plus cecal cuff) is removed. If the cecal wall involvement is extensive, conversion to open surgery with formal ileocecal resection (resection of the terminal ileum, cecum, and appendix with ileocolic anastomosis) may be necessary. The decision between simple appendectomy, partial cecectomy, and ileocecal resection is made intraoperatively based on the extent of cecal wall involvement and tissue viability.

THE OPERATIVE DANGER ZONE ATLAS — Cecal Wall Injury During Appendiceal Base Stapling

The Zone: The junction of the appendiceal base with the cecal wall during laparoscopic appendectomy — specifically the moment of stapler application across the appendiceal base, where the stapler jaws must encompass only the appendiceal wall and not incorporate adjacent cecal wall tissue.

The Structure at Risk: The cecal wall at the appendiceal base. If the endoscopic stapler is applied too close to the cecum (incorporating cecal wall tissue in the staple line), the resulting staple line may narrow the cecal lumen, obstruct the ileocecal valve, or create a defect in the cecal wall (cecal perforation from stapler misfire or tissue pull-through on inflamed, edematous cecal tissue).

The Consequence: Cecal wall incorporation in the staple line produces a postoperative cecal leak or fistula (presenting as peritonitis, abscess, or enterocutaneous fistula on postoperative day 3 to 7) or ileocecal obstruction (from luminal narrowing). Cecal leak after appendectomy carries significant morbidity and often requires reoperation with ileocecal resection.

The Safe Maneuver: Apply the stapler across the appendiceal base at a point where the appendiceal wall is clearly distinct from the cecal wall — at least 5 mm from the cecal-appendiceal junction. Ensure both jaws of the stapler encompass only appendiceal tissue and that the cecal wall is free of the jaws. When the appendiceal base is necrotic or the appendiceal-cecal junction is obliterated by inflammation, convert to partial cecectomy (staple through viable cecal wall around the appendiceal base) rather than attempting to staple across non-viable tissue.

Open Appendectomy

McBurney Incision and Muscle-Splitting Technique

Open appendectomy is performed through a McBurney (muscle-splitting) incision centered at McBurney point (one-third of the distance from the anterior superior iliac spine to the umbilicus). A 3 to 5 cm oblique incision is made in the skin along Langer lines, and the abdominal wall muscles are split (not cut) in the direction of their fibers — the external oblique aponeurosis is split in the direction of its fibers, the internal oblique and transversus abdominis muscles are split along their fibers perpendicular to the external oblique split, and the peritoneum is opened. Muscle splitting preserves the integrity of the abdominal wall musculature and reduces the risk of postoperative incisional hernia compared to a muscle-cutting incision. The cecum is delivered into the wound, and the appendix is identified by following the taeniae coli to their convergence. The mesoappendix is clamped, divided, and ligated with absorbable suture, ligating the appendicular artery. The appendiceal base is crushed with a Kelly clamp, the clamp is removed and reapplied 1 cm distally, and a 0-Vicryl or chromic suture is tied in the crushed groove (the crushed tissue holds the suture and prevents it from slipping). The appendix is divided between the clamp and the ligature, and the stump mucosa is cauterized with electrocautery to destroy the mucosal epithelium (reducing the risk of mucocele formation from the stump).

Retrograde Appendectomy for the Retrocecal Appendix

When the appendix is retrocecal and adherent to the posterior cecal wall or the retroperitoneum, antegrade dissection (from tip to base) is not possible because the tip cannot be mobilized. In this situation, the retrograde technique is used: the appendiceal base is identified first (by following the taeniae coli), the base is ligated and divided, and then the appendix is dissected from base to tip, dividing the mesoappendix and the retroperitoneal attachments in a retrograde fashion. This technique allows the surgeon to work from the known anatomy (the appendiceal base at the cecum) toward the unknown (the retrocecal tip), rather than attempting to free the tip blindly behind the cecum. The retroperitoneal lateral peritoneal attachments of the cecum (the white line of Toldt) may need to be divided to mobilize the cecum medially and expose the retrocecal appendix.

Stump Management and Inversion

After appendiceal ligation and division, the stump may be left as a simple ligated stump (the current standard practice — evidence shows no benefit of inversion over simple ligation) or inverted into the cecum using a purse-string or Z-suture. The historical rationale for stump inversion was to bury the contaminated stump and reduce the risk of intra-abdominal infection, but prospective studies and meta-analyses have shown that simple ligation produces equivalent infection rates, is faster, and avoids the potential complication of intussusception caused by the inverted stump acting as a lead point. Simple ligation is therefore the preferred technique in contemporary practice. In laparoscopic appendectomy, stump inversion is not performed — the staple line or ligated stump is left exposed on the cecal surface.

Management of the Difficult Appendix (Retrocecal, Perforated, Appendiceal Mass)

Perforated Appendicitis With Diffuse Peritonitis

Perforated appendicitis with diffuse peritonitis requires urgent appendectomy (laparoscopic or open) with thorough peritoneal lavage. At operation, purulent fluid is aspirated from all four quadrants, the appendix is removed using the standard technique (with partial cecectomy if the base is necrotic), and the peritoneal cavity is irrigated with warm saline until the effluent is clear. Drains are not routinely placed for diffuse peritonitis (randomized trials show no benefit of drainage in this setting and may increase wound infection rates). Intravenous antibiotics covering gram-negative and anaerobic organisms (typically a second-generation cephalosporin plus metronidazole, or piperacillin-tazobactam) are continued for 3 to 5 days postoperatively if peritonitis is present. The wound is managed by delayed primary closure or healing by secondary intention in contaminated cases (skin closure increases the wound infection rate in perforated appendicitis from approximately 10% with delayed closure to approximately 30% with primary closure).

Appendiceal Phlegmon and Periappendiceal Abscess

When the patient presents late (more than 5 to 7 days after symptom onset) and CT imaging demonstrates an appendiceal phlegmon (a walled-off inflammatory mass involving the appendix, cecum, terminal ileum, and omentum) or a well-formed periappendiceal abscess, initial non-operative management is preferred over immediate appendectomy. The rationale is that operating in an acute phlegmon carries a significantly higher complication rate — the inflamed tissues are friable, the normal anatomical planes are obliterated, and the risk of inadvertent injury to the cecum, terminal ileum, or mesenteric vessels is substantially increased. Non-operative management consists of intravenous antibiotics and, for abscesses greater than 3 cm, CT-guided percutaneous drainage. Clinical improvement (defervescence, resolution of leukocytosis, resolution of peritoneal signs) is expected within 48 to 72 hours. Failure to improve or clinical deterioration mandates urgent operative intervention.

THE OPERATIVE DANGER ZONE ATLAS — Ileal and Cecal Injury During Appendectomy in a Phlegmon

The Zone: The inflammatory mass (phlegmon) surrounding a perforated appendix — where the appendix, cecal wall, terminal ileum, mesentery, and omentum are fused into a single inflammatory conglomerate with obliterated tissue planes.

The Structure at Risk: Terminal ileum and cecal wall. In a phlegmon, the terminal ileum is adherent to the inflamed appendix and the cecal wall is edematous and friable. Dissection to free the appendix from the phlegmon risks full-thickness injury to the terminal ileum (enterotomy) and tearing of the friable cecal wall (cecotomy) — injuries that may not be apparent at the time of surgery in inflamed, edematous tissue.

The Consequence: Unrecognized ileal enterotomy or cecal wall injury produces postoperative peritonitis, abscess, or enterocutaneous fistula — complications that frequently require reoperation with ileocecal resection, diverting ileostomy, and prolonged recovery. These complications convert a relatively simple disease (appendicitis) into a complex, potentially life-threatening surgical problem.

The Safe Maneuver: In a well-formed phlegmon or abscess presenting more than 5 to 7 days after symptom onset, prefer initial non-operative management (antibiotics plus percutaneous drainage) over immediate appendectomy. If operative intervention is required in a phlegmon, accept an incomplete operation rather than risking major injury — perform a partial appendectomy (divide the appendix at a level where the tissue is safe, leaving the adherent tip in situ) or limit the dissection to drainage of the abscess cavity without attempting to free the appendix from the inflammatory mass. Interval appendectomy is performed 6 to 8 weeks later when inflammation has resolved and tissue planes have reformed.

THE OPERATIVE DANGER ZONE ATLAS — Appendicular Artery Hemorrhage from Inadequate Mesoappendix Control

The Zone: The mesoappendix during division — the triangular mesenteric fold containing the appendicular artery, which supplies the appendix from the ileocolic artery.

The Structure at Risk: The appendicular artery. In acute appendicitis, the mesoappendix is thickened, edematous, and friable. The appendicular artery (which is normally a small vessel, 1 to 2 mm in diameter) becomes engorged in the setting of inflammation and may retract into the thickened mesoappendix when divided without adequate hemostasis.

The Consequence: A divided appendicular artery that retracts into the mesoappendix without ligation produces intra-abdominal hemorrhage that collects in the right lower quadrant (mesenteric hematoma). If not recognized, the hematoma expands, compresses adjacent structures, and may require reoperation for hemostasis. In laparoscopic appendectomy, a retracted bleeding appendicular artery in a thickened mesoappendix can be difficult to identify and control because the bleeding source is hidden within the edematous fat.

The Safe Maneuver: Divide the mesoappendix close to the appendiceal wall (not far from the appendix in the broad mesoappendix, where the artery is larger and higher-pressure). Use an energy device (harmonic scalpel, bipolar sealer) or clip-and-cut technique to ensure hemostasis of the appendicular artery before division. In a thickened, edematous mesoappendix, consider using an endoscopic vascular stapler for the mesoappendix rather than an energy device (the stapler provides secure hemostasis even in edematous tissue). After division, inspect the mesoappendix stump for active bleeding before proceeding to base division.

Special Populations — Appendicitis in Pregnancy, Pediatric, and Elderly Patients

Appendicitis in pregnancy is the most common non-obstetric surgical emergency, occurring in approximately 1 in 1,000 to 1 in 1,500 pregnancies, with peak incidence during the second trimester. Diagnosis is complicated by the physiological changes of pregnancy — the gravid uterus displaces the cecum and appendix superiorly and laterally (the point of maximal tenderness migrates from the right lower quadrant to the right flank or right upper quadrant as gestation advances), physiological leukocytosis of pregnancy (white blood cell counts of 12,000 to 15,000 per microliter are normal) reduces the diagnostic utility of leukocyte counts, and nausea and anorexia overlap with normal pregnancy symptoms. Ultrasound is the initial imaging modality (avoiding ionizing radiation), with MRI as the second-line study when ultrasound is inconclusive — CT is reserved for cases where MRI is unavailable and clinical suspicion is high. Prompt surgical intervention is critical because perforation carries a fetal loss rate of approximately 20 to 35% compared to 1.5 to 4% for uncomplicated appendicitis. Laparoscopic appendectomy is safe and preferred in all trimesters, with the patient positioned in left lateral tilt (to prevent aortocaval compression by the gravid uterus), open Hasson entry (to avoid Veress needle injury to the gravid uterus), and low-pressure pneumoperitoneum (10 to 12 mmHg). Tocolytic therapy is not routinely administered prophylactically but is given if uterine contractions develop postoperatively.

In pediatric patients, the classic history of periumbilical pain migrating to the right lower quadrant is less reliable in children under 5 years, who present with diffuse abdominal pain, irritability, vomiting, and diarrhea. Perforation rates are significantly higher in young children (approaching 80 to 100% in children under 3 years) because of delayed diagnosis, a thinner appendiceal wall, and a less developed omentum that is less effective at walling off perforation. In elderly patients (over 65 years), appendicitis carries a higher morbidity and mortality than in younger patients because of delayed presentation (elderly patients often have blunted inflammatory responses and fewer classic signs), higher perforation rates (50 to 70% at presentation), and a greater burden of comorbid disease. The differential diagnosis in elderly patients must include cecal diverticulitis, cecal carcinoma (which can obstruct the appendiceal lumen and cause secondary appendicitis), mesenteric ischemia, and perforated colonic malignancy — CT imaging is essential in all elderly patients with right lower quadrant pain to exclude these alternative diagnoses.

Interval Appendectomy

Rationale and Timing

Interval appendectomy is the elective removal of the appendix after initial non-operative management of a periappendiceal abscess or phlegmon. The procedure is typically performed 6 to 8 weeks after the initial episode, after the inflammation has resolved, the tissue planes have reformed, and a colonoscopy has been performed (to exclude an underlying cecal malignancy — cecal carcinoma masquerading as a periappendiceal abscess is found in 1 to 2% of patients over age 40 presenting with appendiceal abscess). The necessity of interval appendectomy is debated. Traditional teaching recommended routine interval appendectomy because of a reported recurrence rate of appendicitis of 10 to 20% in patients managed non-operatively. More recent data suggest a lower recurrence rate (5 to 10% at 1 year), and some guidelines now recommend selective interval appendectomy — performing it in patients with recurrent symptoms, in patients under 40 with complicated appendicitis (where the risk of recurrence is higher), and in patients over 40 (where colonoscopy and appendectomy exclude an occult cecal neoplasm) — rather than routine interval appendectomy in all patients.

Operative Considerations

Interval appendectomy is typically performed laparoscopically using the same three-trocar technique as for acute appendectomy. The operative difficulty is usually intermediate — less than operating in an acute phlegmon (the tissue planes have reformed) but more than operating on a non-inflamed appendix (residual adhesions from the prior inflammatory episode are present). The surgeon should expect adhesions between the appendix, cecum, terminal ileum, and omentum from the prior episode and should carefully divide these adhesions to identify the appendix. In most cases, the appendix is found partially or completely fibrosed (the appendiceal lumen may be obliterated by scar tissue). The mesoappendix and appendiceal base are managed using the same technique as for standard laparoscopic appendectomy. Conversion to open surgery is occasionally necessary when dense adhesions prevent safe laparoscopic dissection.

Complications and Long-Term Outcomes

The overall complication rate of appendectomy is approximately 5 to 10% for uncomplicated appendicitis and 15 to 30% for complicated (perforated) appendicitis. Surgical site infection is the most common complication — wound infection rates are approximately 3% for laparoscopic appendectomy and 8% for open appendectomy in uncomplicated cases, rising to 10 to 15% in perforated appendicitis. Intra-abdominal abscess occurs in 2 to 5% of cases, typically presenting on postoperative day 5 to 10 with recurrent fever, leukocytosis, and abdominal pain — CT-guided percutaneous drainage is the first-line treatment. Stump appendicitis is a rare but important late complication (occurring weeks to years after appendectomy) caused by inflammation and obstruction of the residual appendiceal stump — it mimics recurrent appendicitis and is diagnosed by CT showing inflammation at the cecal base. Prevention requires dividing the appendix close to its cecal origin (leaving a stump no longer than 5 mm). Adhesive small bowel obstruction occurs in approximately 1 to 2% of patients after appendectomy (lower after laparoscopic than open surgery) and is managed by the standard principles outlined in Chapter 10. The negative appendectomy rate — removal of a histologically normal appendix — has decreased from 15 to 25% in the era before routine CT imaging to approximately 5 to 8% in the current era, although some authorities accept a negative appendectomy rate of up to 10% as an acceptable trade-off to avoid delayed diagnosis and perforation in equivocal cases.

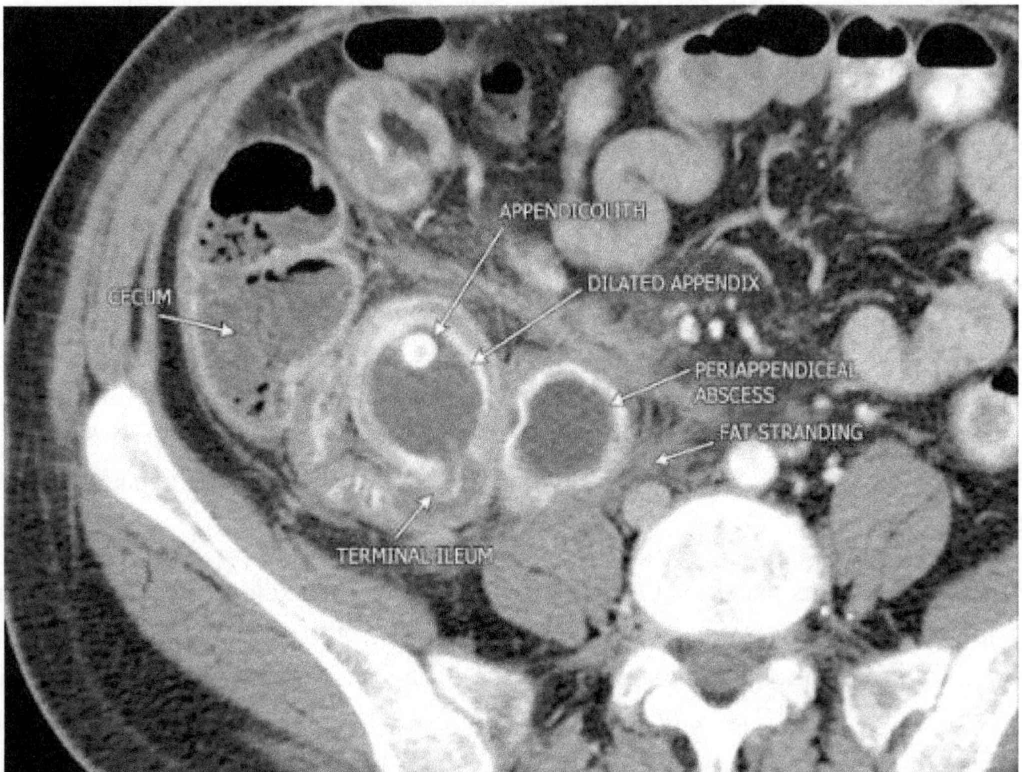

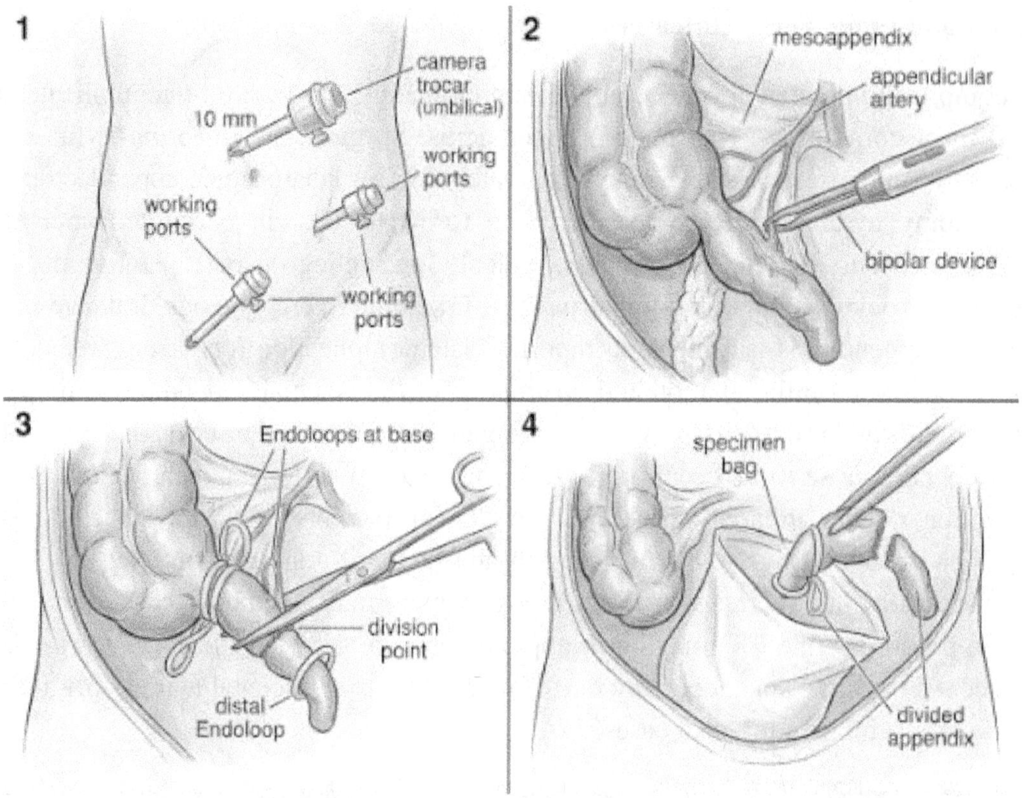

Clinical Case — Complicated Appendicitis With Abscess Requiring Staged Management

A 42-year-old man presents with 7 days of progressively worsening right lower quadrant pain, low-grade fever (38.3 degrees C), and anorexia. On examination, there is a palpable, tender mass in the right iliac fossa. CT demonstrates a 5 cm rim-enhancing periappendiceal abscess with surrounding fat stranding, a thickened, non-opacified appendix, and an appendicolith. There is no free air. Given the duration of symptoms (more than 5 days) and the presence of a well-formed abscess, initial non-operative management is chosen. A 12 French percutaneous drain is placed into the abscess under CT guidance, draining 60 mL of purulent material. The patient is started on intravenous piperacillin-tazobactam. Over 48 hours, the fever resolves, the white blood cell count normalizes, and the abdominal tenderness improves. The drain is removed when output is less than 10 mL per day, and the patient is discharged on oral antibiotics.

At 6 weeks, a colonoscopy is performed (given the patient's age, to exclude a cecal neoplasm) — this is normal. Laparoscopic interval appendectomy is then performed. At operation, dense adhesions are found between the appendix, cecum, and omentum at the site of the prior abscess. The adhesions are carefully divided with sharp dissection. The appendix is identified — it is partially fibrosed and adherent to the posterior cecal wall. The mesoappendix is divided with a harmonic scalpel, and the appendiceal base is secured with an endoscopic stapler. The specimen is retrieved in a bag, and the pelvis is irrigated. Final pathology shows chronic appendicitis with fibrosis and acute-on-chronic inflammation — no malignancy. The patient is discharged the following day. This case illustrates the staged approach to complicated appendicitis: initial non-operative management with percutaneous drainage allows the inflammation to resolve, colonoscopy excludes an underlying neoplasm, and interval appendectomy is performed safely after tissue planes have reformed.

THE OPERATIVE DANGER ZONE ATLAS — Appendiceal Surgery Dangers

Cecal Wall Injury During Appendiceal Base Stapling: Stapler application too close to the cecum incorporates cecal wall tissue, risking postoperative cecal leak, fistula, or ileocecal obstruction. **Safe maneuver:** apply the stapler at least 5 mm from the cecal-appendiceal junction; when the base is necrotic, convert to partial cecectomy through viable cecal wall.

Ileal and Cecal Injury During Appendectomy in a Phlegmon: Obliterated tissue planes in an appendiceal phlegmon make the terminal ileum and friable cecal wall indistinguishable from the appendix, risking enterotomy or cecotomy during dissection. **Safe maneuver:** prefer initial non-operative management (antibiotics plus percutaneous drainage) over immediate appendectomy in a well-formed phlegmon; if operating, accept an incomplete operation rather than risking major injury.

Appendicular Artery Hemorrhage from Inadequate Mesoappendix Control: The engorged appendicular artery retracts into the thickened, edematous mesoappendix when divided without hemostasis, producing a hidden mesenteric hematoma. **Safe maneuver:** divide the mesoappendix close to the appendiceal wall using an energy device or vascular stapler, and inspect the mesoappendix stump for active bleeding before proceeding.

Missed Cecal Neoplasm Masquerading as Appendicitis: Cecal carcinoma is found in 1 to 2% of patients over 40 presenting with appendiceal abscess — a missed diagnosis that delays cancer treatment. **Safe maneuver:** perform colonoscopy before interval appendectomy in all patients over 40 and in any patient with atypical features (mass at the appendiceal base, mucinous material in the abscess, appendiceal mucocele).

Summary and Key Concepts

The three taeniae coli converge at the base of the appendix — tracing the anterior taenia distally from the ascending colon to its convergence on the cecum is the most reliable intraoperative method for locating a difficult appendix.

The retrocecal appendix (65% of patients) produces atypical symptoms (posterior or flank pain, psoas sign) and is more difficult to access laparoscopically — the retrograde technique (dividing the base first, then dissecting toward the tip) is used when the tip cannot be mobilized.

The appendiceal base is secured with Endoloops, an endoscopic stapler, or intracorporeal suture — when the base is necrotic or too friable to hold a ligature, partial cecectomy (stapling through viable cecal wall) is required.

An appendiceal phlegmon or well-formed abscess presenting more than 5 to 7 days after symptom onset is best managed by initial non-operative management (antibiotics plus percutaneous drainage) followed by interval appendectomy at 6 to 8 weeks.

Colonoscopy before interval appendectomy is essential in patients over 40 — cecal carcinoma is found in 1 to 2% of patients presenting with appendiceal abscess.

Perforated appendicitis with diffuse peritonitis requires urgent appendectomy with thorough peritoneal lavage — drains are not routinely placed, and wounds are managed by delayed primary closure or secondary intention.

Simple ligation of the appendiceal stump without inversion is the current standard — prospective studies show no benefit of stump inversion, and the inverted stump may act as a lead point for intussusception.

CHAPTER 12: OPERATIONS OF THE COLON

Learning Objectives

1. Describe the surgical anatomy of the colon, including its segmental arterial supply from the superior and inferior mesenteric arteries, the marginal artery of Drummond, and the anatomical basis for selecting resection margins and ligation points.
2. Perform a right hemicolectomy (open and laparoscopic) with appropriate medial-to-lateral dissection, high ligation of the ileocolic pedicle, and extracorporeal ileocolic anastomosis.
3. Perform a left hemicolectomy, sigmoid colectomy, and Hartmann procedure, including splenic flexure mobilization, identification of the left ureter, and management of the rectal stump.
4. Manage acute colonic emergencies (obstruction, perforation, massive hemorrhage) with the appropriate choice of subtotal colectomy, segmental resection, or damage-control colostomy.
5. Create end, loop, and diverting colostomies with proper site selection, stoma maturation, and management of parastomal complications.

Surgical Anatomy of the Colon and Colonic Vasculature

Gross Anatomy and Peritoneal Attachments

The colon extends from the ileocecal valve to the rectosigmoid junction, measuring approximately 150 cm in length in adults. It is divided into the cecum, ascending colon, hepatic flexure, transverse colon, splenic flexure, descending colon, sigmoid colon, and rectosigmoid junction. The ascending and descending colon are retroperitoneal structures fixed to the posterior abdominal wall by the white line of Toldt (the lateral peritoneal reflection) — mobilization of these segments requires incision along the white line of Toldt and elevation of the colon off the retroperitoneal structures (the right or left ureter, gonadal vessels, duodenum on the right, and the kidney and its Gerota fascia). The transverse colon and sigmoid colon are intraperitoneal, suspended by their respective mesenteries (the transverse mesocolon and sigmoid mesocolon), which contain the vascular supply and lymphatic drainage. The colon is distinguished from the small intestine by three external features: the taeniae coli (three longitudinal muscle bands), the haustra (sacculations between the taeniae), and the appendices epiploicae (fat-filled peritoneal projections along the taeniae).

Arterial Supply — Superior and Inferior Mesenteric Systems

The arterial supply of the colon derives from two major systems. The superior mesenteric artery (SMA) supplies the cecum, ascending colon, hepatic flexure, and proximal two-thirds of the transverse colon through three branches: the ileocolic artery (the most constant branch — supplies the cecum, appendix, and terminal ileum), the right colic artery (supplies the ascending colon — present in only 10 to 40% of the population as a separate branch; when absent, its territory is supplied by branches of the ileocolic and middle colic arteries), and the middle colic artery (supplies the transverse colon, bifurcating into right and left branches within the transverse mesocolon). The inferior mesenteric artery (IMA) supplies the distal third of the transverse colon, splenic flexure, descending colon, sigmoid colon, and upper rectum through three branches: the left colic artery (supplies the splenic flexure and descending colon), the sigmoid arteries (two to four branches supplying the sigmoid colon through its mesocolon), and the superior rectal artery (the terminal branch of the IMA, supplying the upper rectum).

The Marginal Artery of Drummond and the Arc of Riolan

The marginal artery of Drummond is a continuous arterial arcade running along the mesenteric border of the colon, formed by anastomotic connections between the terminal branches of the ileocolic, right colic, middle colic, left colic, and sigmoid arteries. It provides collateral blood supply that allows any segment of the colon to survive after ligation of its named feeding artery, provided the marginal artery is intact. The weakest point of the marginal artery is at the splenic flexure — the watershed zone between the SMA and IMA territories, known as Griffith point — where the marginal artery may be absent or attenuated in up to 5% of the population. The arc of Riolan (the meandering mesenteric artery) is a larger, more proximal anastomotic vessel connecting the SMA and IMA circulations directly, present in a variable proportion of patients and particularly well developed when chronic mesenteric ischemia causes collateral enlargement. The clinical significance of these collateral pathways is critical during colonic surgery: high ligation of the IMA at its origin (as in oncologic left colectomy or sigmoid resection for cancer) removes the primary blood supply to the left colon, and the remaining blood supply to the rectal stump depends entirely on the marginal artery and any collateral vessels — if the marginal artery is absent at Griffith point, the rectal stump may be ischemic, producing anastomotic leak.

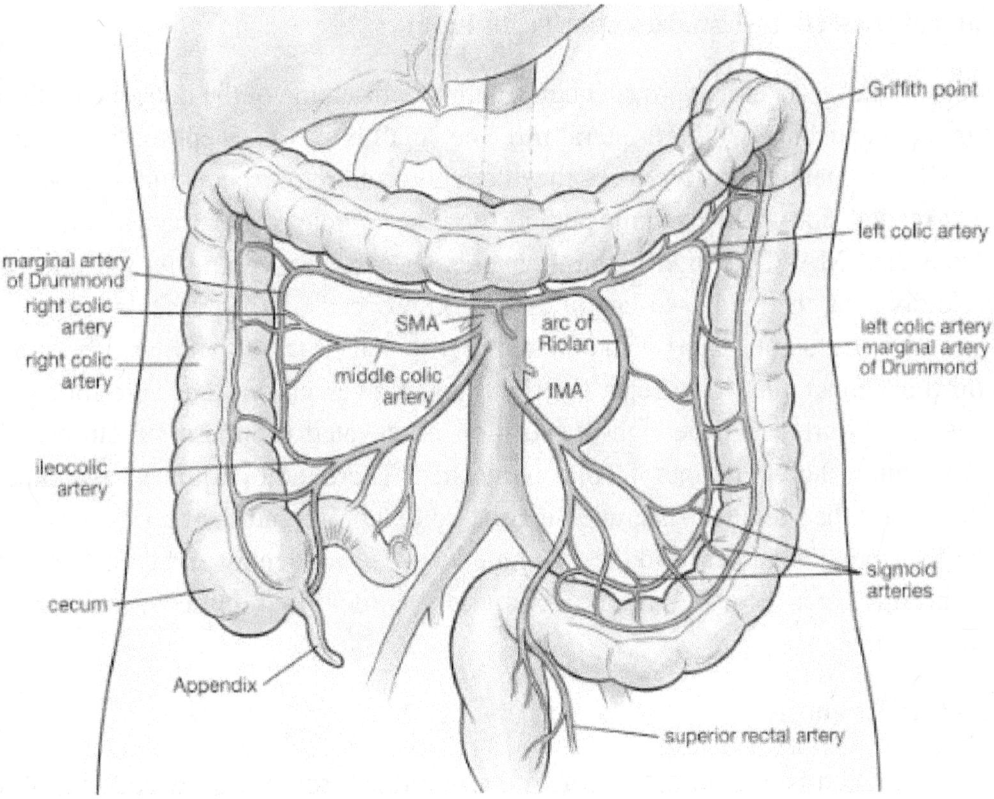

KEY POINT: The marginal artery of Drummond is weakest at the splenic flexure (Griffith point) — when performing high ligation of the IMA for sigmoid or rectal cancer, the surgeon must verify that the marginal artery is intact at Griffith point and that the left colon has adequate perfusion before constructing the anastomosis. If the marginal artery is absent or attenuated, mobilize the splenic flexure to bring well-perfused transverse colon down for a tension-free, well-vascularized anastomosis.

Right Hemicolectomy (Open and Laparoscopic)

Indications and Oncologic Principles

Right hemicolectomy is the standard oncologic resection for malignancies of the cecum, ascending colon, and hepatic flexure. The procedure removes the cecum, ascending colon, and hepatic flexure along with their mesentery and lymphovascular pedicles (the ileocolic and right colic vessels), with margins of at least 5 cm proximal and distal to the tumor. An extended right hemicolectomy includes the transverse colon up to the left branch of the middle colic artery and is indicated for tumors at the hepatic flexure or proximal transverse colon. The minimum adequate lymph node harvest for staging colorectal cancer is 12 nodes — the oncologic adequacy of the resection depends on the extent of mesenteric excision, which is achieved by high ligation of the named vascular pedicles at their origins, harvesting the lymph nodes along the named arteries and their mesenteric drainage basin.

Medial-to-Lateral Dissection (Laparoscopic Technique)

The laparoscopic medial-to-lateral approach begins with identification of the ileocolic pedicle. The patient is positioned in Trendelenburg with left lateral tilt. The small bowel is swept to the left upper quadrant. The ileocolic pedicle is identified as it crosses the duodenum and retroperitoneum — a peritoneal window is created on the medial side of the ileocolic pedicle, and the pedicle is skeletonized, clipped, and divided at its origin from the SMA. This high ligation ensures an adequate central lymph node harvest. After ileocolic pedicle division, the medial-to-lateral dissection proceeds in the avascular embryological plane between the right mesocolon (anteriorly) and the retroperitoneal structures (posteriorly) — the duodenum (second and third portions), the right ureter, the right gonadal vessels, and the anterior surface of Gerota fascia are swept posteriorly, and the right mesocolon is elevated off these structures. The dissection continues laterally until the white line of Toldt is reached. The lateral peritoneal attachments along the white line of Toldt are then divided (lateral-to-medial completion), and the hepatic flexure is mobilized by dividing the hepatocolic ligament and the attachments to the duodenum and the anterior surface of the right kidney. The right branch of the middle colic artery is identified, clipped, and divided within the transverse mesocolon.

Extracorporeal Anastomosis

The mobilized right colon is exteriorized through the umbilical trocar site (extended to 3 to 4 cm). The terminal ileum and transverse colon are divided extracorporeally with a linear stapler, and a side-to-side functional end-to-end stapled ileocolic anastomosis is constructed using two firings of a linear stapler (one creating the anastomotic lumen, the second closing the common enterotomy). The anastomosis is inspected for hemostasis and integrity, the mesenteric defect is closed (to prevent internal hernia), and the specimen is passed off the field. The anastomosis is returned to the abdomen, and the fascia at the extraction site is closed.

THE OPERATIVE DANGER ZONE ATLAS — Duodenal Injury During Right Hemicolectomy Dissection

---

The Zone: The medial-to-lateral dissection plane behind the right mesocolon — where the embryological fusion plane between the ascending mesocolon and the retroperitoneum overlies the second and third portions of the duodenum and the uncinate process of the pancreas.

The Structure at Risk: The duodenum (second and third portions). During medial-to-lateral dissection after ileocolic pedicle division, the duodenum lies directly beneath the posterior surface of the right mesocolon and may be adherent to the mesocolon by inflammatory adhesions (especially in locally advanced cancers) or may be tented anteriorly if excessive traction is applied to the mesocolon.

The Consequence: Full-thickness duodenal injury produces a duodenal leak — one of the most morbid complications in abdominal surgery, carrying significant mortality. A duodenal fistula requires prolonged drainage, parenteral nutrition, and may necessitate reoperation for definitive repair.

The Safe Maneuver: Maintain the dissection plane directly on the anterior surface of the retroperitoneal structures (Gerota fascia, duodenal serosa, gonadal vessels) — the plane is avascular and should separate cleanly with blunt dissection. Visualize the duodenum as a distinct shiny yellow structure and sweep it posteriorly. Never burn blindly in this space with energy devices. If the tumor is adherent to the duodenum, perform en bloc resection of the involved duodenal wall with primary closure rather than attempting to dissect the tumor off the duodenum.

Left Hemicolectomy and Sigmoid Colectomy

Indications and Operative Approach

Left hemicolectomy removes the splenic flexure, descending colon, and sigmoid colon with their mesentery, and is indicated for tumors of the splenic flexure and descending colon. Sigmoid colectomy is the most commonly performed elective colonic resection and is indicated for sigmoid colon cancer, complicated diverticular disease (recurrent diverticulitis, diverticular abscess, fistula, stricture), and sigmoid volvulus. For oncologic resections, the IMA is ligated at its origin from the aorta (high ligation), providing a central lymph node harvest along the IMA trunk. For benign disease (diverticulitis), the IMA can be ligated distal to the left colic artery takeoff (low ligation), preserving left colic artery perfusion to the remaining left colon and reducing the ischemic risk to the anastomosis. The distal resection margin for sigmoid colectomy is at the rectosigmoid junction — identified where the taeniae coli fan out and fuse into a circumferential longitudinal muscle layer (the transition from sigmoid to rectum).

Splenic Flexure Mobilization

Mobilization of the splenic flexure is a critical step in left hemicolectomy, sigmoid colectomy, and anterior resection because it provides the length needed for a tension-free, well-vascularized colorectal or coloanal anastomosis. The splenic flexure is fixed by three attachments: the splenocolic ligament (connecting the splenic flexure to the lower pole of the spleen), the phrenocolic ligament (connecting the splenic flexure to the left hemidiaphragm), and the greater omentum (fused to the anterior surface of the transverse mesocolon at the splenic flexure). Mobilization proceeds by dividing the lateral peritoneal attachments of the descending colon along the white line of Toldt upward toward the splenic flexure, then dividing the splenocolic and phrenocolic ligaments under direct vision. The greater omentum is separated from the transverse colon in the avascular plane along the inferior border of the omentum at the level of the transverse mesocolon. The tail of the pancreas lies in the immediate posterior vicinity of the splenic flexure and must be identified and protected during mobilization — injury to the pancreatic tail produces a postoperative pancreatic fistula.

THE OPERATIVE DANGER ZONE ATLAS — Splenic Injury During Splenic Flexure Mobilization

---

The Zone: The splenocolic ligament and the peritoneal attachments between the splenic flexure of the colon and the lower pole of the spleen — the operative field during splenic flexure mobilization for left hemicolectomy, sigmoid colectomy, or anterior resection.

The Structure at Risk: The spleen (lower pole and hilum). The splenocolic ligament is often short and places the splenic capsule in direct proximity to the operative dissection. Excessive traction on the splenic flexure transmits force to the splenocolic ligament, which pulls on the splenic capsule and may cause capsular avulsion, lower pole laceration, or hilar avulsion.

The Consequence: Iatrogenic splenic injury during left-sided colonic resection is the most common indication for unplanned splenectomy during colorectal surgery, occurring in 1 to 8% of cases. Splenectomy adds the morbidity of asplenia (lifelong infection risk from encapsulated organisms, need for vaccination) to a colonic resection and significantly increases operative blood loss and transfusion requirements.

The Safe Maneuver: Divide the splenocolic ligament under direct vision, close to the colonic wall and away from the splenic capsule. Avoid medial (downward) traction on the splenic flexure, which transmits force to the splenocolic ligament and the lower pole of the spleen. Mobilize the splenic flexure by approaching from the inferior direction (dividing the lateral peritoneal attachments of the descending colon first, then working upward) rather than pulling the splenic flexure down and away from the spleen. If the splenocolic ligament is short or densely adherent, divide it sharply in small increments, keeping the energy device away from the splenic capsule.

Identification and Protection of the Left Ureter

The left ureter is at risk of injury during sigmoid colectomy and left hemicolectomy because it courses in the retroperitoneum directly beneath the sigmoid mesocolon, crossing the common iliac artery at its bifurcation into the external and internal iliac arteries. The ureter is identified by elevating the sigmoid mesocolon and looking for the characteristic peristaltic vermicular movement of the ureter in the retroperitoneum. In elective cases, the ureter is typically easily identified in the avascular retroperitoneal plane after the sigmoid mesocolon is elevated off the retroperitoneum. In complicated cases (diverticular abscess, locally advanced cancer with retroperitoneal extension, redo surgery with scarring), the ureter may be displaced, encased in inflammatory tissue, or adherent to the sigmoid mesocolon — preoperative ureteral stent placement may be considered in high-risk cases to facilitate intraoperative identification by palpation.

Total Abdominal Colectomy With Ileorectal Anastomosis

Indications and Technique

Total abdominal colectomy with ileorectal anastomosis removes the entire colon from cecum to rectosigmoid junction, preserving the rectum, and reconstructs intestinal continuity with an anastomosis between the terminal ileum and the upper rectum. Indications include synchronous colon cancers (two or more primary tumors in separate colonic segments), hereditary non-polyposis colorectal cancer (Lynch syndrome) with a colonic malignancy (where the risk of metachronous colon cancer is 40 to 50% within 10 years, making subtotal colectomy oncologically superior to segmental resection), medically refractory ulcerative colitis (when rectal sparing allows ileorectal anastomosis rather than proctocolectomy with ileal pouch), colonic inertia (slow-transit constipation refractory to medical therapy), and attenuated familial adenomatous polyposis (when the rectum has a low polyp burden amenable to surveillance). The operative technique involves mobilization of the entire colon by dividing the lateral peritoneal attachments along the white line of Toldt bilaterally, dividing the hepatic and splenic flexure attachments, ligating and dividing the ileocolic, right colic, middle colic, and IMA pedicles, transecting the terminal ileum and rectosigmoid, and constructing a stapled or handsewn ileorectal anastomosis.

Functional Outcomes and Patient Selection

Ileorectal anastomosis preserves the rectum and its reservoir function, which results in better functional outcomes (fewer bowel movements per day, less urgency, and less nocturnal incontinence) than proctocolectomy with ileal pouch-anal anastomosis. However, the retained rectum remains at risk for cancer and requires lifelong endoscopic surveillance. Patients must understand this commitment to ongoing rectal surveillance before selecting ileorectal anastomosis over proctocolectomy. In patients with ulcerative colitis, ileorectal anastomosis is appropriate only when the rectum is relatively spared by inflammation — a severely diseased, noncompliant rectum will produce urgency, frequency, and incontinence regardless of the proximal reconstruction. Bowel frequency after ileorectal anastomosis typically stabilizes at 3 to 5 semiformed stools per day, compared to 4 to 8 stools per day after ileal pouch-anal anastomosis.

Hartmann Procedure and Reversal

Indications and Technique

The Hartmann procedure is a sigmoid colectomy with formation of an end colostomy and closure of the rectal stump — performed without anastomosis. It is the standard emergency operation for complicated sigmoid diverticulitis (Hinchey III and IV — purulent or feculent peritonitis), perforated sigmoid colon cancer, sigmoid volvulus with gangrenous bowel, and any left-sided colonic emergency where the patient's physiological status (septic shock, hemodynamic instability, malnutrition, immunosuppression) makes primary anastomosis unsafe. The sigmoid colon is resected, the proximal end is brought out as a mature end colostomy in the left lower quadrant through a pre-marked stoma site, and the distal rectal stump is closed with a linear stapler, oversewn, and dropped back into the pelvis. The rectal stump staple line is left long (the anvil of the stapler should protrude from the stump to facilitate future identification during

Hartmann reversal). The abdominal cavity is irrigated thoroughly, and drains are placed at the surgeon's discretion.

Hartmann Reversal — Timing and Technical Challenges

Reversal of a Hartmann procedure (restoration of intestinal continuity by anastomosing the end colostomy to the rectal stump) is one of the most technically demanding operations in colorectal surgery. Reversal is typically performed 3 to 6 months after the index operation, after the patient has recovered from the acute illness, nutritional status has been optimized, and intra-abdominal adhesions have partially matured. The principal technical challenge is identification of the rectal stump — which may be buried in dense pelvic adhesions, retracted deep into the pelvis, or difficult to distinguish from surrounding structures. Preoperative localization of the stump is aided by flexible sigmoidoscopy (to determine the length and accessibility of the stump) and intraoperative use of a rigid proctoscope or EEA sizer inserted transanally to identify the stump by palpation and transillumination. The colostomy is taken down, the proximal colon is mobilized to reach the pelvis without tension, the rectal stump is identified and opened, and a circular stapled colorectal anastomosis is constructed. Hartmann reversal carries a complication rate of 15 to 30% — including anastomotic leak (5 to 12%), wound infection, and adhesive small bowel obstruction — and approximately 20 to 30% of patients who undergo a Hartmann procedure never undergo reversal (due to comorbidity, patient preference, or recurrent disease).

CLINICAL PEARL: During a Hartmann procedure, leave the rectal stump staple line intentionally long and mark it with a non-absorbable suture or clip. This seemingly minor step dramatically simplifies identification of the rectal stump during subsequent Hartmann reversal — without a marker, the stump can be impossible to find in a pelvis filled with dense adhesions.

Subtotal Colectomy for Acute Colonic Emergencies

Lower Gastrointestinal Hemorrhage Requiring Operative Intervention

Acute massive lower gastrointestinal hemorrhage requires operative intervention in approximately 10 to 15% of cases — when bleeding does not stop with endoscopic therapy, angiographic embolization is unsuccessful or unavailable, and the patient requires ongoing transfusion. When preoperative localization of the bleeding source has been achieved (by CT angiography, mesenteric angiography, or tagged red blood cell scan), a directed segmental colectomy is performed — right hemicolectomy for a right-sided source, left hemicolectomy or sigmoid colectomy for a left-sided source. When the bleeding source has NOT been localized despite all preoperative investigations — which occurs in approximately 10 to 25% of patients taken to surgery for massive lower GI hemorrhage — subtotal colectomy with ileostomy or ileorectal anastomosis is the operation of choice. Subtotal colectomy removes the entire colon (the most likely source of hemorrhage — diverticular disease, angiodysplasia, and mucosal lesions), eliminates the risk of rebleeding from an unresected colonic segment, and avoids the unacceptable rebleeding rate (approximately 30 to 75%) that occurs when a blind segmental colectomy is performed without localization.

Fulminant Colitis and Toxic Megacolon

Subtotal colectomy with end ileostomy is the standard emergency operation for fulminant colitis (ulcerative colitis or Crohn colitis) refractory to maximal medical therapy, and for toxic megacolon (transverse colon diameter greater than 6 cm with systemic toxicity) that fails to improve within 24 to 72 hours of medical management or demonstrates clinical deterioration (worsening sepsis, perforation, hemorrhage). The subtotal colectomy removes the entire diseased colon while preserving the rectum for potential future reconstruction (ileal pouch-anal anastomosis in ulcerative colitis, performed as a second or third stage after the patient has recovered). The rectal stump is managed by Hartmann closure (stapled and dropped into the pelvis) or by creating a mucous fistula (bringing the proximal rectal stump to the skin surface as a non-functioning stoma). A primary anastomosis is never constructed in the emergency setting for fulminant colitis or toxic megacolon — the combination of malnutrition, immunosuppression (from corticosteroids and biologics), and active colonic inflammation makes anastomotic leak rates prohibitively high.

THE OPERATIVE DANGER ZONE ATLAS — Left Ureteral Injury During Emergency Sigmoid Resection

---

The Zone: The retroperitoneum beneath the sigmoid mesocolon during emergency sigmoid colectomy (for perforation, obstruction, or volvulus) — where the left ureter courses from the pelvic brim, crossing the common iliac bifurcation, toward the bladder.

The Structure at Risk: The left ureter. In emergency sigmoid resection for perforated diverticulitis or locally advanced sigmoid cancer, the sigmoid mesocolon is thickened by inflammation and edema, and the normal retroperitoneal tissue planes are obliterated. The left ureter may be displaced medially by a diverticular abscess, encased in a phlegmon, or adherent to the inflammatory mass — making it indistinguishable from the surrounding tissue.

The Consequence: Ureteral ligation produces silent hydronephrosis and progressive renal damage, which may not be recognized for days to weeks postoperatively (presenting as flank pain, rising creatinine, or urosepsis). Ureteral transection produces a urinary leak (urinoma) presenting as peritonitis, abscess, or a drain output with elevated creatinine. Both injuries require reoperation or interventional nephrostomy and ureteral stenting, with a small but real risk of permanent renal loss.

The Safe Maneuver: Identify the left ureter early in the operation, before dividing the sigmoid mesocolon — elevate the sigmoid mesocolon off the retroperitoneum and look for the characteristic peristaltic movement. In cases where the ureter cannot be identified due to inflammation or abscess, consider preoperative ureteral stent placement (in elective cases) or intraoperative cystoscopy with ureteral catheter placement. Maintain the dissection plane anterior to the ureter at all times. When dividing the mesocolon, control each vessel individually close to the colonic wall rather than placing blind mass clamps through the thickened, inflamed mesocolon.

Colostomy Creation (End, Loop, and Diverting)

Stoma Site Selection and Preoperative Marking

Proper stoma site selection is the single most important factor in determining long-term stoma function and patient quality of life. The ideal stoma site is within the rectus abdominis muscle (to reduce the risk of parastomal hernia), at a flat area of skin away from skin folds, scars, bony prominences, and the belt line (to allow secure appliance adhesion), and at a site that the patient can see and reach (for self-care). Preoperative stoma marking by an enterostomal therapy nurse is the standard of care for all elective stoma creation — the patient is assessed in sitting, standing, and lying positions, and the site is marked on the skin with indelible ink. In emergency surgery when preoperative marking is not possible, the surgeon selects a site through the rectus muscle at the junction of the lateral one-third and medial two-thirds of a line from the umbilicus to the anterior superior iliac spine, adjusting for the patient's body habitus.

End Colostomy Construction

An end colostomy is created by bringing the divided end of the proximal colon through the abdominal wall at the pre-marked stoma site. A 2 to 3 cm circular disc of skin is excised at the stoma site, the subcutaneous fat is divided to the anterior rectus sheath, a cruciate incision is made in the anterior rectus sheath, the rectus muscle fibers are split (not cut), the posterior rectus sheath and peritoneum are opened, and a two-finger-width opening is created in the abdominal wall. The proximal colon is delivered through this opening without tension or twist, ensuring the mesentery lies in its natural orientation. The stoma is matured by everting the bowel wall and suturing the full-thickness bowel edge to the dermal layer of the skin with absorbable sutures (3-0 Vicryl), creating a budded stoma that protrudes 1 to 2 cm above the skin surface. Adequate protrusion is essential for appliance function — a flush or retracted stoma leads to appliance leakage, peristomal skin breakdown, and poor quality of life.

Loop Colostomy and Diverting Stoma Techniques

A loop colostomy is created by bringing a loop of intact colon (typically transverse or sigmoid) through the abdominal wall over a supporting rod or bridge. A longitudinal incision is made in the antimesenteric taenia of the exteriorized loop, opening the bowel lumen without dividing it completely. The proximal (functioning) limb is matured as a budded stoma, while the distal (defunctioning) limb is flush with the skin. The supporting rod is removed after 7 to 10 days when adhesions have formed between the bowel and the abdominal wall, preventing retraction. A diverting loop ileostomy (rather than loop colostomy) is the preferred method of fecal diversion in most modern colorectal practice — particularly for protecting a low colorectal or coloanal anastomosis after anterior resection for rectal cancer — because loop ileostomy achieves more complete diversion, has lower rates of prolapse and parastomal hernia, and is easier to reverse than loop colostomy.

Stoma Type	Construction	Common Indications	Key Complications
End colostomy	Divided colon brought through abdominal wall; distal end closed (Hartmann) or removed	Hartmann procedure, APR, sigmoid perforation, obstructing left-sided cancer	Parastomal hernia (30-50% at 2 years), stoma retraction, prolapse
Loop colostomy	Loop of intact colon brought through abdominal wall over rod; opened on antimesenteric surface	Fecal diversion for perineal wounds, protection of distal anastomosis, palliation of obstructing rectal cancer	Prolapse (more common than end colostomy), incomplete diversion, difficult appliance management
Loop ileostomy	Loop of terminal ileum brought through abdominal wall; proximal limb budded, distal limb flush	Protection of low colorectal or coloanal anastomosis, fecal diversion in colitis, perineal wound management	High-output dehydration, peristomal skin excoriation (alkaline ileal effluent), SBO at reversal

THE OPERATIVE DANGER ZONE ATLAS — Parastomal Vascular Compromise During Colostomy Creation

The Zone: The abdominal wall opening for stoma creation — where the colon is delivered through a circular fasciotomy in the rectus sheath, traversing the rectus muscle, subcutaneous tissue, and skin.

The Structure at Risk: The mesenteric blood supply to the stoma. The colon must pass through the abdominal wall opening with its mesentery in the correct orientation and without compression. If the fascial opening is too tight (less than two finger-breadths), the mesentery is compressed as it passes through the abdominal wall, producing venous congestion (the stoma appears dusky and edematous) progressing to arterial ischemia (the stoma turns dark purple to black). The inferior epigastric artery may also be injured if the fasciotomy extends too far laterally.

The Consequence: Stomal ischemia from mesenteric compression produces stoma necrosis — if the necrosis extends below the fascial level (assessed by inserting a lighted test tube into the stoma to visualize the mucosal color at the fascial level), urgent stoma revision is required because the ischemic segment is intra-abdominal and may perforate. Superficial necrosis above the fascial level can be observed and will heal by secondary intention with eventual stenosis requiring revision.

The Safe Maneuver: Create an abdominal wall opening that admits two fingers (approximately 2.5 to 3 cm) comfortably — large enough for the bowel and its mesentery to pass without compression but not so large as to create a wide fascial defect (which predisposes to parastomal hernia). Ensure the mesentery lies in its natural orientation without twist (180-degree rotation of the mesentery occludes the vascular supply). After maturation, assess the stoma color — a healthy stoma is beefy red and bleeds when scratched. If dusky, enlarge the fascial opening or revise the stoma.

Clinical Case — Emergency Hartmann Procedure for Perforated Diverticulitis

A 68-year-old woman with a history of diverticular disease presents with sudden-onset diffuse abdominal pain, fever of 39.1 degrees C, and hemodynamic instability (heart rate 118, blood pressure 88/52 mmHg). CT demonstrates free intraperitoneal air, a sigmoid perforation at the apex of a diverticular segment, and diffuse free fluid consistent with feculent peritonitis (Hinchey IV). After fluid resuscitation and broad-spectrum antibiotics (piperacillin-tazobactam plus vancomycin), the patient is taken to the operating room for emergency laparotomy. At operation, feculent peritonitis is confirmed with gross contamination of all four quadrants. The sigmoid colon is densely inflamed and thickened with a 2 cm perforation at the antimesenteric border. The sigmoid colon is resected from the descending-sigmoid junction to the rectosigmoid junction after identifying and protecting the left ureter. The proximal descending colon is brought out as an end colostomy through a site in the left lower quadrant within the rectus muscle. The rectal stump is closed with a linear stapler and marked with a long polypropylene suture for future identification during reversal. The peritoneal cavity is irrigated with 6 liters of warm saline. Two closed-suction drains are placed in the pelvis.

Postoperatively, the patient requires 48 hours of vasopressor support in the intensive care unit for septic shock. She is transitioned to oral antibiotics on day 5, the drains are removed on day 7, and the stoma begins functioning on day 3. She is discharged on day 12 with enterostomal therapy nurse follow-up for stoma management education. At 4 months, having recovered nutritionally and physiologically, she undergoes Hartmann reversal — the rectal stump is identified with the aid of a rigid proctoscope inserted transanally, dense pelvic adhesions are divided, and a circular stapled colorectal anastomosis is constructed. Final pathology from the original specimen confirms diverticular disease with perforation and no evidence of malignancy.

THE OPERATIVE DANGER ZONE ATLAS — Colonic Surgery Dangers

Duodenal Injury During Right Hemicolectomy Dissection: The duodenum lies directly beneath the right mesocolon in the medial-to-lateral dissection plane and may be injured if the dissection strays into the retroperitoneum. **Safe maneuver:** maintain the avascular embryological plane on the anterior surface of the retroperitoneal structures, visualize the duodenum, and sweep it posteriorly — never burn blindly with energy devices in this space.

Splenic Injury During Splenic Flexure Mobilization: The splenocolic ligament transmits traction force to the splenic capsule during splenic flexure mobilization, risking capsular avulsion or lower pole laceration — the most common cause of unplanned splenectomy during colorectal surgery. **Safe maneuver:** divide the splenocolic ligament under direct vision close to the colonic wall, approach from the inferior direction, and avoid downward traction on the splenic flexure.

Left Ureteral Injury During Emergency Sigmoid Resection: The left ureter courses beneath the sigmoid mesocolon and may be displaced or encased by a diverticular phlegmon, making it indistinguishable from surrounding inflammatory tissue during emergency sigmoid colectomy. **Safe maneuver:** identify the ureter early before dividing the mesocolon, consider preoperative ureteral stents in high-risk cases, and control each mesenteric vessel individually rather than placing mass clamps.

Parastomal Vascular Compromise During Colostomy Creation: A tight fascial opening compresses the colonic mesentery, producing venous congestion progressing to arterial ischemia and stoma necrosis. **Safe maneuver:** create a two-finger-width fascial opening, ensure the mesentery is not twisted, and assess stoma color after maturation — a dusky stoma requires immediate fascial enlargement or revision.

Summary and Key Concepts

The marginal artery of Drummond is weakest at the splenic flexure (Griffith point) — high ligation of the IMA requires verification that the marginal artery is intact at Griffith point to ensure adequate perfusion of the rectal stump before anastomosis construction.

Right hemicolectomy uses medial-to-lateral dissection beginning with high ligation of the ileocolic pedicle, developing the avascular embryological plane between the mesocolon and retroperitoneum while protecting the duodenum, right ureter, and gonadal vessels.

The left ureter crosses the common iliac bifurcation beneath the sigmoid mesocolon and must be identified before sigmoid mesenteric division — in emergency cases with inflammation, it may be displaced or encased in phlegmon.

Subtotal colectomy with ileostomy is the operation of choice for massive lower GI hemorrhage when the bleeding source has not been localized preoperatively — blind segmental resection carries an unacceptable rebleeding rate of 30 to 75%.

Hartmann reversal is one of the most technically demanding colorectal operations — preoperative stump localization with sigmoidoscopy and intraoperative use of a transanally placed rigid proctoscope are essential for identifying a buried rectal stump.

Stoma site selection within the rectus muscle, away from skin folds and bony prominences, is the single most important factor in long-term stoma function — preoperative marking by an enterostomal nurse is the standard of care.

In fulminant colitis with toxic megacolon, subtotal colectomy with end ileostomy and rectal stump preservation is the standard emergency operation — primary anastomosis is never constructed in this setting due to prohibitively high leak rates from malnutrition, immunosuppression, and active inflammation.

CHAPTER 13: OPERATIONS OF THE RECTUM AND ANUS

Learning Objectives

1. Describe the surgical anatomy of the rectum, anal canal, and pelvic floor, including the mesorectal envelope, the fascial planes of the pelvis, the internal and external anal sphincter complex, and the autonomic nerve supply.
2. Perform a low anterior resection with total mesorectal excision (TME) for mid and low rectal cancer, preserving the autonomic pelvic nerves and achieving negative circumferential resection margins.
3. Perform an abdominoperineal resection for low rectal cancer not amenable to sphincter-preserving surgery.
4. Manage common anorectal conditions operatively — hemorrhoids, anorectal abscess and fistula, anal fissure, and rectal prolapse — using appropriate technique and anatomical knowledge.

Surgical Anatomy of the Rectum, Anal Canal, and Pelvic Floor

The Rectum and Mesorectum

The rectum begins at the rectosigmoid junction (approximately 15 cm from the anal verge) and extends to the anorectal ring (the junction of the rectum with the anal canal, palpable as the upper border of the puborectalis muscle sling on digital rectal examination). The rectum follows the curve of the sacrum and has three lateral deflections marked by the valves of Houston (mucosal folds visible on proctoscopy). The rectum is surrounded by a fatty tissue envelope called the mesorectum, which is bounded by the mesorectal fascia (fascia propria of the rectum) — a thin but distinct fascial layer that encases the mesorectal fat, the superior rectal artery and vein, and the perirectal lymph nodes. The mesorectal fascia is the key anatomical landmark for total mesorectal excision: sharp dissection in the areolar tissue plane between the mesorectal fascia (enveloping the rectum) and the parietal pelvic fascia (covering the pelvic sidewalls, sacrum, and pelvic autonomic nerves) produces a complete, intact mesorectal specimen — the oncologic standard for rectal cancer surgery.

Autonomic Nerve Supply of the Pelvis

The pelvic autonomic nerves control urinary and sexual function and lie in the plane between the mesorectal fascia and the parietal pelvic fascia — the exact plane of TME dissection. The superior hypogastric plexus (presacral nerves) lies on the anterior surface of the aortic bifurcation and the sacral promontory, and bifurcates into the right and left hypogastric nerves, which descend along the pelvic sidewalls in the parietal pelvic fascia. The hypogastric nerves join the pelvic splanchnic nerves (parasympathetic fibers from S2-S4, the nervi erigentes) at the inferior hypogastric plexus (pelvic plexus) on the lateral pelvic sidewall at the level of the seminal vesicles in males or the uterosacral ligaments in females. From the pelvic plexus, the neurovascular bundles of Walsh course anterolaterally along the rectum at the 2 and 10 o'clock positions to innervate the bladder, prostate, seminal vesicles, and corpora cavernosa. Injury to these nerves during rectal dissection produces urinary retention (30 to 50% with nerve damage), erectile dysfunction (15 to 45%), and retrograde ejaculation.

The Anal Canal and Sphincter Complex

The anal canal extends from the anorectal ring to the anal verge (approximately 3 to 4 cm). It is divided by the dentate line (pectinate line) into an upper and lower half. Above the dentate line, the canal is lined by columnar epithelium, has visceral sensory innervation (insensitive to pain), and drains to the internal iliac lymph nodes. Below the dentate line, the canal is lined by squamous epithelium, has somatic sensory innervation (exquisitely sensitive to pain — the basis for the severe pain of anal fissure, thrombosed external hemorrhoids, and perianal abscess), and drains to the inguinal lymph nodes. The internal anal sphincter is an involuntary smooth muscle ring (the thickened terminal portion of the circular muscle layer of the rectum) responsible for approximately 80% of resting anal tone. The external anal sphincter is a voluntary striated muscle ring that surrounds the internal sphincter and provides the squeeze pressure for voluntary continence. The intersphincteric groove between the internal and external sphincters is palpable on digital rectal examination and is the anatomical landmark for intersphincteric dissection during abdominoperineal resection and intersphincteric resection.

Epidemiology and Risk Factors for Rectal Cancer

Rectal cancer accounts for approximately 30% of all colorectal cancers, with an estimated 45,000 new cases annually in the United States. The incidence is rising in adults under 50 (early-onset colorectal cancer), a trend observed worldwide over the past two decades, with the most rapid increase in the 20 to 34 age group. Risk factors include hereditary syndromes (Lynch syndrome — hereditary non-polyposis colorectal cancer, accounting for 2 to 4% of rectal cancers; familial adenomatous polyposis, accounting for less than 1%), inflammatory bowel disease (ulcerative colitis and Crohn colitis with longstanding colonic inflammation), prior pelvic irradiation, obesity, red and processed meat consumption, tobacco use, and alcohol consumption. Protective factors include regular physical activity, aspirin use (which reduces adenoma recurrence and colorectal cancer incidence by approximately 20%), fiber intake, and screening colonoscopy with polypectomy. The adenoma-carcinoma sequence remains the dominant pathway — progression from normal mucosa through adenomatous polyp to invasive carcinoma occurs over approximately 10 to 15 years, providing the basis for colonoscopic screening and polypectomy as cancer prevention.

Low Anterior Resection With Total Mesorectal Excision

Oncologic Principles and Dissection Technique

Total mesorectal excision is the oncologic standard for mid and low rectal cancer (tumors within 12 cm of the anal verge). TME involves sharp dissection under direct vision in the areolar tissue plane between the mesorectal fascia and the parietal pelvic fascia, circumferentially around the rectum, removing the rectum and its intact mesorectal envelope as a single surgical specimen. The quality of the TME specimen directly determines oncologic outcomes — an incomplete mesorectum (with tears, defects, or coning of the mesorectal fat exposing the muscularis propria) is associated with a three-fold increase in local recurrence compared to a complete, intact mesorectal specimen. The posterior dissection proceeds along the presacral fascia, the lateral dissection stays on the medial surface of the parietal pelvic fascia (preserving the hypogastric nerves and the pelvic plexus on the pelvic sidewall), and the anterior dissection follows the plane of Denonvilliers fascia (between the rectum and the prostate or vagina). The distal margin for rectal cancer is a minimum of 1 cm below the tumor (2 cm margins have been shown to be oncologically equivalent to 5 cm margins in rectal cancer, unlike colon cancer) — for very low tumors, intersphincteric resection preserves the external sphincter while achieving a negative distal margin.

Anastomotic Technique and Diverting Stoma

After TME and rectal transection, intestinal continuity is restored with a stapled colorectal or coloanal anastomosis. For mid-rectal tumors, a double-stapled technique is used — the rectal stump is closed with a linear stapler from below, the anvil of a circular stapler (EEA) is secured in the proximal colon, and the EEA is inserted transanally, docked to the anvil through the stapled rectal stump, and fired to create the anastomosis. For very low tumors, a handsewn coloanal anastomosis is performed at the level of the dentate line. A colonic J-pouch (a 5 to 6 cm pouch formed by folding the distal colon on itself and stapling the common wall) improves functional outcomes (reduced frequency, less urgency, improved continence) compared to a straight coloanal anastomosis and is the preferred reconstruction for low anastomoses. A diverting loop ileostomy is constructed to protect the anastomosis — standard practice for all anastomoses at or below 6 cm from the anal verge, reducing the clinical consequences of an anastomotic leak from peritonitis to a manageable pelvic collection.

THE OPERATIVE DANGER ZONE ATLAS — Autonomic Nerve Injury During Total Mesorectal Excision

The Zone: The lateral pelvic sidewall during TME dissection — where the hypogastric nerves and the inferior hypogastric plexus (pelvic plexus) lie on the medial surface of the parietal pelvic fascia, in the immediate plane of dissection between the mesorectal fascia and the parietal fascia.

The Structure at Risk: The hypogastric nerves and the neurovascular bundles of Walsh. The hypogastric nerves course along the pelvic sidewall and are at risk during lateral TME dissection — if the dissection strays laterally beyond the mesorectal fascia onto the pelvic sidewall, the hypogastric nerves are divided. The neurovascular bundles of Walsh lie at the anterolateral aspect of the rectum at the 2 and 10 o'clock positions and are at risk during the anterior dissection at the level of the seminal vesicles or vagina.

The Consequence: Bilateral hypogastric nerve injury produces urinary retention requiring long-term catheterization, complete erectile dysfunction (loss of both tumescence and ejaculation), and loss of bladder sensation. Unilateral injury produces partial dysfunction — retrograde ejaculation and reduced bladder contractility on the affected side. The incidence of urogenital dysfunction after TME with nerve-sparing technique is 10 to 30%, rising to 50% or more without nerve preservation.

The Safe Maneuver: Maintain the dissection plane strictly between the mesorectal fascia and the parietal pelvic fascia — the hypogastric nerves lie on the parietal side and are preserved when the dissection stays on the mesorectal side. Use sharp dissection under direct vision (not blunt or energy-device dissection) in the lateral and anterolateral planes where the nerves lie closest. Identify the hypogastric nerves at the sacral promontory at the beginning of the posterior dissection and trace them distally. At the anterolateral dissection, identify the neurovascular bundles of Walsh at the 2 and 10 o'clock positions and dissect them off the mesorectal fascia under direct vision.

Neoadjuvant Therapy and Perioperative Management

Neoadjuvant chemoradiation is the standard of care for locally advanced rectal cancer (clinical stage T3-4 or node-positive disease) and is administered before surgery to downstage the tumor, reduce local recurrence, and improve sphincter preservation rates. The standard regimen is long-course chemoradiation (50.4 Gy in 28 fractions over 5.5 weeks with concurrent fluoropyrimidine-based chemotherapy), with surgery performed 6 to 10 weeks after completion to allow maximum tumor response. Total neoadjuvant therapy (TNT) — delivering all chemotherapy (both radiosensitizing and systemic doses) before surgery — has shown improved complete pathologic response rates (approximately 25 to 30%) and is increasingly adopted. Patients achieving a clinical complete response (no residual tumor on digital rectal examination, endoscopy, and MRI) may be offered a watch-and-wait strategy (organ preservation) with intensive surveillance rather than immediate surgery, avoiding the morbidity of radical resection. The low anterior resection syndrome (LARS) — a constellation of urgency, frequency, clustering, and incontinence after low anterior resection — occurs in 50 to 90% of patients after low colorectal or coloanal anastomosis and significantly impacts quality of life. Colonic J-pouch reconstruction, avoiding anastomoses below 4 cm from the anal verge when possible, and pelvic floor rehabilitation are strategies to mitigate LARS.

Abdominoperineal Resection

Indications and Combined Approach

Abdominoperineal resection (APR) is indicated for low rectal cancers that cannot be treated with sphincter-preserving surgery — specifically, tumors involving or within 1 cm of the external anal sphincter, tumors with direct invasion of the levator ani muscles, and tumors in patients with pre-existing fecal incontinence where a functional anastomosis is not achievable. APR is a two-stage procedure performed either synchronously (two surgical teams working simultaneously on the abdominal and perineal phases) or sequentially. The abdominal phase is identical to a low anterior resection with TME — mobilization of the sigmoid colon, high ligation of the IMA, TME dissection in the pelvis down to the level of the levator ani muscles. An end sigmoid colostomy is created in the left lower quadrant. The perineal phase involves circumferential incision around the anus, dissection through the ischiorectal fat, division of the levator ani muscles, and removal of the entire anus, distal rectum, and mesorectum as a single specimen. The perineal wound is closed primarily with reconstruction of the pelvic floor (using omentum or a biological mesh to fill the pelvic dead space) or, in irradiated patients, with a myocutaneous flap (vertical rectus abdominis myocutaneous flap — VRAM — or gracilis flap) to bring vascularized tissue into the irradiated pelvis.

Cylindrical (Extralevator) Abdominoperineal Excision

The extralevator APR (cylindrical APR) was developed to reduce the high rate of positive circumferential resection margins (CRM) associated with the conventional APR performed in the prone jack-knife position. In a conventional APR, the perineal dissection tapers inward along the levator muscles toward the anus, producing a waisted specimen with the thinnest tissue margin at the level of the levator muscles — exactly where the tumor often extends in low rectal cancers. The extralevator technique removes the levator muscles en bloc with the specimen rather than dissecting along their surface, producing a cylindrical specimen with a wider circumferential margin at the levator level. The perineal dissection is performed with the patient in the prone position (or lithotomy with steep Trendelenburg), entering the pelvis outside the levator muscles, taking the coccyx if necessary, and removing the levators with the specimen. This technique reduces the CRM-positive rate from 15 to 30% (conventional) to 5 to 10% (extralevator) and reduces local recurrence rates.

Transanal Excision and Transanal Minimally Invasive Surgery (TAMIS)

Patient Selection and Technique

Transanal excision is the local excision of early rectal neoplasms through the anus without abdominal surgery. It is appropriate only for carefully selected early-stage rectal cancers (T1 lesions without lymphovascular invasion, well or moderately differentiated, less than 3 cm in size, involving less than 30% of the rectal circumference, without nodal involvement on imaging). Transanal excision achieves local control for these favorable T1 lesions while avoiding the morbidity of radical resection (including the risk of permanent colostomy, urogenital dysfunction, and anastomotic complications). However, it does NOT address the mesorectal lymph nodes — the risk of occult nodal metastasis in T1 rectal cancer is 6 to 12%, and the recurrence rate after transanal excision for unfavorable T1 or any T2 lesion is unacceptably high (approximately 25 to 40%). TAMIS uses a transanal access platform (GelPOINT Path or similar) and standard laparoscopic instruments, providing superior visualization and more precise dissection than conventional transanal excision performed through a rigid operating anoscope. A full-thickness excision of the rectal wall is performed with a 1 cm circumferential margin, and the specimen is pinned for orientation and sent for formal pathological analysis. If pathology reveals unfavorable features (T2 depth, lymphovascular invasion, positive margins, poor differentiation), the patient is counseled for radical resection (TME) or neoadjuvant chemoradiation.

Hemorrhoidectomy (Excisional and Stapled)

Classification and Operative Indications

Internal hemorrhoids are classified by the Goligher classification: grade I (bleeding without prolapse), grade II (prolapse with spontaneous reduction), grade III (prolapse requiring manual reduction), and grade IV (irreducible prolapse). Office-based procedures (rubber band ligation, injection sclerotherapy, infrared coagulation) are first-line for grades I and II. Operative hemorrhoidectomy is indicated for grade III and IV hemorrhoids, mixed internal-external hemorrhoids, hemorrhoids that have failed conservative and office-based treatment, acutely thrombosed circumferential hemorrhoids, and hemorrhoids associated with additional anorectal pathology (fissure, fistula, skin tags) requiring operative management.

Excisional Hemorrhoidectomy — Milligan-Morgan and Ferguson Techniques

Excisional hemorrhoidectomy (the Milligan-Morgan open technique or Ferguson closed technique) removes the hemorrhoidal tissue at the three primary hemorrhoidal positions (left lateral, right anterior, and right posterior — the 3, 7, and 11 o'clock positions). Each hemorrhoidal complex is grasped, a V-shaped incision is made in the perianal skin at the base of the external component, the dissection proceeds cephalad in the submucosal plane to separate the hemorrhoidal plexus from the underlying internal sphincter muscle, and the pedicle is suture-ligated at its apex (above the dentate line). The critical technical rule is to preserve adequate mucosal and skin bridges between the three excision sites — excising too much tissue (confluent excisions without intervening skin and mucosal bridges) produces anal stenosis, which is the most significant long-term complication of hemorrhoidectomy and may require anoplasty for correction. The Milligan-Morgan technique leaves the wounds open (healing by secondary intention over 4 to 6 weeks), while the Ferguson technique closes the wounds with running absorbable suture — both produce equivalent long-term outcomes, although the Ferguson technique may produce less postoperative pain and faster healing.

Operative Management of Anorectal Abscess and Fistula

Anorectal Abscess — Classification and Drainage

Anorectal abscesses arise from infection of the anal glands (cryptoglandular theory) — the anal glands, located in the intersphincteric space at the level of the dentate line, become obstructed, and the resulting abscess tracks through the anatomical tissue planes of the anorectal region. Abscesses are classified by their location: perianal (the most common, 60% — located in the perianal skin and subcutaneous tissue), ischiorectal (20 to 25% — located in the ischiorectal fossa between the external sphincter and the ischial tuberosity), intersphincteric (2 to 5% — located in the intersphincteric space between the internal and external sphincters), and supralevator (2 to 3% — located above the levator ani muscles). The treatment of anorectal abscess is incision and drainage — antibiotics alone are insufficient. Perianal abscesses are drained through a cruciate skin incision directly over the point of maximal fluctuance, excising the skin corners to prevent premature closure. Ischiorectal abscesses require a deeper incision with digital exploration of the abscess cavity to break up loculations. A fistula tract (connecting the abscess to the anal canal) is present in approximately 30 to 50% of anorectal abscesses at the time of drainage — if identified, it is managed at the same sitting with a draining seton (a vessel loop threaded through the fistula tract to maintain drainage and prevent recurrent abscess).

Fistula-in-Ano — Goodsall Rule and Operative Management

Fistula-in-ano is a chronic epithelialized tract connecting the anal canal (internal opening at the dentate line) to the perianal skin (external opening). The Goodsall rule predicts the location of the internal opening based on the position of the external opening: external openings anterior to the transverse anal line (the line drawn between the ischial tuberosities through the center of the anus) track radially to the nearest crypt at the dentate line, while external openings posterior to the transverse anal line curve posteriorly to the posterior midline. Fistulas are classified by the Parks classification based on their relationship to the sphincter complex: intersphincteric (track through the intersphincteric space — the most common), transsphincteric (track through both the internal and external sphincters), suprasphincteric (track above the puborectalis and then down through the ischiorectal fossa), and extrasphincteric (track from the rectum through the levator ani muscles to the perianal skin, bypassing the sphincter complex entirely). Simple low fistulas (intersphincteric, low transsphincteric involving less than 30% of the external sphincter) are treated by fistulotomy — laying open the tract and allowing it to heal by secondary intention. Complex fistulas (high transsphincteric, suprasphincteric, extrasphincteric, recurrent, or those in patients with Crohn disease or pre-existing incontinence) require sphincter-sparing techniques: a cutting seton (a silk suture tied progressively tighter to slowly cut through the sphincter while allowing it to heal and scar behind the seton), a ligation of intersphincteric fistula tract (LIFT) procedure, an endorectal advancement flap, or fibrin glue or collagen plug insertion.

THE OPERATIVE DANGER ZONE ATLAS — Sphincter Injury During Fistulotomy or Abscess Drainage

The Zone: The anorectal sphincter complex during operative management of anorectal abscess and fistula — specifically during fistulotomy (laying open the fistula tract), where the knife or electrocautery divides all tissue between the fistula tract and the anal canal.

The Structure at Risk: The external anal sphincter. In fistulotomy, the tract is laid open by dividing the tissue between the external opening and the internal opening — if the tract passes through a significant portion of the external sphincter (a high transsphincteric fistula), fistulotomy divides that portion of the sphincter, producing a keyhole deformity and incontinence to gas and liquid stool.

The Consequence: Iatrogenic fecal incontinence from excessive sphincter division during fistulotomy is the most serious complication of fistula surgery. Incontinence after fistulotomy correlates directly with the proportion of external sphincter divided — fistulotomy for a fistula involving more than 30% of the external sphincter carries an incontinence risk of 30 to 50%. Anterior fistulas in women are particularly high risk because the anterior external sphincter is shorter and thinner in females.

The Safe Maneuver: Before performing fistulotomy, assess the proportion of external sphincter that the tract traverses by examining under anesthesia with a probe in the tract and a finger in the anal canal. If more than 30% of the external sphincter would be divided, do NOT perform fistulotomy — use a sphincter-sparing technique (seton drainage, LIFT procedure, or advancement flap) instead. In anterior fistulas in women, the threshold for a sphincter-sparing approach is even lower. Always classify the fistula (Parks classification) before choosing the operative technique.

Complications of Anorectal Surgery

Urinary retention is the most common early complication after anorectal surgery, occurring in 10 to 25% of patients and attributed to reflex inhibition of detrusor function from perineal pain and sympathetic stimulation. Risk factors include older age, spinal anesthesia, excessive intravenous fluid administration (bladder distension), and higher grades of hemorrhoidal disease. Limiting intravenous fluids to less than 1 liter intraoperatively and encouraging early voiding reduce the incidence. Postoperative hemorrhage after hemorrhoidectomy occurs in 2 to 6% of patients, typically between postoperative day 7 and 14 (secondary hemorrhage from sloughing of the eschar over the ligated pedicle), and may require return to the operating room for suture ligation under anesthesia. Perianal sepsis (abscess formation) after fistula surgery occurs when inadequate drainage or premature closure of the wound allows reaccumulation of infected material. Fecal incontinence after anorectal surgery varies by procedure — 5 to 15% minor incontinence (to flatus) after lateral internal sphincterotomy, 10 to 40% after fistulotomy depending on the proportion of sphincter divided, and 5 to 10% after hemorrhoidectomy when excessive sphincter stretch from the operating anoscope causes temporary sphincter weakness.

Lateral Internal Sphincterotomy

Indications and Technique

Lateral internal sphincterotomy (LIS) is the definitive operative treatment for chronic anal fissure that has failed conservative management (stool softeners, topical nitroglycerin, topical calcium channel blockers, and botulinum toxin injection). A chronic fissure is defined by the presence of a sentinel tag (a skin tag at the distal end of the fissure), exposed internal sphincter fibers in the base of the fissure, and hypertrophied anal papilla at the proximal end. The pathophysiology of chronic anal fissure involves internal sphincter spasm that reduces blood flow to the posterior midline of the anal canal (the watershed zone of the inferior rectal artery), perpetuating ischemia and preventing healing. LIS divides the distal portion of the internal anal sphincter in the lateral position (left lateral — the 3 o'clock position), reducing internal sphincter tone and restoring blood flow to the fissure bed. The open technique involves a 1 cm radial incision at the intersphincteric groove at the 3 o'clock position, identification of the distal edge of the internal sphincter, and division of the internal sphincter under direct vision up to the level of the dentate line (not above — division above the dentate line risks excessive sphincter division and incontinence). The closed technique uses a narrow-blade knife inserted through a small stab incision at the intersphincteric groove, directed between the internal and external sphincters, and swept medially to divide the internal sphincter. The healing rate for chronic anal fissure after LIS exceeds 95%. The principal risk is minor incontinence to flatus (5 to 15%), which is usually transient.

Operative Management of Rectal Prolapse

Classification and Surgical Options

Full-thickness rectal prolapse (procidentia) is the circumferential, full-thickness intussusception of the rectal wall through the anal canal. It occurs most commonly in elderly women and is associated with chronic constipation, straining, multiparity, pudendal neuropathy, and pelvic floor weakness. Operative repair is the definitive treatment and can be performed via abdominal or perineal approach. Abdominal approaches include laparoscopic ventral mesh rectopexy (the current preferred approach in many centers — a mesh is sutured to the anterior rectum and fixed to the sacral promontory, suspending the rectum without posterior mobilization, which avoids division of the lateral ligaments and preserves autonomic nerve function and rectal reservoir compliance) and laparoscopic suture rectopexy (fixation of the mobilized rectum to the presacral fascia without mesh). Perineal approaches include the Delorme procedure (mucosal sleeve resection with muscular plication — the rectal mucosa is excised circumferentially from the prolapsing segment, the denuded muscular wall is plicated with concertina-like absorbable sutures, and the mucosal edges are re-anastomosed) and the Altemeier procedure (perineal rectosigmoidectomy — full-thickness resection of the prolapsing rectum and sigmoid through the perineum with primary coloanal anastomosis, with or without concurrent levatorplasty to repair the pelvic floor). Perineal approaches are preferred for high-risk elderly patients who are poor candidates for general anesthesia and laparotomy because they can be performed under regional anesthesia.

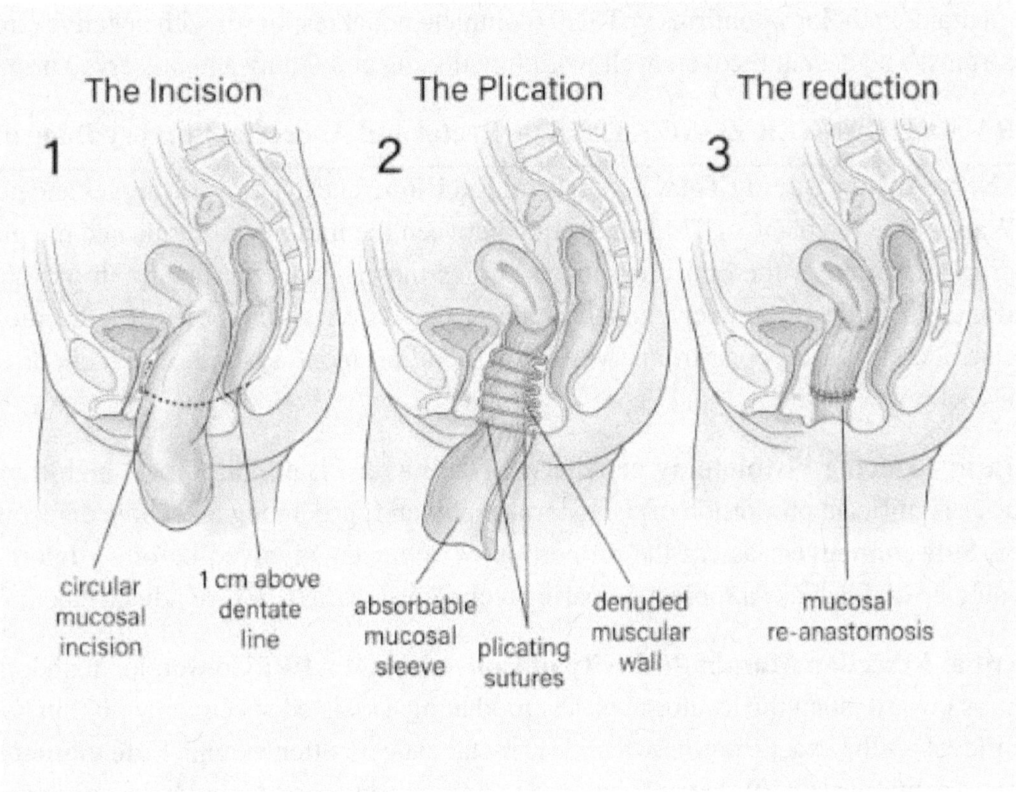

CLINICAL PEARL: The concentric circular fold pattern of full-thickness rectal prolapse (procidentia) distinguishes it from mucosal-only prolapse, which produces radial folds. This distinction is critical because full-thickness prolapse requires operative repair (Delorme, Altemeier, or rectopexy), while mucosal prolapse can often be managed with rubber band ligation or mucosal excision alone.

Clinical Case — Locally Advanced Low Rectal Cancer Requiring Abdominoperineal Resection

A 58-year-old man presents with rectal bleeding, tenesmus, and a palpable mass on digital rectal examination at 3 cm from the anal verge. MRI demonstrates a T3N1 low rectal cancer involving the anterior rectal wall with extension into the intersphincteric space but no invasion of the external sphincter. The tumor's proximity to the anal verge (3 cm) and involvement of the intersphincteric space precludes sphincter-preserving surgery (a coloanal anastomosis requires at least 1 cm of normal rectum below the tumor, and intersphincteric involvement makes intersphincteric resection unsafe). The patient receives neoadjuvant long-course chemoradiation (5-FU-based chemotherapy with 50.4 Gy radiation over 5.5 weeks). Restaging MRI at 8 weeks shows partial response with persistent T3 tumor. The decision is made for extralevator abdominoperineal excision (cylindrical APR). The abdominal phase is performed laparoscopically — the IMA is ligated at its origin, and TME is performed in the nerve-sparing plane down to the level of the levator ani muscles. A permanent end sigmoid colostomy is created at a pre-marked site in the left lower quadrant. The patient is turned prone, and the perineal phase is performed — a circumferential incision is made wide of the external sphincter, the ischiorectal fat is divided, the levator muscles are divided flush with the pelvic sidewall (not along their surface), and the specimen is delivered from below. The pelvic floor is reconstructed with a biological mesh, and the perineal wound is closed over a suction drain. Pathology confirms ypT3N0 (complete nodal response) with negative circumferential and distal margins. The patient recovers well, with functioning colostomy and preserved urinary function.

THE OPERATIVE DANGER ZONE ATLAS — Rectal and Anorectal Surgery Dangers

Autonomic Nerve Injury During Total Mesorectal Excision: The hypogastric nerves and neurovascular bundles of Walsh lie in the plane of TME dissection between the mesorectal fascia and the parietal pelvic fascia — lateral deviation of the dissection plane injures these nerves, producing urinary retention and erectile dysfunction. **Safe maneuver:** maintain sharp dissection strictly between the mesorectal and parietal fasciae, identify the hypogastric nerves at the sacral promontory, and trace them distally through the lateral dissection.

Sphincter Injury During Fistulotomy or Abscess Drainage: Fistulotomy for a high transsphincteric fistula divides a significant proportion of the external sphincter, producing a keyhole deformity and fecal incontinence. **Safe maneuver:** assess the proportion of sphincter involved before fistulotomy; if more than 30% would be divided, use a sphincter-sparing technique (seton, LIFT, or advancement flap) instead.

Circumferential Resection Margin Positivity in Conventional APR: Conventional abdominoperineal resection tapers inward along the levator muscles, producing a waisted specimen with thin tissue margins at the levator level — the exact location where low rectal cancers often extend. **Safe maneuver:** perform an extralevator (cylindrical) APR that removes the levator muscles en bloc with the specimen, producing a wider circumferential margin and reducing local recurrence.

Anal Stenosis from Excessive Hemorrhoidectomy: Confluent hemorrhoid excisions without adequate mucosal and skin bridges between excision sites produce cicatricial anal stenosis requiring anoplasty for correction. **Safe maneuver:** preserve mucosal and skin bridges between all three primary hemorrhoid excision sites (3, 7, and 11 o'clock); never allow excision sites to become confluent.

Summary and Key Concepts

Total mesorectal excision (TME) is the oncologic standard for mid and low rectal cancer — sharp dissection in the plane between the mesorectal fascia and parietal pelvic fascia produces an intact mesorectal specimen and preserves the pelvic autonomic nerves that control urinary and sexual function.

The pelvic autonomic nerves (hypogastric nerves and neurovascular bundles of Walsh) lie in the TME dissection plane — nerve-sparing technique reduces the incidence of urogenital dysfunction from 50% to 10 to 30%.

Extralevator (cylindrical) APR removes the levator muscles en bloc with the specimen, reducing CRM-positive rates from 15 to 30% (conventional APR) to 5 to 10% and is the preferred technique for tumors involving the levator muscles.

Transanal excision (TAMIS) is appropriate only for carefully selected early T1 rectal cancers without unfavorable histological features — unfavorable pathology mandates radical resection (TME) because the 6 to 12% risk of occult nodal metastasis is not addressed by local excision.

Fistulotomy is safe only for fistulas involving less than 30% of the external sphincter — complex or high fistulas require sphincter-sparing techniques (seton, LIFT, advancement flap) to preserve continence.

The Goodsall rule predicts internal opening location: anterior external openings track radially to the nearest crypt, posterior external openings curve to the posterior midline.

Full-thickness rectal prolapse shows concentric circular folds (distinguishing it from mucosal prolapse with radial folds) and requires operative repair — laparoscopic ventral mesh rectopexy or perineal approaches (Delorme or Altemeier) depending on patient fitness.

CHAPTER 14: OPERATIONS OF THE BREAST

Learning Objectives

1. Describe the surgical anatomy of the breast, including the fascial boundaries, lymphatic drainage pathways, axillary nodal levels (I–III), and the neurovascular structures at risk during breast and axillary surgery.
2. Perform breast-conserving surgery (lumpectomy) with negative margins and oncoplastic closure techniques, and explain the oncologic equivalence of breast conservation with radiation to mastectomy for early-stage breast cancer.
3. Perform sentinel lymph node biopsy with dual-tracer technique and apply the results to guide axillary management decisions.
4. Select the appropriate mastectomy type (simple, modified radical, skin-sparing, nipple-sparing) and reconstruction modality based on tumor characteristics, patient anatomy, and oncologic safety.

Surgical Anatomy of the Breast and Axilla

Breast Anatomy and Fascial Boundaries

The breast is a modified apocrine gland situated on the anterior chest wall between the second and sixth ribs, extending from the lateral border of the sternum to the anterior axillary line. It rests on the pectoralis major muscle (upper two-thirds) and the serratus anterior muscle (lower one-third), separated from the underlying muscle by the retromammary (deep) fascia — a loose areolar layer that permits the breast to move freely over the chest wall and provides the dissection plane for mastectomy. The breast parenchyma is organized into 15 to 20 lobes, each draining through a lactiferous duct to the nipple. The breast receives its blood supply from three sources: the internal mammary artery perforators (medial breast — the dominant supply, providing approximately 60% of total blood flow), the lateral thoracic artery (lateral breast), and the intercostal perforators (posterior breast). The sensory innervation of the nipple-areola complex derives primarily from the lateral cutaneous branch of the fourth intercostal nerve (T4), which courses from the lateral chest wall through the breast parenchyma to reach the nipple — this nerve is at risk during oncoplastic dissection and mastectomy, and its division produces nipple numbness.

Axillary Anatomy and Lymph Node Levels

The axilla is a pyramidal space bounded by the pectoralis major and minor muscles anteriorly, the subscapularis and latissimus dorsi muscles posteriorly, the serratus anterior muscle medially, the convergence of the anterior and posterior walls superiorly, and the axillary skin inferiorly. The axillary lymph nodes are classified into three levels relative to the pectoralis minor muscle: level I (lateral to the lateral border of the pectoralis minor — the low axilla), level II (behind the pectoralis minor — the mid axilla), and level III (medial to the medial border of the pectoralis minor — the apical axilla, including the subclavicular nodes). Lymphatic drainage from the breast follows a sequential pattern from level I to level II to level III — skip metastases (involvement of level II or III with negative level I nodes) occur in approximately 1 to 3% of cases. The axilla contains several critical structures that must be identified and preserved during axillary dissection: the axillary vein (the superior boundary of the dissection), the long thoracic nerve of Bell (running on the medial surface of the serratus anterior muscle — injury produces a winged scapula), the thoracodorsal nerve and vessels (running along the posterior axillary wall to the latissimus dorsi muscle), and the intercostobrachial nerve (the lateral cutaneous branch of T2, crossing the axilla from medial to lateral — division produces numbness of the medial upper arm and axilla).

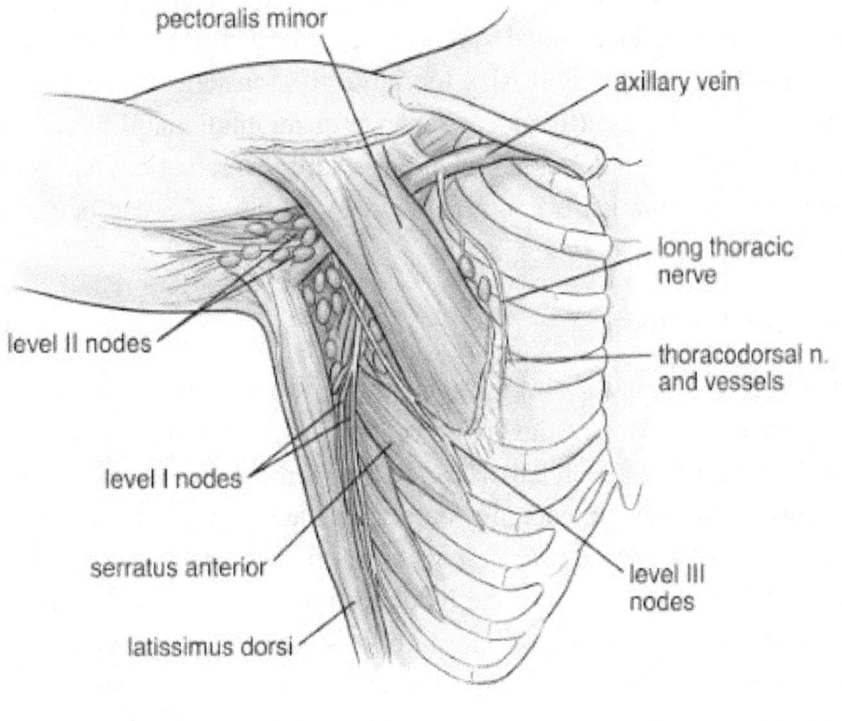

Epidemiology and Staging Considerations

Breast cancer is the most commonly diagnosed cancer in women worldwide, with approximately 2.3 million new cases annually and approximately 300,000 new cases annually in the United States. The lifetime risk for women is approximately 1 in 8 (12.5%). The majority of breast cancers are diagnosed at early stage (stage I or II) due to screening mammography — early-stage disease is amenable to breast-conserving surgery or mastectomy with equivalent long-term survival. The surgical approach is determined by tumor size relative to breast volume, tumor multifocality or multicentricity, margin status, patient preference, genetic risk factors (BRCA1/BRCA2 mutations, which confer a lifetime breast cancer risk of 45 to 80% and often influence the decision toward bilateral mastectomy), and the availability of radiation therapy (breast-conserving surgery requires adjuvant whole-breast radiation). The shift toward less radical surgery has been one of the defining trends in surgical oncology — from the Halsted radical mastectomy through modified radical mastectomy to breast-conserving surgery, and from complete axillary lymph node dissection to sentinel lymph node biopsy — driven by randomized controlled trials demonstrating oncologic equivalence with less morbidity.

Breast-Conserving Surgery (Lumpectomy With Oncoplastic Techniques)

Oncologic Principles and Margin Requirements

Breast-conserving surgery (BCS) removes the primary tumor with a surrounding margin of normal tissue while preserving the remaining breast. Multiple randomized controlled trials with 20-year follow-up (NSABP B-06, Milan I) have demonstrated equivalent overall survival between BCS with whole-breast radiation and mastectomy for stage I and II breast cancer. The current margin standard is no tumor on ink (a negative margin defined as no cancer cells touching the inked surgical specimen surface) — wider margins do not further reduce local recurrence when followed by whole-breast radiation. Contraindications to BCS include tumor size too large for cosmetically acceptable excision relative to breast volume, multicentric disease (tumors in separate quadrants), inability to achieve negative margins after re-excision, prior chest wall radiation precluding additional radiation, and pregnancy during the first or second trimester (where radiation is contraindicated, although BCS can be performed if radiation can be delivered postpartum).

Oncoplastic Closure Techniques

Oncoplastic surgery integrates plastic surgical techniques into the lumpectomy to allow excision of larger volumes of tissue (up to 30 to 40% of the breast volume) while maintaining breast shape and symmetry. Level I oncoplastic techniques use local tissue rearrangement (advancement flaps, rotation flaps, or glandular reshaping) to fill the lumpectomy defect and are appropriate for smaller defects. Level II oncoplastic techniques use volume displacement (breast reduction or mastopexy patterns — such as the Wise pattern, vertical mammaplasty, or round block technique) to excise the tumor within a reduction or lift pattern, reshaping the remaining tissue into a smaller but well-formed breast. Contralateral symmetrization (reduction or lift of the opposite breast) is performed at the same sitting or as a delayed procedure. Oncoplastic techniques have expanded the indications for breast conservation into tumors previously considered too large for lumpectomy — enabling breast conservation in 25 to 30% of patients who would otherwise require mastectomy — while maintaining equivalent oncologic outcomes and local recurrence rates.

THE OPERATIVE DANGER ZONE ATLAS — Positive Margin After Lumpectomy Due to Inadequate Specimen Orientation

The Zone: The lumpectomy cavity — the tissue bed remaining after excision of the primary breast cancer, where the adequacy of surgical margins is determined by pathological assessment of the specimen surfaces.

The Structure at Risk: The surgical margin. Inadequate specimen orientation (failure to orient the excised specimen with sutures or clips marking the six surfaces — superior, inferior, medial, lateral, anterior, posterior) prevents the pathologist from identifying which specific margin is positive, forcing the surgeon to perform a wider, non-directed re-excision rather than a targeted re-excision of only the involved margin. This results in unnecessary tissue loss and poorer cosmetic outcomes.

The Consequence: A positive margin (tumor on ink) requires re-excision, which is performed in 20 to 30% of patients after initial lumpectomy. Without specimen orientation, the re-excision must encompass the entire lumpectomy cavity rather than the specific involved margin, increasing tissue loss and potentially converting a cosmetically acceptable breast conservation to a mastectomy.

The Safe Maneuver: Orient every lumpectomy specimen with a minimum of two sutures (short stitch = superior, long stitch = lateral, or a three-suture system adding anterior), communicate the orientation to the pathologist, and obtain intraoperative margin assessment (frozen section or touch preparation cytology) for all margins. If a specific margin is close or positive, perform a directed cavity shaving of that margin at the same sitting. Clip the lumpectomy cavity walls with metallic clips to guide future radiation boost targeting.

Intraoperative Margin Assessment and Re-Excision Strategies

Intraoperative margin assessment reduces the rate of positive margins requiring return to the operating room for re-excision. Three techniques are available: frozen section analysis (the gold standard — provides immediate histological assessment but is time-consuming and may miss small foci of tumor), touch preparation (imprint) cytology (faster but less sensitive for DCIS), and gross inspection with cavity shaving (the surgeon excises additional thin slices of tissue from the walls of the lumpectomy cavity — anterior, posterior, medial, lateral, superior, and inferior — regardless of frozen section results). The cavity shaving technique has been shown in randomized trials to reduce the positive margin rate from approximately 20% to 10% and significantly reduces the need for re-excision surgery. When a directed re-excision is needed (positive or close margin on a specific surface identified by specimen orientation), a targeted cavity shaving of only the involved margin is performed — this is why meticulous specimen orientation at the time of initial excision is critical. The re-excision rate after initial lumpectomy varies by institution from 15% to 35% — centers using routine cavity shaving and intraoperative frozen section have the lowest re-excision rates. Each re-excision degrades cosmetic outcome, increases cost, delays adjuvant therapy, and increases patient anxiety — the goal is to achieve negative margins at the first operation.

Mastectomy (Simple, Modified Radical, and Skin-Sparing)

Types of Mastectomy

Simple (total) mastectomy removes all breast tissue, including the nipple-areola complex, without axillary lymph node dissection. It is indicated for ductal carcinoma in situ (DCIS) not amenable to breast conservation, prophylactic mastectomy for high-risk patients (BRCA carriers), phyllodes tumor, and invasive cancer when sentinel lymph node biopsy is performed separately. Modified radical mastectomy (the Patey or Auchincloss modification) removes all breast tissue plus the nipple-areola complex and performs an axillary lymph node dissection (levels I and II) — it is indicated when axillary dissection is required (clinically positive axilla, positive sentinel lymph node biopsy meeting criteria for completion dissection). The Halsted radical mastectomy (which removes the pectoralis major and minor muscles in addition to the breast and axillary nodes) is rarely performed today — reserved only for tumors directly invading the pectoralis major muscle. Skin-sparing mastectomy preserves the breast skin envelope (removing only the nipple-areola complex and biopsy scars) to facilitate immediate reconstruction — the oncologic safety of skin-sparing mastectomy has been established by multiple studies showing equivalent local recurrence rates to conventional mastectomy. Nipple-sparing mastectomy preserves both the breast skin and the nipple-areola complex and is appropriate for prophylactic mastectomy and selected cancers located more than 2 cm from the nipple with no involvement of the retroareolar tissue (confirmed by frozen section of the retroareolar margin).

Mastectomy Technique — Skin Flap Dissection

The critical technical step in all mastectomy types is the development of thin, well-vascularized skin flaps. The dissection plane is between the subcutaneous fat and the breast parenchyma — a plane that is often indistinct because breast tissue is interdigitated with subcutaneous fat. Flaps that are too thin (dissecting within or close to the dermis) risk skin flap necrosis (because the subdermal plexus is interrupted), while flaps that are too thick leave residual breast tissue behind (which defeats the oncologic purpose of the mastectomy and may produce residual palpable breast tissue in the mastectomy skin flaps). The incidence of mastectomy skin flap necrosis ranges from 5 to 30% and is increased by smoking, obesity, diabetes, prior radiation, and the extent of skin flap undermining in skin-sparing and nipple-sparing mastectomy. Intraoperative assessment of skin flap perfusion using indocyanine green (ICG) fluorescence angiography allows real-time visualization of flap vascularity and has been shown to reduce mastectomy skin flap necrosis by identifying areas of marginal perfusion before wound closure.

Perioperative Considerations and Complications

Preoperative planning for mastectomy includes genetic counseling and testing (BRCA1/BRCA2 and other breast cancer susceptibility genes) when indicated, multidisciplinary tumor board discussion to determine the sequence of systemic therapy and surgery, and consultation with plastic surgery for reconstruction planning. When immediate reconstruction is planned, the mastectomy surgeon and the reconstructive surgeon must coordinate the skin incision, the extent of skin preservation, and the planned reconstructive technique. Postoperative complications include seroma (the most common — occurring in 20 to 50% of patients; managed by serial aspiration), wound infection (5 to 10%), skin flap necrosis (5 to 30%, higher in skin-sparing and nipple-sparing mastectomy), hematoma (2 to 5%), and chronic pain at the surgical site (20 to 30%, attributed to intercostal nerve injury during flap dissection). Drain management is a key postoperative issue — closed-suction drains are placed at the time of mastectomy and removed when output falls below 30 mL per 24 hours. Early drain removal reduces patient discomfort and the risk of drain-associated infection, while premature removal increases seroma rates. Post-mastectomy radiation therapy, when indicated (T3-4 tumors, four or more positive lymph nodes, positive margins), complicates reconstruction — it increases capsular contracture rates around implants and may compromise flap healing. When post-mastectomy radiation is anticipated, delayed reconstruction (after completion of radiation) or autologous reconstruction (which tolerates radiation better than implants) is often preferred.

Sentinel Lymph Node Biopsy and Axillary Lymph Node Dissection

Sentinel Lymph Node Biopsy — Technique and Indications

Sentinel lymph node biopsy (SLNB) is the standard axillary staging procedure for clinically node-negative invasive breast cancer. The sentinel lymph node is the first lymph node receiving lymphatic drainage from the tumor — identified intraoperatively using a dual-tracer technique: technetium-99m sulfur colloid (injected preoperatively and localized with a handheld gamma probe) and isosulfan blue dye or indocyanine green (injected at the time of surgery). The combination of radiotracer and blue dye achieves a sentinel node identification rate exceeding 95% and a false-negative rate of approximately 5 to 10%. SLNB has replaced routine axillary lymph node dissection (ALND) for axillary staging because it provides equivalent staging information with dramatically less morbidity — SLNB carries a lymphedema rate of 5 to 7% compared to 20 to 30% for ALND, and avoids the shoulder dysfunction, chronic pain, and sensory loss associated with ALND. The ACOSOG Z0011 trial demonstrated that patients with one or two positive sentinel lymph nodes undergoing BCS with whole-breast radiation do NOT require completion ALND — a paradigm-shifting finding that has further reduced the need for ALND.

Axillary Lymph Node Dissection — Technique and Boundaries

When ALND is required (clinically positive axilla, three or more positive sentinel nodes, positive sentinel nodes after neoadjuvant chemotherapy without nodal response), the dissection removes levels I and II lymph nodes. The boundaries of the dissection are the axillary vein superiorly (the dissection proceeds along the inferior surface of the axillary vein, sweeping the fatty lymphatic tissue inferiorly), the latissimus dorsi muscle posteriorly, the pectoralis minor muscle anteriorly, and the chest wall (serratus anterior muscle) medially. The long thoracic nerve must be identified on the medial surface of the serratus anterior and preserved — it is vulnerable during medial dissection when the lymphatic tissue is swept off the chest wall. The thoracodorsal nerve and vessels are identified on the posterior axillary wall and preserved — the thoracodorsal vessels are the blood supply for the latissimus dorsi muscle flap, which may be needed for future reconstruction. The intercostobrachial nerve is sacrificed in most ALND procedures (it crosses the field and is usually inseparable from the specimen), producing numbness of the medial upper arm — the patient should be counseled about this expected sensory change preoperatively.

THE OPERATIVE DANGER ZONE ATLAS — Long Thoracic Nerve Injury During Axillary Dissection

The Zone: The medial wall of the axilla during axillary lymph node dissection — where the long thoracic nerve (nerve of Bell) runs on the surface of the serratus anterior muscle beneath the fascial investing layer.

The Structure at Risk: The long thoracic nerve. It courses along the lateral surface of the serratus anterior muscle from the neck to the inferior angle of the scapula. During axillary dissection, the nerve is at risk when the lymphatic tissue is swept off the medial chest wall — particularly when an energy device is used close to the serratus anterior surface, or when the nerve is not identified before beginning the medial dissection.

The Consequence: Division or thermal injury to the long thoracic nerve denervates the serratus anterior muscle, producing a winged scapula — the medial border of the scapula protrudes posteriorly, and the patient loses the ability to elevate the arm above the horizontal plane (loss of overhead reach). This is a permanent, functionally debilitating deficit.

The Safe Maneuver: Identify the long thoracic nerve at the beginning of the medial dissection — it runs vertically on the surface of the serratus anterior muscle, identifiable as a glistening white cord. Maintain all dissection superficial (lateral) to the nerve. Do not use energy devices directly on the serratus anterior surface in the vicinity of the nerve — use blunt dissection to sweep lymphatic tissue off the chest wall medially. If the nerve cannot be clearly identified, palpate the serratus anterior muscle and dissect on its surface under direct vision until the nerve is visualized.

Lymphedema — Prevention, Risk, and Management

Lymphedema of the ipsilateral upper extremity is the most functionally significant long-term complication of axillary surgery and occurs when surgical disruption of axillary lymphatic channels exceeds the capacity of remaining lymphatic pathways to drain interstitial fluid from the arm. The incidence after sentinel lymph node biopsy alone is 5 to 7%, rising to 20 to 30% after axillary lymph node dissection, and further increasing to 30 to 50% when ALND is combined with axillary radiation. Risk factors include the extent of axillary surgery (number of nodes removed), concurrent axillary radiation, obesity (body mass index greater than 30), postoperative wound complications (seroma, infection), and lack of early mobilization. Prevention strategies include limiting the extent of axillary surgery when oncologically safe (the Z0011 paradigm), performing reverse axillary mapping (identifying and preserving the arm-draining lymphatic channels during ALND — which are distinct from the breast-draining sentinel lymphatic channels), early postoperative arm mobilization and physiotherapy, patient education about risk reduction (avoiding blood draws, blood pressure measurements, and venipuncture in the ipsilateral arm), and prospective surveillance with volumetric arm measurements (bioimpedance spectroscopy) to detect subclinical lymphedema before it becomes clinically apparent. Treatment of established lymphedema includes complete decongestive therapy (manual lymphatic drainage, multilayer compression bandaging, exercise, and skin care), compression garments for maintenance, and, for refractory cases, microsurgical lymphovenous anastomosis or vascularized lymph node transfer — techniques that create new lymphatic drainage pathways and can produce sustained volume reduction.

Axillary Management After Neoadjuvant Chemotherapy

Neoadjuvant chemotherapy (NACT) is increasingly used for locally advanced breast cancer (stage IIB-III) and for aggressive subtypes (triple-negative, HER2-positive) to downstage the primary tumor and the axilla before surgery. In patients who are clinically node-positive at diagnosis and convert to clinically node-negative after NACT, sentinel lymph node biopsy can be performed after chemotherapy to assess axillary response. However, the false-negative rate of SLNB after NACT is higher than in the upfront surgery setting (approximately 10 to 15% versus 5 to 10%) — strategies to reduce this false-negative rate include removing three or more sentinel nodes (reduces false-negative rate to less than 10%), using dual-tracer technique, and clipping the biopsied positive node at the time of diagnosis for targeted axillary dissection (TAD — the clipped node is localized and removed at surgery along with the sentinel nodes, ensuring that the index positive node is included in the specimen). Patients who achieve a pathologic complete response (pCR) in the axilla (no residual cancer in the sentinel nodes after NACT) have excellent prognosis, and axillary dissection is omitted. Patients with residual axillary disease after NACT typically require completion ALND and regional radiation.

Breast Reconstruction (Immediate and Delayed Options)

Implant-Based and Autologous Reconstruction

Breast reconstruction is offered to all patients undergoing mastectomy and may be performed immediately (at the time of mastectomy) or in a delayed fashion (months to years after mastectomy). Immediate reconstruction is preferred when oncologically safe because it preserves the breast skin envelope (in skin-sparing or nipple-sparing mastectomy), reduces the number of operations, and produces superior aesthetic outcomes. Implant-based reconstruction uses a tissue expander placed beneath the pectoralis major muscle (or in a prepectoral position with acellular dermal matrix coverage), which is gradually expanded with saline injections over 6 to 12 weeks and then exchanged for a permanent silicone or saline implant. Direct-to-implant reconstruction (placing the permanent implant at the time of mastectomy without a tissue expander stage) is appropriate when the mastectomy skin flaps have adequate perfusion and sufficient tissue coverage. Autologous (flap-based) reconstruction transfers the patient's own tissue to create a breast mound — options include the deep inferior epigastric perforator (DIEP) flap (abdominal tissue transferred as a free flap with microvascular anastomosis), the transverse rectus abdominis myocutaneous (TRAM) flap (pedicled or free), and the latissimus dorsi myocutaneous flap (often combined with an implant for volume). Autologous reconstruction provides a more natural-appearing breast that ages with the patient and does not require implant replacement, but involves longer operative time, donor site morbidity, and microsurgical expertise.

Complications of Breast Reconstruction

Implant-based reconstruction complications include capsular contracture (the most common long-term complication — fibrotic scar tissue forms around the implant, producing firmness, distortion, and pain; graded by the Baker classification from I to IV), implant infection (requiring implant removal in 1 to 5% of cases), implant rupture (silicone gel migration or saline deflation), implant malposition, and breast implant-associated anaplastic large cell lymphoma (BIA-ALCL — a rare T-cell lymphoma associated with textured implants, with an estimated incidence of 1 in 3,000 to 30,000 patients with textured implants; presenting as a late seroma or mass around the implant; cured by implant and capsule removal in most cases). Autologous flap reconstruction complications include flap loss (partial or complete — 1 to 5% for free flaps, often due to microvascular thrombosis requiring emergent re-exploration), donor site complications (abdominal wall weakness or hernia after TRAM flap, seroma, wound dehiscence), and fat necrosis within the flap (producing a palpable mass that may mimic recurrence on imaging and require biopsy for confirmation).

Management of Breast Abscess and Benign Breast Disease

Breast Abscess — Lactational and Non-Lactational

Breast abscess is most commonly a complication of lactational mastitis (caused by Staphylococcus aureus entering through cracked nipple skin during breastfeeding) but also occurs in non-lactating women (periareolar abscess associated with smoking, squamous metaplasia of lactiferous ducts, and duct ectasia). Lactational breast abscess is managed by ultrasound-guided aspiration (for abscesses less than 5 cm — repeated aspiration may be necessary) or by incision and drainage (for abscesses greater than 5 cm, multiloculated abscesses, or failed aspiration). The incision is placed over the point of maximal fluctuance, avoiding the areolar complex when possible to protect the lactiferous ducts. Breastfeeding should continue from both breasts during treatment — continued drainage of the affected breast reduces milk stasis and promotes resolution. Non-lactational periareolar abscess is a chronic, recurrent condition associated with squamous metaplasia of the lactiferous duct lining (Zuska disease). Treatment of the acute episode is drainage, but definitive management requires excision of the involved duct and its associated fistula tract (central duct excision or Hadfield procedure) — without duct excision, recurrence rates approach 50%.

Excisional Biopsy and Management of Benign Lesions

Excisional biopsy (open surgical biopsy) has largely been replaced by image-guided core needle biopsy for the diagnosis of breast lesions. However, excisional biopsy remains indicated when core needle biopsy results are discordant with imaging findings (the pathology does not explain the imaging abnormality), for lesions that cannot be adequately sampled by core needle biopsy (papillary lesions, radial scars, atypical ductal hyperplasia where upgrade to DCIS on excision occurs in 15 to 30%), and for definitive excision of palpable benign lesions (fibroadenomas greater than 3 cm, phyllodes tumors, or symptomatic cysts that have not resolved with aspiration). Wire-guided localization or radioactive seed localization is used to guide excision of non-palpable mammographic abnormalities — a localizing wire or seed is placed into the lesion under mammographic or ultrasound guidance preoperatively, and the surgeon excises the tissue surrounding the wire or seed with a margin of normal tissue. Specimen radiography confirms that the target lesion (the mammographic abnormality or the localizing seed) is contained within the excised specimen.

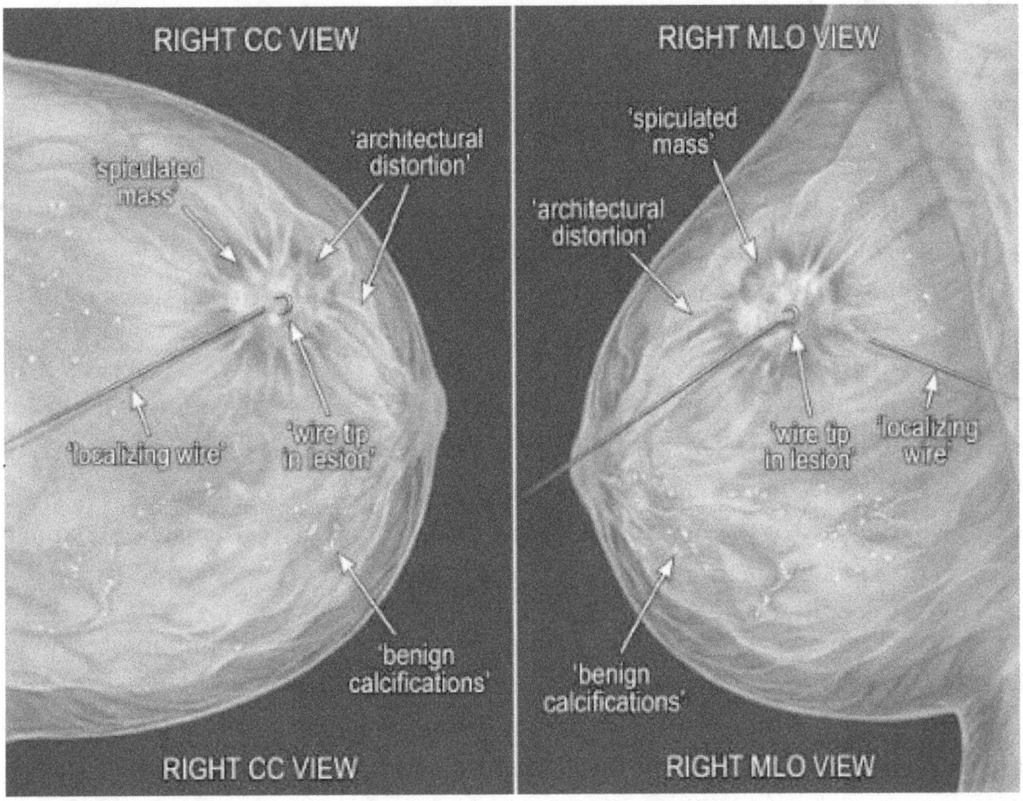

KEY POINT: The ACOSOG Z0011 trial demonstrated that patients with one or two positive sentinel lymph nodes undergoing breast-conserving surgery with whole-breast radiation do NOT benefit from completion axillary lymph node dissection — equivalent survival and axillary recurrence rates were observed with sentinel lymph node biopsy alone, fundamentally changing axillary management and sparing thousands of patients the morbidity of ALND.

Clinical Case — Stage IIA Breast Cancer With Positive Sentinel Node Managed by Breast Conservation

A 52-year-old woman presents with a 2.2 cm palpable mass in the upper outer quadrant of the left breast. Core needle biopsy reveals invasive ductal carcinoma, ER-positive, PR-positive, HER2-negative (Luminal A subtype). Staging CT and bone scan show no distant metastases. The tumor-to-breast ratio is favorable for breast conservation. At operation, a wire-guided lumpectomy is performed with oncoplastic tissue rearrangement — the specimen is oriented with sutures, and specimen radiography confirms the clip marking the biopsy site is within the specimen. Sentinel lymph node biopsy with dual-tracer technique identifies three sentinel nodes — two are negative, and one contains a 4 mm macrometastasis. Per ACOSOG Z0011 criteria (BCS with whole-breast radiation, one to two positive sentinel nodes, no extranodal extension), completion ALND is not performed. Final pathology confirms a 2.1 cm invasive ductal carcinoma with negative margins (no tumor on ink) and one of three sentinel nodes positive. Adjuvant therapy includes whole-breast radiation with tumor bed boost, endocrine therapy (aromatase inhibitor for 5 years), and a 21-gene recurrence score (Oncotype DX) to determine whether adjuvant chemotherapy is indicated.

THE OPERATIVE DANGER ZONE ATLAS — Breast Surgery Dangers

Positive Margin After Lumpectomy Due to Inadequate Specimen Orientation: Without proper specimen orientation (sutures marking six surfaces), a positive margin forces a wider non-directed re-excision rather than a targeted shaving, increasing tissue loss and potentially converting breast conservation to mastectomy. **Safe maneuver:** orient every specimen with at least two sutures, obtain intraoperative margin assessment, and perform directed cavity shavings for close or positive margins at the same sitting.

Long Thoracic Nerve Injury During Axillary Dissection: The long thoracic nerve runs on the medial axillary wall surface of the serratus anterior and is at risk when lymphatic tissue is swept off the chest wall — injury produces a permanent winged scapula with loss of overhead arm elevation. **Safe maneuver:** identify the nerve at the start of the medial dissection, maintain all dissection superficial to it, and avoid energy devices on the serratus anterior surface near the nerve.

Mastectomy Skin Flap Necrosis from Inadequate Perfusion: Thin mastectomy flaps risk devascularization of the subdermal plexus, producing skin flap necrosis in 5 to 30% of cases — rates are higher in skin-sparing and nipple-sparing mastectomy and in patients who smoke, are obese, or have diabetes. **Safe maneuver:** use intraoperative ICG fluorescence angiography to assess flap perfusion before closure, and excise any non-viable skin edges at the time of mastectomy rather than closing over ischemic tissue.

Axillary Vein Injury During Level II Dissection: The axillary vein forms the superior boundary of the axillary dissection — overzealous dissection above the vein or failure to identify venous tributaries crossing the surgical field risks major venous hemorrhage. **Safe maneuver:** identify the axillary vein at the beginning of the dissection, maintain all dissection below its inferior surface, and individually control all venous tributaries before division.

Summary and Key Concepts

Breast-conserving surgery with whole-breast radiation produces equivalent long-term survival to mastectomy for stage I and II breast cancer — the current margin standard is no tumor on ink, and oncoplastic techniques extend breast conservation to tumors previously considered too large for lumpectomy.

Sentinel lymph node biopsy with dual-tracer technique (radiotracer plus blue dye) has replaced routine axillary dissection for staging — achieving a sentinel node identification rate exceeding 95% with lymphedema rates of 5 to 7% compared to 20 to 30% for ALND.

The ACOSOG Z0011 trial established that completion ALND is not required for patients with one or two positive sentinel nodes undergoing BCS with whole-breast radiation — this paradigm-shifting finding has reduced ALND and its associated morbidity.

The long thoracic nerve (on the serratus anterior surface) and thoracodorsal nerve (on the posterior axillary wall) must be identified and preserved during axillary dissection — long thoracic nerve injury produces a winged scapula.

Skin-sparing and nipple-sparing mastectomy provide equivalent oncologic safety to conventional mastectomy while enabling superior immediate reconstruction — nipple-sparing mastectomy requires frozen section confirmation of a negative retroareolar margin.

Autologous reconstruction (DIEP flap, TRAM flap, latissimus dorsi flap) provides a more natural result that ages with the patient, while implant-based reconstruction is faster with less donor site morbidity.

Non-lactational periareolar abscess (Zuska disease) requires central duct excision for definitive management — drainage alone carries a recurrence rate approaching 50%.

CHAPTER 15: OPERATIONS OF THE THYROID AND PARATHYROID

Learning Objectives

1. Describe the surgical anatomy of the thyroid and parathyroid glands, including the relationship of the recurrent laryngeal nerve (RLN) to the ligament of Berry, the blood supply, and the anatomical variations that place structures at risk during thyroid and parathyroid surgery.
2. Perform a total thyroidectomy with systematic identification and preservation of the recurrent laryngeal nerves and the parathyroid glands.
3. Perform a focused (minimally invasive) parathyroidectomy for a localized parathyroid adenoma, and a four-gland exploration when preoperative localization is discordant or negative.
4. Manage the complications of thyroid and parathyroid surgery, including recurrent laryngeal nerve injury, hypoparathyroidism, and postoperative hematoma.

Surgical Anatomy of the Thyroid, Parathyroid, and Recurrent Laryngeal Nerve

Thyroid Gland — Gross Anatomy and Blood Supply

The thyroid gland consists of two lateral lobes connected by an isthmus overlying the second and third tracheal rings. A pyramidal lobe (a midline cephalad extension from the isthmus, representing the embryological remnant of the thyroglossal duct) is present in approximately 30 to 50% of patients. The thyroid is enclosed within a true capsule (the surgical capsule) and is surrounded by a loose perithyroidal fascia (the surgical dissection plane). The arterial supply is dual: the superior thyroid artery (the first branch of the external carotid artery) supplies the upper pole and is ligated close to the thyroid capsule during thyroidectomy to avoid injury to the external branch of the superior laryngeal nerve (EBSLN), and the inferior thyroid artery (a branch of the thyrocervical trunk from the subclavian artery) supplies the lower pole and crosses the recurrent laryngeal nerve in a variable relationship. The thyroid ima artery (an unpaired artery arising directly from the aortic arch or brachiocephalic trunk and ascending to the thyroid isthmus) is present in 1 to 4% of the population and may cause unexpected bleeding during isthmus division or low tracheostomy. The venous drainage consists of the superior thyroid veins (draining to the internal jugular vein), the middle thyroid veins (draining directly to the internal jugular vein — these are short, fragile veins that may be avulsed during lateral retraction of the thyroid lobe if not ligated early), and the inferior thyroid veins (draining from the lower poles to the brachiocephalic veins).

The Recurrent Laryngeal Nerve — Course and Variations

The recurrent laryngeal nerve (RLN) is the most important structure at risk during thyroid surgery. It courses in the tracheoesophageal groove between the trachea and the esophagus and enters the larynx at the cricothyroid joint, posterior to the inferior cornu of the thyroid cartilage, to innervate all intrinsic muscles of the larynx except the cricothyroid (which is innervated by the EBSLN). The RLN has a variable relationship to the inferior thyroid artery — it may pass anterior to, posterior to, or between the branches of the inferior thyroid artery, and this variability means that the artery CANNOT be used as a reliable landmark for finding the nerve. The ligament of Berry (the posterior suspensory ligament) is the dense connective tissue attachment between the thyroid gland and the trachea — the RLN passes through or immediately adjacent to the ligament of Berry as it enters the larynx, and this is the point of greatest danger to the nerve during thyroidectomy. A non-recurrent laryngeal nerve (the nerve courses directly from the vagus to the larynx without descending into the chest and looping around the subclavian artery or aortic arch) is a rare but critical anatomical variant, present in approximately 0.5 to 1% of patients on the right side and associated with an aberrant retroesophageal right subclavian artery (arteria lusoria). A non-recurrent nerve is at extreme risk because it enters the operative field from a lateral direction where it is not expected.

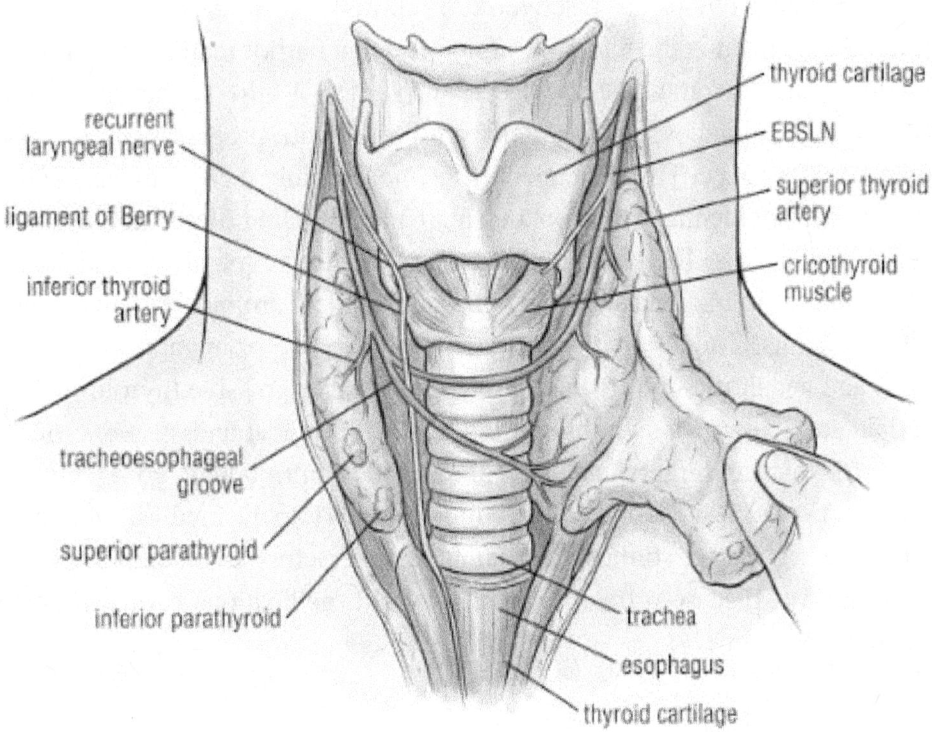

Parathyroid Gland Anatomy and Embryology

There are typically four parathyroid glands — two superior and two inferior — although supernumerary glands (five or more glands) are present in approximately 5 to 15% of the population. The superior parathyroid glands derive from the fourth pharyngeal pouch and have a relatively constant position on the posterior surface of the upper thyroid lobe at the level of the cricoid cartilage, posterior to the RLN. The inferior parathyroid glands derive from the third pharyngeal pouch (migrating with the thymus during embryological descent) and have a more variable position — they may be located at the lower pole of the thyroid, within the thymic tongue, in the anterior mediastinum (having descended with the thymus into the chest), or rarely within the thyroid parenchyma (intrathyroidal parathyroid). The vascular supply of all parathyroid glands derives primarily from the inferior thyroid artery — because the inferior thyroid artery provides the dominant blood supply to both the superior and inferior parathyroid glands, the artery should be ligated close to the thyroid capsule (distal ligation) rather than at its trunk (proximal ligation) to preserve the parathyroid blood supply. Inadvertent devascularization of the parathyroid glands during thyroidectomy is the most common cause of postoperative hypoparathyroidism.

Epidemiology and Clinical Indications for Thyroid Surgery

Thyroid nodules are exceedingly common — palpable nodules are found in 4 to 7% of adults on physical examination, and incidental nodules are discovered by ultrasound in 20 to 76% of the population. The clinical challenge is distinguishing the 5 to 15% of nodules that harbor malignancy from the vast majority that are benign. Fine-needle aspiration (FNA) biopsy, guided by the Bethesda System for Reporting Thyroid Cytopathology (six diagnostic categories from I to VI with progressively increasing malignancy risk), is the primary tool for triage. Thyroid cancer is the most rapidly increasing cancer diagnosis in many countries, largely due to incidental detection of small papillary microcarcinomas on imaging studies performed for other indications. Differentiated thyroid carcinomas (papillary and follicular) constitute approximately 90% of thyroid malignancies and carry an excellent prognosis (10-year survival exceeding 90% for papillary carcinoma). Medullary thyroid carcinoma (arising from parafollicular C-cells, 5 to 10% of thyroid cancers) and anaplastic thyroid carcinoma (the most aggressive thyroid malignancy, less than 2% of cases, median survival 4 to 6 months) require distinct surgical and systemic treatment strategies. Benign indications for thyroid surgery include compressive multinodular goiter producing dysphagia, dyspnea, or stridor (particularly substernal goiter, which extends into the mediastinum through the thoracic inlet), toxic multinodular goiter or solitary toxic adenoma refractory to or inappropriate for radioactive iodine therapy, and Graves disease refractory to antithyroid medications or in patients who decline or cannot receive radioactive iodine.

Total and Subtotal Thyroidectomy

Indications and Operative Technique

Total thyroidectomy (removal of the entire thyroid gland) is indicated for differentiated thyroid cancer (papillary and follicular carcinoma) greater than 1 cm with adverse features, bilateral multinodular goiter with compressive symptoms, Graves disease refractory to medical therapy, and any indication where bilateral thyroid pathology necessitates complete removal. The patient is positioned supine with neck extension (a shoulder roll is placed to extend the neck, but excessive extension should be avoided in elderly patients with cervical spondylosis). A low collar (Kocher) incision is made 1 to 2 cm above the sternal notch in a natural skin crease. Subplatysmal flaps are raised superiorly to the thyroid notch and inferiorly to the sternal notch. The strap muscles (sternohyoid and sternothyroid) are divided in the midline raphe and retracted laterally. The middle thyroid veins are ligated and divided early to allow lateral mobilization of the thyroid lobe. The superior pole is dissected by individually ligating the branches of the superior thyroid artery close to the thyroid capsule — care is taken to identify and preserve the EBSLN, which runs with or near the superior thyroid artery and can be injured during superior pole ligation (injury produces loss of the high-pitched voice and vocal fatigue, particularly noticeable in professional voice users). The inferior thyroid artery is identified, and its branches are ligated individually on the thyroid capsule (distal ligation) to preserve parathyroid blood supply. The RLN is identified in the tracheoesophageal groove (inferior approach — the nerve is found caudal to the inferior thyroid artery where it enters the groove), and the dissection proceeds along the nerve superiorly, under direct vision, through the ligament of Berry to its entry into the larynx.

Intraoperative Nerve Monitoring

Intraoperative nerve monitoring (IONM) uses an endotracheal tube with surface electrodes in contact with the vocal cords and a nerve stimulator to provide real-time electromyographic feedback during thyroidectomy. IONM does not replace visual identification of the RLN (which remains the gold standard for nerve preservation) but serves as an adjunct that confirms the anatomical identification of the nerve (stimulation of the identified structure produces a characteristic electromyographic waveform), predicts postoperative nerve function (loss of signal after dissection predicts vocal cord palsy), and guides the decision to proceed with contralateral thyroidectomy in bilateral procedures — if the RLN on the first side has lost its signal (suggesting injury), the surgeon may choose to defer the contralateral thyroidectomy to a second stage rather than risking bilateral vocal cord paralysis (which produces airway obstruction requiring tracheostomy). The rate of RLN injury during thyroidectomy by experienced thyroid surgeons is 1 to 2% for temporary palsy (neuropraxia that recovers within 6 to 12 months) and 0.5 to 1% for permanent palsy.

THE OPERATIVE DANGER ZONE ATLAS — Recurrent Laryngeal Nerve Injury at the Ligament of Berry

The Zone: The ligament of Berry (posterior suspensory ligament of the thyroid) — the dense connective tissue attachment between the posteromedial surface of the thyroid gland and the second and third tracheal rings. The RLN passes through or immediately adjacent to this ligament as it enters the larynx.

The Structure at Risk: The recurrent laryngeal nerve at its point of entry into the larynx. The ligament of Berry is the tightest attachment of the thyroid to the trachea and is the last tissue divided when mobilizing the thyroid lobe. The nerve is at maximal risk at this point because the ligament may contain or be closely adherent to the nerve, and the dissection requires sharp division close to the tracheal wall.

The Consequence: Unilateral RLN injury produces ipsilateral vocal cord paralysis — hoarseness, breathy voice, aspiration of thin liquids, and weak cough. Bilateral RLN injury produces bilateral vocal cord paralysis with the cords fixed in the paramedian position — airway obstruction requiring emergent reintubation and tracheostomy. Bilateral injury is a catastrophic complication that produces a permanent tracheostomy in approximately 30% of cases.

The Safe Maneuver: Identify the RLN in the tracheoesophageal groove before reaching the ligament of Berry and trace it superiorly, under direct vision, to its laryngeal entry point. Divide the ligament of Berry sharply (with a scalpel, not energy device) in small increments while directly visualizing the nerve. Never use monopolar electrocautery or an energy device within 2 mm of the identified nerve — thermal spread from energy devices can cause delayed neuropraxia or permanent thermal injury. If using IONM, confirm the nerve signal is intact after ligament division.

Postoperative Monitoring and Management of Complications

After total thyroidectomy, the two most critical postoperative complications requiring vigilant monitoring are hematoma and hypocalcemia. Post-thyroidectomy hematoma occurs in 1 to 2% of cases, typically within the first 6 hours, and presents with rapidly progressive neck swelling, dyspnea, stridor, and hemodynamic changes. Because the expanding hematoma occupies the confined anterior cervical space beneath the strap muscles and cervical fascia, even small volumes of blood can produce airway compromise by compressing the trachea and causing laryngeal edema from venous and lymphatic congestion. The emergency treatment is bedside wound opening — the skin sutures or staples are removed, the strap muscles are separated, and the hematoma is evacuated manually at the bedside before attempting reintubation or transport to the operating room. This maneuver can be lifesaving and must not be delayed for formal airway management. Hypocalcemia from hypoparathyroidism is monitored by serial serum calcium levels at 6-hour intervals for the first 24 hours. Symptoms of hypocalcemia (perioral numbness, paresthesias of the fingertips, muscle cramps, Chvostek sign — facial muscle twitching on tapping the facial nerve, Trousseau sign — carpopedal spasm with blood pressure cuff inflation) should prompt immediate measurement of ionized calcium and initiation of intravenous calcium gluconate for symptomatic hypocalcemia. Prophylactic oral calcium and vitamin D supplementation is initiated in all patients after total thyroidectomy, with the dose titrated based on postoperative calcium levels and PTH trends.

Thyroid Lobectomy and Isthmusectomy

Indications and Technical Considerations

Thyroid lobectomy (hemithyroidectomy) with isthmusectomy removes one thyroid lobe and the isthmus and is indicated for solitary thyroid nodules requiring excisional biopsy (follicular neoplasm or Bethesda IV cytology on fine-needle aspiration, where the distinction between follicular adenoma and carcinoma requires histological examination of the nodule capsule), well-differentiated thyroid cancer less than 1 cm without adverse features (microcarcinoma), unilateral toxic adenoma, and unilateral compressive goiter. The operative technique is identical to one side of a total thyroidectomy — the RLN and parathyroid glands on the operative side must be identified and preserved with the same rigor as during total thyroidectomy. The advantage of lobectomy over total thyroidectomy is preservation of the contralateral lobe with its parathyroid glands and RLN, eliminating the risk of bilateral RLN injury and reducing the risk of permanent hypoparathyroidism (which requires lifelong calcium and vitamin D supplementation) from approximately 2 to 5% after total thyroidectomy to essentially zero after lobectomy. Approximately 50 to 70% of patients who undergo lobectomy maintain sufficient thyroid function from the remaining lobe to avoid the need for lifelong thyroid hormone replacement therapy.

Parathyroidectomy (Focused and Four-Gland Exploration)

Primary Hyperparathyroidism — Localization and Operative Strategy

Primary hyperparathyroidism is caused by a single parathyroid adenoma in approximately 85% of cases, multigland hyperplasia in 10 to 15%, double adenoma in 2 to 5%, and parathyroid carcinoma in less than 1%. Preoperative localization using two concordant imaging modalities — sestamibi scintigraphy (technetium-99m sestamibi scan, with or without SPECT/CT) and high-resolution ultrasound — identifies a single adenoma and guides focused (minimally invasive) parathyroidectomy. When both modalities localize the same abnormal gland, a focused approach is used: a small (2 to 3 cm) incision directly over the localized gland, identification and excision of the adenoma, and confirmation of cure by measuring intraoperative parathyroid hormone (ioPTH) levels — a drop of 50% or more from the pre-excision baseline within 10 minutes of excision (the Miami criterion) confirms successful removal of the hyperfunctioning tissue and allows the operation to be concluded without exploring the remaining glands. When preoperative localization is discordant (the two modalities point to different glands) or negative (neither modality localizes an adenoma), a bilateral neck exploration (four-gland exploration) is performed — all four parathyroid glands are identified, each is assessed by size and color (adenomas are enlarged, typically greater than 60 mg, and darker in color than normal glands), the adenoma is excised, and the remaining glands are confirmed as normal. For multigland hyperplasia, subtotal parathyroidectomy (3.5-gland resection, leaving a vascularized remnant of approximately 50 mg from one gland) or total parathyroidectomy with autotransplantation (all four glands removed, with a portion of one gland implanted into the sternocleidomastoid muscle or forearm) is performed.

Ectopic Parathyroid Glands — Locations and Approach

When preoperative imaging localizes an adenoma to an ectopic location, or when four-gland exploration fails to identify all four glands in their expected positions, the surgeon must be familiar with the common ectopic locations. The most frequent ectopic site for the inferior parathyroid gland (derived from the third pharyngeal pouch, which descends with the thymus) is within the thymic tongue or the anterior mediastinum — accessed by transcervical thymectomy (pulling the thymus up through the cervical incision) or, for deep mediastinal glands, by thoracoscopic or median sternotomy approach. The most frequent ectopic site for the superior parathyroid gland is the tracheoesophageal groove (where it may descend posteriorly into the posterior mediastinum), the retroesophageal space, or within the posterior thyroid capsule (intrathyroidal parathyroid — found in approximately 1 to 3% of patients and identified only by thyroid lobectomy with serial sectioning of the specimen). An undescended parathyroid gland may be found near the carotid bifurcation or high in the neck along the course of the embryological pharyngeal pouch migration pathway.

THE OPERATIVE DANGER ZONE ATLAS — Parathyroid Devascularization During Thyroidectomy

---

The Zone: The posterior surface of the thyroid lobe during total thyroidectomy — where the parathyroid glands are located on or near the thyroid capsule and receive their blood supply from the terminal branches of the inferior thyroid artery.

The Structure at Risk: The parathyroid glands and their blood supply. The inferior thyroid artery provides the dominant arterial supply to both the superior and inferior parathyroid glands on each side. If the inferior thyroid artery is ligated at its trunk (proximal ligation) rather than at its individual branches on the thyroid capsule (distal ligation), the blood supply to both parathyroid glands on that side is interrupted.

The Consequence: Devascularization of the parathyroid glands produces postoperative hypoparathyroidism — hypocalcemia presenting as perioral numbness, tingling, carpopedal spasm, Chvostek sign, Trousseau sign, and, if severe, laryngospasm, seizures, and cardiac arrhythmias. Permanent hypoparathyroidism (lasting more than 6 months) occurs in 2 to 5% of total thyroidectomies and requires lifelong calcium and vitamin D supplementation. Temporary hypoparathyroidism (recovering within 6 months) occurs in 10 to 30%.

The Safe Maneuver: Ligate the branches of the inferior thyroid artery individually on the thyroid capsule (distal ligation), not at the arterial trunk. Identify each parathyroid gland during the dissection and preserve its vascular pedicle. If a parathyroid gland is inadvertently devascularized (it turns dark and fails to pink up after 15 minutes), perform immediate autotransplantation — mince the gland into 1 mm fragments and implant them into a pocket in the sternocleidomastoid muscle, marking the site with a non-absorbable suture or clip.

Secondary and Tertiary Hyperparathyroidism

Secondary hyperparathyroidism develops in patients with chronic kidney disease as a compensatory response to chronic hypocalcemia and hyperphosphatemia — all four parathyroid glands undergo diffuse hyperplasia. Surgical intervention (subtotal parathyroidectomy or total parathyroidectomy with autotransplantation) is indicated when severe secondary hyperparathyroidism becomes refractory to medical management (calcimimetics, phosphate binders, vitamin D analogs) and produces symptomatic bone disease (renal osteodystrophy), pathological fractures, intractable pruritus, soft tissue calcification (calciphylaxis — a life-threatening condition of widespread arterial and soft tissue calcification producing painful ischemic skin necrosis), or persistent hypercalcemia after renal transplantation (tertiary hyperparathyroidism — where chronically hyperplastic parathyroid tissue continues to produce excess PTH autonomously despite correction of renal failure by transplantation). Subtotal parathyroidectomy (3.5-gland resection) is preferred when the patient may undergo future renal transplantation (the remaining parathyroid remnant can reduce its function post-transplant), while total parathyroidectomy with forearm autotransplantation is preferred in patients unlikely to receive a transplant (the forearm graft site allows easy access for future reduction if the graft becomes hyperplastic). Intraoperative PTH monitoring is essential to confirm adequate resection.

Minimally Invasive and Endoscopic Thyroid and Parathyroid Surgery

Minimally Invasive Video-Assisted Thyroidectomy and Remote-Access Approaches

Minimally invasive video-assisted thyroidectomy (MIVAT) uses a 1.5 to 2 cm central neck incision with endoscopic assistance to perform thyroid lobectomy or total thyroidectomy — it provides excellent cosmesis with a nearly invisible scar while maintaining direct visualization of the RLN and parathyroid glands. Patient selection for MIVAT requires a thyroid nodule less than 3 cm, thyroid lobe volume less than 30 mL, and the absence of thyroiditis (which produces adhesions that make the dissection difficult through a small incision). Remote-access thyroidectomy (the transoral or transaxillary approach, including robotic-assisted transaxillary thyroidectomy) eliminates the cervical incision entirely by approaching the thyroid through a distant access site — the transaxillary approach uses an incision in the axilla, and the transoral approach uses incisions inside the lower lip (transoral endoscopic thyroidectomy vestibular approach — TOETVA). These remote-access approaches are most popular in East Asia where keloid-prone skin and cultural preference against neck scars drive demand. The oncologic and functional outcomes appear equivalent to conventional open thyroidectomy in experienced centers, although operative times are longer and the learning curve is substantial.

Central Neck Dissection for Thyroid Cancer

Central neck dissection (level VI lymph node dissection) removes the lymph nodes in the central compartment of the neck — bounded by the hyoid bone superiorly, the innominate artery inferiorly, and the carotid sheaths laterally. The central compartment contains the paratracheal, pretracheal, and prelaryngeal (Delphian) lymph nodes and is the most common site of lymph node metastasis from differentiated thyroid cancer (involvement in 20 to 60% of papillary thyroid carcinoma, often micrometastatic and not detectable on preoperative imaging). Prophylactic (elective) central neck dissection at the time of total thyroidectomy for papillary thyroid cancer remains controversial — proponents argue it provides accurate staging, may reduce recurrence and the need for reoperative surgery in an irradiated field, and has minimal additional morbidity when performed at the time of the initial thyroidectomy. Opponents cite the low reoperation rate for central neck recurrence, the increased rate of temporary and permanent hypoparathyroidism when central neck dissection is added to thyroidectomy (because the parathyroid glands lie within the central compartment and must be meticulously identified and preserved or autotransplanted during the dissection), and the absence of randomized trial evidence demonstrating a survival benefit. Therapeutic central neck dissection (for clinically apparent or imaging-detected central neck lymph node metastases) is performed routinely when involved nodes are identified preoperatively on ultrasound or are discovered intraoperatively. Lateral neck dissection (levels II through V) is performed for clinically apparent lateral cervical lymph node metastases from thyroid cancer, identified preoperatively by ultrasound and confirmed by FNA with thyroglobulin washout.

Completion Thyroidectomy and Reoperation in the Central Neck

Indications and Technical Challenges

Completion thyroidectomy (removal of the remaining thyroid lobe after a prior lobectomy) is indicated when final pathology from a thyroid lobectomy reveals a cancer that requires total thyroidectomy (differentiated thyroid cancer greater than 1 cm, aggressive histological variants, lymph node metastases, or vascular invasion identified on final pathology). Reoperation in the central neck (for persistent or recurrent thyroid cancer, or for remedial parathyroidectomy after a failed initial exploration) is technically challenging because the normal tissue planes are obliterated by scar tissue from the prior surgery, and the RLN and remaining parathyroid glands are at significantly higher risk of injury than during a virgin operation. The rate of RLN injury during reoperative thyroid surgery is 3 to 12% (compared to 1 to 2% for primary thyroidectomy), and the rate of permanent hypoparathyroidism is 5 to 15% (compared to 2 to 5% for primary total thyroidectomy). Key technical principles for central neck reoperation include approaching the thyroid bed through a lateral approach (entering the surgical field lateral to the scar tissue and identifying the RLN in virgin tissue below the scar before dissecting into the central compartment), using intraoperative nerve monitoring (which is particularly valuable in reoperative cases where the nerve course may be distorted by scar tissue), and performing the operation in a high-volume center with experienced endocrine surgeons.

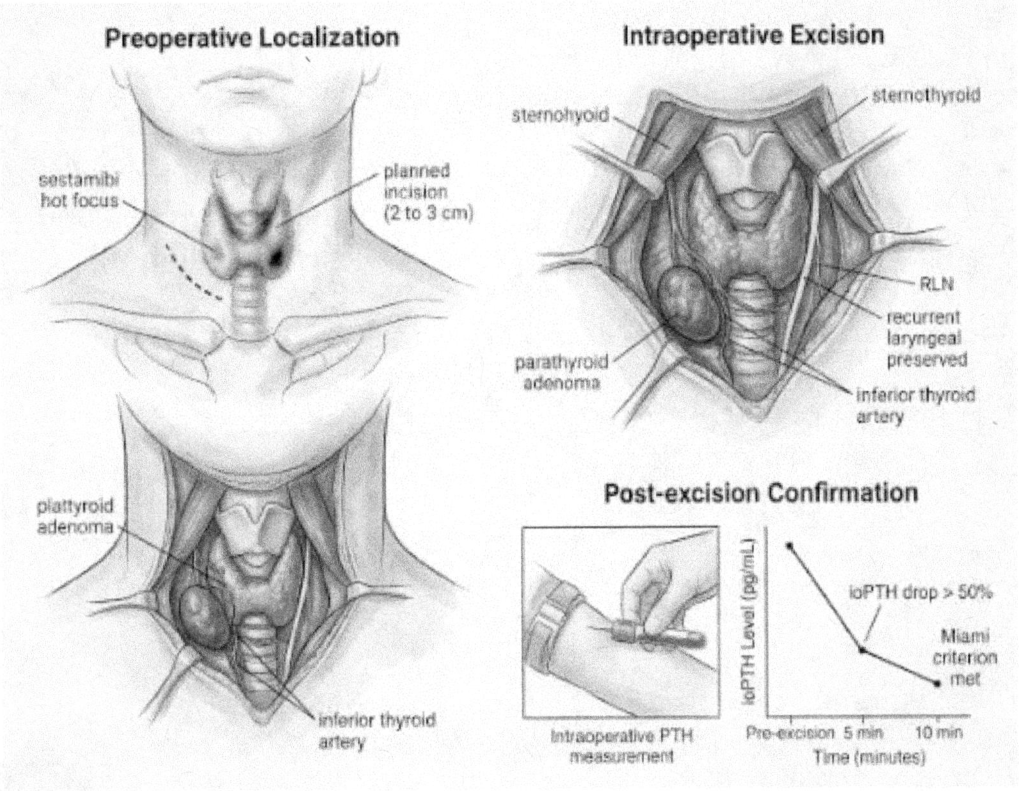

CLINICAL PEARL: If a parathyroid gland is inadvertently devascularized during thyroidectomy (it turns dark and fails to pink up after 15 minutes despite warm saline irrigation), perform immediate autotransplantation: mince the gland into 1 mm fragments and implant them into a sternocleidomastoid muscle pocket, marking the site with a non-absorbable suture. Autotransplanted parathyroid tissue functions in approximately 85 to 90% of cases, typically within 4 to 6 weeks.

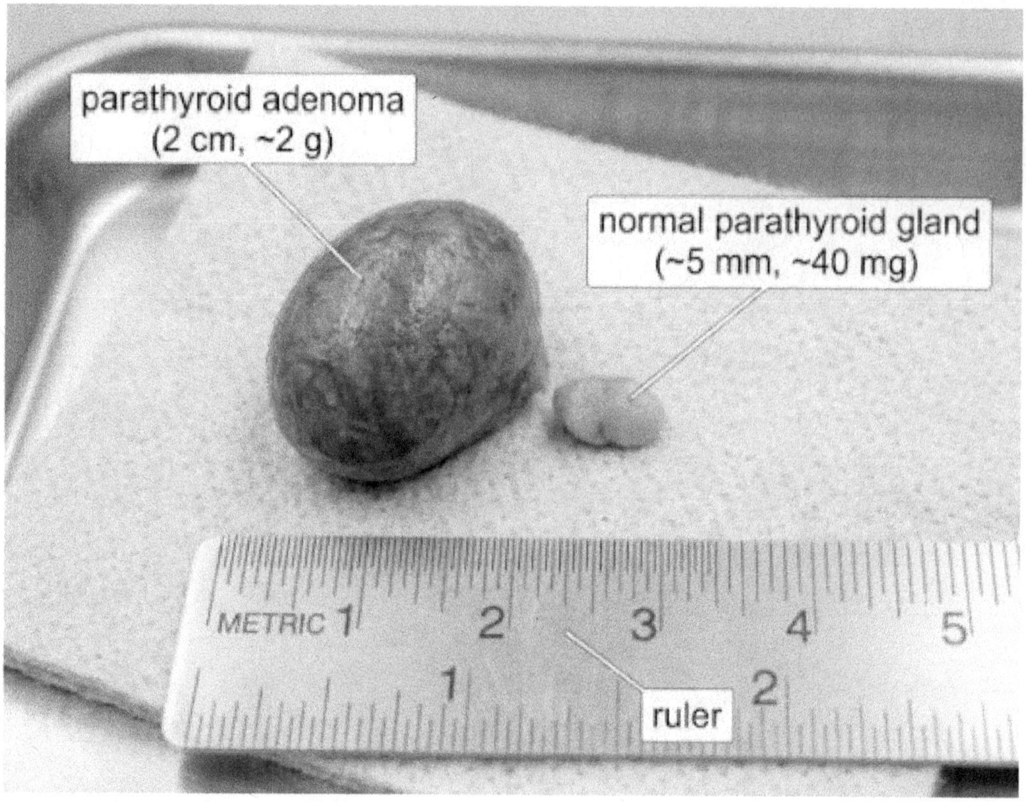

Clinical Case — Substernal Goiter Requiring Total Thyroidectomy With Cervical Approach

A 62-year-old woman presents with progressive dyspnea on exertion, orthopnea, and a sensation of pressure in the anterior neck over the past year. CT reveals a large multinodular goiter with substernal extension — the right thyroid lobe extends into the anterior mediastinum to the level of the aortic arch, displacing the trachea to the left and compressing it to a diameter of 8 mm (normal greater than 15 mm). Pulmonary function testing shows an extrathoracic airway obstruction pattern. The patient undergoes total thyroidectomy through a cervical collar incision. The substernal component is delivered through the cervical incision by blunt digital dissection of the retrosternal space and gentle traction — approximately 95% of substernal goiters can be removed through a cervical approach because the substernal component receives its blood supply from the cervical thyroid vessels and is not adherent to mediastinal structures. The right RLN is identified in the tracheoesophageal groove and traced superiorly through the ligament of Berry under direct vision with intraoperative nerve monitoring. Both superior parathyroid glands are identified and preserved with their vascular pedicles. The left inferior parathyroid gland is devascularized during dissection — it is autotransplanted into the left sternocleidomastoid muscle. The specimen weighs 380 grams. Postoperatively, the patient's dyspnea resolves immediately. Serum calcium is checked at 6 hours and is mildly low (8.1 mg/dL) with an intact PTH of 12 pg/mL — the patient is started on oral calcium and calcitriol supplementation. At 6 weeks, the PTH has recovered to 28 pg/mL (the autotransplanted gland is functioning), and calcium supplementation is weaned.

Recurrent Laryngeal Nerve Injury at the Ligament of Berry: The RLN passes through or immediately adjacent to the ligament of Berry as it enters the larynx — this is the point of maximal danger because the ligament is the tightest thyroid-tracheal attachment and requires sharp division close to the tracheal wall. **Safe maneuver:** identify the RLN in the tracheoesophageal groove and trace it superiorly under direct vision to its laryngeal entry; divide the ligament with a scalpel (not energy device) in small increments while directly visualizing the nerve.

Parathyroid Devascularization During Thyroidectomy: The inferior thyroid artery is the dominant blood supply to both superior and inferior parathyroid glands — proximal ligation at the trunk interrupts blood flow to all parathyroid glands on that side, producing hypoparathyroidism. **Safe maneuver:** ligate branches individually on the thyroid capsule (distal ligation); if a gland is devascularized, perform immediate autotransplantation into the sternocleidomastoid muscle.

External Branch of the Superior Laryngeal Nerve Injury During Superior Pole Ligation: The EBSLN courses with or near the superior thyroid artery and innervates the cricothyroid muscle — injury eliminates cricothyroid function, producing loss of vocal pitch range and projection, particularly debilitating for professional voice users. **Safe maneuver:** ligate the branches of the superior thyroid artery individually on the thyroid capsule (not the trunk), identifying the EBSLN before applying clips or ties.

Postoperative Hematoma with Airway Compromise: Post-thyroidectomy hematoma is a rare (1 to 2%) but life-threatening emergency — expanding hematoma in the confined anterior cervical space compresses the trachea and produces airway obstruction within minutes. **Safe maneuver:** the wound must be opened emergently at the bedside (remove sutures or staples, evacuate the hematoma) before attempting reintubation or transport to the operating room — delay for definitive airway management risks complete airway loss.

Summary and Key Concepts

The recurrent laryngeal nerve is at greatest risk at the ligament of Berry — its point of entry into the larynx through the dense posterior suspensory ligament. Visual identification of the nerve before and during ligament division, combined with intraoperative nerve monitoring, minimizes injury risk.

The inferior thyroid artery provides the dominant blood supply to both superior and inferior parathyroid glands — distal ligation (on the thyroid capsule) preserves parathyroid perfusion, while proximal ligation devascularizes all parathyroid glands on that side.

A non-recurrent laryngeal nerve (present in 0.5 to 1% of patients on the right, associated with aberrant retroesophageal subclavian artery) enters the operative field from a lateral direction — failure to recognize this variant places the nerve at extreme risk.

Focused parathyroidectomy requires concordant localization on two imaging modalities and intraoperative PTH monitoring — a 50% drop in PTH within 10 minutes of excision (the Miami criterion) confirms cure and allows completion of a minimally invasive procedure.

If a parathyroid gland is inadvertently devascularized, immediate autotransplantation into the sternocleidomastoid muscle preserves function in approximately 85 to 90% of cases.

Post-thyroidectomy hematoma is a life-threatening emergency requiring bedside wound opening to relieve airway compression — delay for transport or formal airway management risks fatal airway obstruction.

Completion thyroidectomy and central neck reoperation carry significantly higher rates of RLN injury (3 to 12%) and permanent hypoparathyroidism (5 to 15%) compared to primary thyroidectomy, and should be performed in experienced high-volume centers.

CHAPTER 16: OPERATIONS OF THE ADRENAL GLAND

Learning Objectives

1. Describe the surgical anatomy of the adrenal glands, including the arterial supply, venous drainage (the critical difference between right and left adrenal veins), and the relationship of each adrenal gland to surrounding retroperitoneal structures.
2. Perform a laparoscopic transabdominal adrenalectomy using the lateral decubitus approach, with safe identification and control of the adrenal vein.
3. Apply the principles of preoperative alpha-blockade and volume expansion for pheochromocytoma before operative resection.
4. Select the appropriate operative approach (laparoscopic transabdominal, posterior retroperitoneoscopic, or open) based on tumor size, histological suspicion, and functional status.

Surgical Anatomy of the Adrenal Glands and Retroperitoneum

Gross Anatomy and Anatomical Relationships

The adrenal glands are paired retroperitoneal organs situated on the superomedial aspect of each kidney, within the perirenal (Gerota) fascia. Each gland weighs approximately 4 to 6 grams and consists of a cortex (the outer layer, producing glucocorticoids, mineralocorticoids, and adrenal androgens) and a medulla (the inner layer, producing catecholamines — epinephrine and norepinephrine). The right adrenal gland is pyramidal in shape and lies between the right kidney inferiorly, the inferior vena cava (IVC) medially, the right diaphragmatic crus posteriorly, and the bare area of the liver anteriorly. The intimate relationship of the right adrenal gland to the IVC is the principal surgical concern on the right side — the right adrenal vein (a short, 2 to 5 mm vessel draining directly into the posterolateral surface of the IVC) is the most dangerous structure encountered during right adrenalectomy. The left adrenal gland is crescentic (semilunar) in shape and lies between the left kidney inferiorly, the aorta medially, the left diaphragmatic crus posteriorly, the tail of the pancreas and the splenic vessels anteriorly, and the spleen superolaterally. The left adrenal vein is longer (2 to 4 cm) and drains into the left renal vein, often joining the inferior phrenic vein before entering the renal vein — this longer length makes the left adrenal vein easier to control than the right.

Arterial Supply and Venous Drainage

Each adrenal gland receives a rich arterial supply from three sources: the superior adrenal arteries (multiple small branches from the inferior phrenic artery), the middle adrenal artery (a direct branch from the aorta), and the inferior adrenal artery (a branch from the renal artery). Despite the triple arterial supply, there is a single dominant vein on each side — the right adrenal vein draining directly into the IVC and the left adrenal vein draining into the left renal vein. The venous drainage is the key to the operation: early identification and ligation of the adrenal vein is the first priority of adrenalectomy because it prevents systemic release of catecholamines during manipulation of a pheochromocytoma (catecholamine surge from tumor manipulation with an intact venous drainage produces hypertensive crisis) and because inadvertent avulsion of the right adrenal vein from the IVC produces hemorrhage that is difficult to control. The multiple small arterial branches are ligated during circumferential dissection of the gland after the vein has been secured.

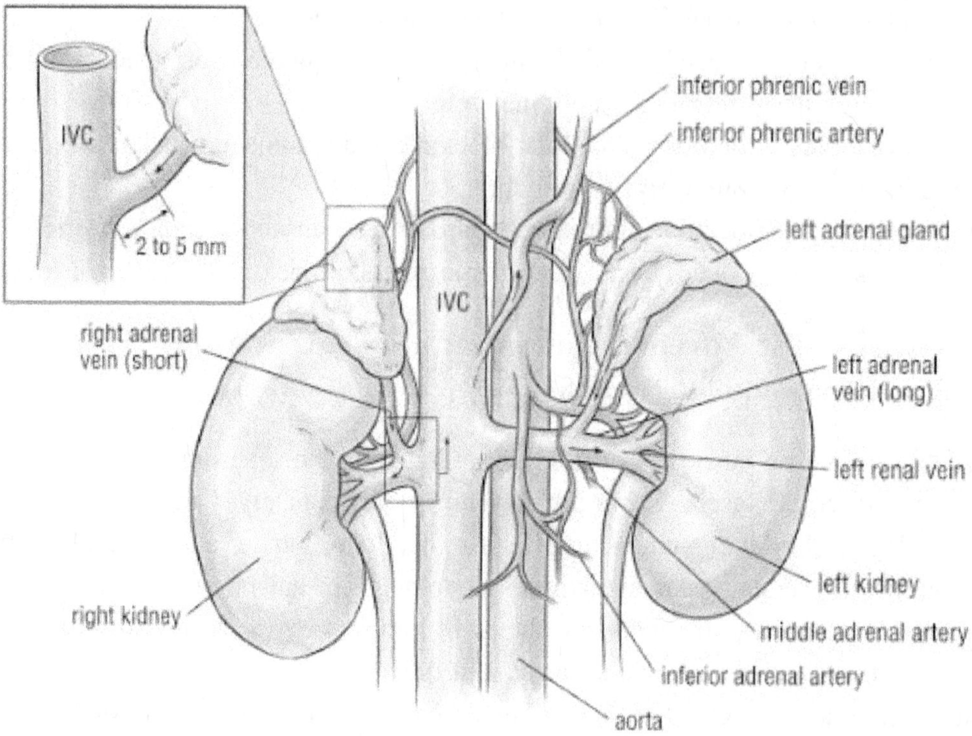

Epidemiology and Indications for Adrenalectomy

Adrenal incidentalomas (adrenal masses discovered incidentally on imaging studies performed for unrelated indications) are found in approximately 4 to 5% of abdominal CT scans. The two critical questions in evaluating any adrenal mass are whether it is functional (producing hormones) and whether it is malignant. All incidentalomas undergo biochemical evaluation for subclinical Cushing syndrome (overnight 1 mg dexamethasone suppression test), pheochromocytoma (plasma free metanephrines or 24-hour urine fractionated catecholamines and metanephrines), and primary hyperaldosteronism (aldosterone-to-renin ratio, if hypertensive or hypokalemic). Indications for adrenalectomy include functional tumors of any size (pheochromocytoma, aldosterone-producing adenoma, cortisol-producing adenoma, sex-steroid-producing tumor), non-functional tumors greater than 4 cm (due to increasing malignancy risk — the risk of adrenocortical carcinoma rises from 2% for tumors less than 4 cm to 25% for tumors greater than 6 cm), imaging characteristics suspicious for malignancy (irregular borders, heterogeneous enhancement, calcification, growth on serial imaging), and known or suspected adrenocortical carcinoma. Bilateral adrenalectomy is performed for bilateral pheochromocytoma (in hereditary syndromes — MEN 2, von Hippel-Lindau), ACTH-independent bilateral macronodular adrenal hyperplasia, and as a last resort for Cushing disease refractory to pituitary surgery (bilateral adrenalectomy produces iatrogenic Addison disease requiring lifelong glucocorticoid and mineralocorticoid replacement and carries the risk of Nelson syndrome — enlargement of a residual ACTH-producing pituitary adenoma due to loss of cortisol feedback suppression).

KEY POINT: Every adrenal incidentaloma must be biochemically evaluated for function (subclinical Cushing syndrome, pheochromocytoma, hyperaldosteronism) regardless of size. Failure to diagnose a pheochromocytoma preoperatively can produce a lethal intraoperative catecholamine crisis if the tumor is manipulated without appropriate alpha-blockade.

Laparoscopic Transabdominal Adrenalectomy

Patient Positioning and Approach

Laparoscopic transabdominal adrenalectomy in the lateral decubitus position is the standard approach for adrenal tumors less than 6 cm without suspicion for adrenocortical carcinoma or local invasion. The patient is placed in the lateral decubitus position with the operative side up, and the table is flexed to open the space between the costal margin and the iliac crest. Three or four trocars are placed in the ipsilateral flank. On the right side, the liver is retracted superiorly to expose the right adrenal gland between the liver and the kidney — the peritoneum lateral to the IVC is incised, and the right adrenal vein is identified on the posterolateral surface of the IVC, clip-ligated (two clips on the IVC side, one clip on the adrenal side), and divided. After vein control, the gland is dissected circumferentially off the IVC, the diaphragmatic crus, and the upper pole of the kidney, ligating the small arterial branches with clips or an energy device. On the left side, the splenic flexure of the colon and the tail of the pancreas are mobilized medially to expose the left adrenal gland — the left adrenal vein is identified draining into the left renal vein, clip-ligated, and divided. The dissection then proceeds circumferentially. The specimen is placed in a retrieval bag to prevent tumor spillage and extracted through the largest trocar site.

Technical Principles for Safe Dissection

The critical technical principles of laparoscopic adrenalectomy are early venous control (the adrenal vein is the first structure identified and ligated — this is paramount for pheochromocytoma, where tumor manipulation with an intact venous outflow produces catecholamine release into the systemic circulation, causing hypertensive crisis and cardiac arrhythmias), careful circumferential dissection on the gland surface (dissecting in the plane between the adrenal capsule and the surrounding fat, keeping the yellow adrenal cortex visible on the specimen side to ensure complete excision), and avoidance of morcellation (the gland is removed intact in a retrieval bag — morcellation prevents accurate pathological assessment of margin status and tumor capsule integrity, which is essential for distinguishing benign adenoma from adrenocortical carcinoma). For pheochromocytoma specifically, the anesthesia team must be prepared for catecholamine surges during gland manipulation (even after vein ligation, catecholamine release from the gland into the venous stump and small venous tributaries can produce brief hypertensive episodes) — intravenous phentolamine, nitroprusside, nicardipine, or esmolol should be immediately available for acute blood pressure management.

THE OPERATIVE DANGER ZONE ATLAS — Right Adrenal Vein Avulsion from the Inferior Vena Cava

The Zone: The junction of the right adrenal vein with the posterolateral surface of the inferior vena cava during right laparoscopic adrenalectomy — the area where the short (2 to 5 mm) right adrenal vein emerges from the adrenal gland and enters the IVC.

The Structure at Risk: The inferior vena cava at the right adrenal vein insertion. The right adrenal vein is uniquely dangerous because of its extremely short length — there is almost no distance between the adrenal gland and the IVC wall, and any lateral traction on the adrenal gland during dissection before the vein has been controlled transmits force directly to the IVC wall, risking avulsion of the vein from the cava.

The Consequence: Avulsion of the right adrenal vein from the IVC produces a defect in the caval wall — a hole in the low-pressure, high-volume IVC that causes rapid, brisk venous hemorrhage (dark, non-pulsatile, high-volume blood loss). Under pneumoperitoneum, the gas pressure may initially tamponade the bleeding, but desufflation for conversion to open surgery releases this tamponade and produces torrential hemorrhage. This injury can be rapidly fatal if not immediately controlled.

The Safe Maneuver: Identify the right adrenal vein BEFORE mobilizing the adrenal gland — do not apply lateral traction to the gland until the vein is secured. Dissect directly on the posterolateral surface of the IVC to identify the vein at its insertion point. Clip-ligate the vein with at least two clips on the IVC side and one on the adrenal side before division. If avulsion occurs, immediately apply direct pressure with a laparoscopic instrument, maintain pneumoperitoneum (which helps tamponade the bleeding), and convert to open surgery with pressure maintained on the IVC until the vascular surgeon can place a side-biting Satinsky clamp and repair the defect with a 5-0 polypropylene suture.

Posterior Retroperitoneoscopic Adrenalectomy

Technique and Advantages

Posterior retroperitoneoscopic adrenalectomy (PRA) approaches the adrenal gland directly through the retroperitoneum via a prone (jackknife) position, avoiding the peritoneal cavity entirely. Three trocars are placed in the posterior flank below the twelfth rib. The retroperitoneal space is developed with balloon dissection, and the adrenal gland is identified on the superomedial surface of the kidney within Gerota fascia. The adrenal vein is identified, clipped, and divided, and the gland is dissected circumferentially. PRA offers several advantages over the lateral transabdominal approach: it avoids intraperitoneal adhesions (ideal for patients with prior abdominal surgery), provides direct access to the adrenal gland without the need to mobilize the liver, spleen, colon, or pancreas, allows bilateral adrenalectomy without repositioning (both sides are accessed from the same prone position), and may produce shorter operative times and faster recovery for experienced surgeons. The principal limitations are the small working space (which limits PRA to tumors less than 6 cm and makes the approach difficult in obese patients with excessive retroperitoneal fat) and the steep learning curve for surgeons accustomed to transabdominal laparoscopy.

Open Adrenalectomy for Large Tumors and Adrenocortical Carcinoma

Indications and Oncologic Principles

Open adrenalectomy is indicated for tumors greater than 6 cm (where the risk of adrenocortical carcinoma is substantial and complete oncologic resection requires wide margins and en bloc resection of involved adjacent structures), for known or suspected adrenocortical carcinoma (ACC — where the goal is R0 resection with an intact tumor capsule, without rupture or spillage), and for tumors with imaging evidence of local invasion (into the kidney, IVC, liver, or diaphragm). The approach depends on tumor size, location, and extent of invasion: a subcostal or chevron incision provides excellent exposure for most adrenal tumors; a thoracoabdominal incision may be needed for very large right-sided tumors with IVC involvement extending to the hepatic veins or right atrium. For ACC specifically, the operative principles include en bloc resection (removing the adrenal gland, surrounding periadrenal fat, and any adherent or invaded structures — the ipsilateral kidney, the tail of pancreas on the left, a segment of the diaphragm, or a portion of the liver — as a single specimen without violating the tumor capsule), regional lymph node dissection (periaortic and pericaval nodes), and avoidance of tumor rupture or morcellation (which converts a potentially curable localized cancer into a disseminated peritoneal disease). IVC involvement is present in approximately 10 to 25% of large right-sided ACCs — resection may require IVC thrombectomy under vascular control (suprahepatic and infrarenal IVC clamping) or, for intracardiac tumor extension, cardiopulmonary bypass.

Prognosis and Adjuvant Therapy for Adrenocortical Carcinoma

Adrenocortical carcinoma is rare (1 to 2 per million population per year) but aggressive — the overall 5-year survival is approximately 35 to 50% for localized disease and less than 15% for metastatic disease. Complete surgical resection (R0) is the only curative treatment, and the quality of the initial operation (margin status, capsule integrity, absence of tumor spillage) is the single most important prognostic factor for long-term survival. Adjuvant mitotane (an adrenolytic drug that destroys adrenocortical cells) is recommended for all patients after complete resection of ACC, with target serum levels of 14 to 20 micrograms per mL. For unresectable or metastatic ACC, the combination of etoposide, doxorubicin, cisplatin, and mitotane (the EDP-M regimen) is the standard systemic therapy based on the FIRM-ACT trial. Debulking surgery may be considered for recurrent or metastatic ACC to reduce tumor burden and control hormone excess (functional ACCs producing cortisol, aldosterone, or androgens cause significant systemic morbidity from hormone overproduction).

THE OPERATIVE DANGER ZONE ATLAS — Tumor Capsule Rupture During Adrenocortical Carcinoma Resection

The Zone: The dissection plane between a large adrenocortical carcinoma and its adjacent structures — the IVC, the ipsilateral kidney, the liver (right side), the tail of the pancreas and spleen (left side), and the diaphragm. The danger is greatest where the tumor is adherent to or invading an adjacent organ, because the natural impulse to dissect the tumor off the surface of the adjacent organ risks entering the tumor pseudocapsule.

The Structure at Risk: The tumor capsule itself. Adrenocortical carcinoma is surrounded by a pseudocapsule that is often thin and friable — disruption of this capsule spills viable tumor cells into the operative field, peritoneal cavity, and retroperitoneal space. Unlike benign adenomas, ACC cells implant readily on peritoneal surfaces and grow aggressively.

The Consequence: Capsule rupture or morcellation converts a potentially curable localized ACC (ENSAT stage I or II, 5-year survival 60 to 80%) into peritoneal carcinomatosis — upstaging the tumor to stage IV with a 5-year survival below 15%. Tumor spillage is an independent adverse prognostic factor and eliminates the possibility of curative-intent surgery, because microscopic peritoneal implants are not amenable to complete resection.

The Safe Maneuver: Commit to en bloc resection at the outset — if the tumor is adherent to the kidney, resect the kidney en bloc with the adrenal gland rather than attempting to peel the tumor off the renal surface. Apply the same principle to the diaphragm, the tail of the pancreas, and the liver capsule. Use a specimen retrieval bag even in open surgery to prevent contact between the tumor surface and the wound. Never morcellate an adrenal mass of unknown histology — the pathologist needs the intact capsule to distinguish adenoma from carcinoma. If a laparoscopic approach was planned but intraoperative findings suggest ACC (firm, adherent, irregular tumor), convert to open surgery immediately rather than attempting a technically difficult laparoscopic dissection that risks capsule breach.

Hereditary Pheochromocytoma and Paraganglioma Syndromes

Approximately 30 to 40% of pheochromocytomas and paragangliomas are hereditary, associated with germline mutations in at least 20 susceptibility genes. The most clinically relevant syndromes are multiple endocrine neoplasia type 2 (MEN 2A and MEN 2B — RET proto-oncogene mutations, autosomal dominant), von Hippel-Lindau disease (VHL gene mutations — associated with bilateral pheochromocytomas, renal cell carcinomas, hemangioblastomas, and pancreatic neuroendocrine tumors), neurofibromatosis type 1 (NF1 gene — pheochromocytoma in 1 to 5% of patients), and the succinate dehydrogenase (SDH) complex mutations (SDHB, SDHD, SDHC, SDHA — particularly SDHB, which carries the highest malignancy risk, with 30 to 70% of SDHB-mutated pheochromocytomas and paragangliomas developing metastatic disease). Hereditary pheochromocytomas are more frequently bilateral (up to 50% in MEN 2 and VHL), more frequently multifocal (extra-adrenal paragangliomas in SDH mutations), diagnosed at a younger age, and more likely to recur after initial resection. Current guidelines recommend genetic testing for all patients diagnosed with pheochromocytoma or paraganglioma, regardless of age or family history, because the high prevalence of germline mutations fundamentally changes surveillance and surgical planning.

The surgical implications of hereditary pheochromocytoma are distinct from sporadic disease. Bilateral pheochromocytoma (common in MEN 2 and VHL) requires a decision between bilateral total adrenalectomy (which cures the pheochromocytoma but produces lifelong adrenal insufficiency with permanent glucocorticoid and mineralocorticoid dependence and the risk of adrenal crisis during intercurrent illness) and cortical-sparing adrenalectomy (partial adrenalectomy, removing the medullary tumor while preserving a rim of functioning adrenal cortex to maintain endogenous cortisol production). Cortical-sparing adrenalectomy preserves adrenal function in approximately 60 to 80% of patients but carries a recurrence risk of 10 to 20% in the retained adrenal remnant, requiring lifelong biochemical surveillance with annual plasma free metanephrines and imaging. For SDHB-mutated pheochromocytomas, the high malignancy risk warrants more aggressive initial surgery and closer postoperative surveillance — annual whole-body functional imaging (MIBG scintigraphy or gallium-68 DOTATATE PET/CT) is recommended in addition to biochemical testing.

THE OPERATIVE DANGER ZONE ATLAS — Catecholamine Crisis During Pheochromocytoma Resection

The Zone: The operative field during any manipulation of a pheochromocytoma — from the initial peritoneal incision to specimen extraction. The catecholamine-producing medullary tissue releases epinephrine and norepinephrine in response to mechanical pressure, traction, and compression of the tumor.

The Structure at Risk: The cardiovascular system. Catecholamine release from a manipulated pheochromocytoma produces acute hypertensive crisis (systolic blood pressure exceeding 250 mmHg), tachyarrhythmias (ventricular tachycardia, supraventricular tachycardia), and, if severe, myocardial infarction, stroke, or cardiac arrest. After adrenal vein ligation and tumor removal, the sudden cessation of catecholamine production may produce rebound hypotension and cardiovascular collapse.

The Consequence: Intraoperative hypertensive crisis from uncontrolled catecholamine release produces end-organ damage — hypertensive encephalopathy, intracerebral hemorrhage, acute pulmonary edema, or myocardial ischemia. The mortality rate of pheochromocytoma surgery without adequate preoperative preparation historically exceeded 30% and remains 1 to 3% even with modern alpha-blockade protocols.

The Safe Maneuver: Preoperative alpha-blockade (phenoxybenzamine 10 to 20 mg two to three times daily, titrated upward over 10 to 14 days until orthostatic hypotension is achieved, or doxazosin as a selective alpha-1 blocker alternative) for a minimum of 7 to 14 days before surgery. Liberal salt and fluid loading (high-sodium diet plus 2 to 3 liters of fluid daily) to expand the contracted intravascular volume. Beta-blockade (propranolol or atenolol) is added ONLY AFTER adequate alpha-blockade — beta-blockade alone (without alpha-blockade) is contraindicated because it produces unopposed alpha-mediated vasoconstriction and worsens hypertension. Intraoperatively, ligate the adrenal vein as the first step to minimize catecholamine release during subsequent gland manipulation. The anesthesiologist must have intravenous phentolamine, nitroprusside, and magnesium sulfate available for acute blood pressure management.

Preoperative Preparation for Pheochromocytoma and Functional Adrenal Tumors

Alpha-Blockade Protocol and Volume Expansion

Preoperative preparation for pheochromocytoma is one of the most critical perioperative protocols in endocrine surgery because inadequate preparation carries a mortality risk that dwarfs the technical risks of the operation itself. The standard protocol begins with alpha-adrenergic blockade 10 to 14 days before surgery: phenoxybenzamine (a non-selective, irreversible alpha-blocker) is started at 10 mg twice daily and titrated upward by 10 mg increments every 2 to 3 days until the target endpoints are achieved — seated blood pressure below 130/80 mmHg, orthostatic hypotension (a systolic drop of at least 10 to 15 mmHg on standing, indicating adequate alpha-blockade and volume depletion that needs correction), no ST-segment or T-wave changes on electrocardiography, and no more than one premature ventricular contraction every 5 minutes on telemetry. The alternative selective alpha-1 blocker doxazosin (starting at 2 mg daily, titrated up to 16 mg or higher) is increasingly used because of its availability and lower side effect profile, although it does not provide the irreversible, long-acting blockade of phenoxybenzamine. Volume expansion with a high-sodium diet and liberal oral fluids (2 to 3 liters daily) is initiated simultaneously with alpha-blockade — patients with pheochromocytoma are chronically volume-depleted due to sustained catecholamine-mediated vasoconstriction, and failure to expand the intravascular volume before surgery produces severe rebound hypotension after the tumor is removed and catecholamine levels abruptly fall.

Preparation for Other Functional Adrenal Tumors

Cortisol-producing adenomas (causing Cushing syndrome) require perioperative stress-dose glucocorticoid coverage because the contralateral adrenal gland is suppressed by chronic cortisol excess and cannot mount a normal cortisol response to surgical stress. Hydrocortisone 100 mg intravenously is given at induction, followed by a taper over 48 to 72 hours, with transition to oral hydrocortisone replacement that is gradually weaned over months as the contralateral adrenal recovers. Recovery of the hypothalamic-pituitary-adrenal axis may take 6 to 18 months. Aldosterone-producing adenomas (causing primary hyperaldosteronism — Conn syndrome) require preoperative correction of hypokalemia with potassium supplementation and spironolactone (a mineralocorticoid receptor antagonist) for 4 to 6 weeks before surgery. Blood pressure improvement after unilateral adrenalectomy for aldosteronoma is seen in approximately 70 to 80% of patients, but complete cure of hypertension occurs in only 30 to 50% (the remainder have essential hypertension coexisting with the aldosteronoma). Adrenal sex-steroid-producing tumors (virilizing or feminizing tumors — rare, more commonly adrenocortical carcinomas) do not require specific preoperative endocrine preparation but require the oncologic approach described for ACC.

THE OPERATIVE DANGER ZONE ATLAS — Adrenal Cortical Insufficiency After Cortisol-Producing Adenoma Resection

The Zone: The immediate postoperative period following unilateral adrenalectomy for a cortisol-producing adenoma (Cushing syndrome). The danger zone is not an anatomical location but a physiological window — the interval between removal of the autonomously functioning adenoma and recovery of the suppressed contralateral adrenal gland and hypothalamic-pituitary-adrenal axis.

The Structure at Risk: The hypothalamic-pituitary-adrenal axis. Chronic cortisol hypersecretion from the adenoma suppresses CRH production by the hypothalamus and ACTH secretion by the anterior pituitary through negative feedback — this in turn causes atrophy of the contralateral adrenal cortex, which cannot produce cortisol when the adenoma is removed. The patient is left in a state of iatrogenic secondary adrenal insufficiency.

The Consequence: Acute adrenal crisis (addisonian crisis) — characterized by refractory hypotension unresponsive to fluids and vasopressors, hyponatremia, hyperkalemia, hypoglycemia, nausea, vomiting, and cardiovascular collapse. If unrecognized and untreated, adrenal crisis is fatal. The risk is highest during the first 48 hours after surgery when surgical stress maximally demands cortisol production that the suppressed adrenal cannot provide.

The Safe Maneuver: Administer stress-dose hydrocortisone 100 mg intravenously at the time of anesthetic induction, before the adrenal vein is ligated. Continue hydrocortisone 50 mg IV every 8 hours for the first 24 hours, then taper to 25 mg every 8 hours for 24 hours, transitioning to oral hydrocortisone 20 mg morning and 10 mg evening. Taper the oral dose gradually over months, guided by serial morning cortisol levels and cosyntropin stimulation testing — do not discontinue replacement until the 250 microgram cosyntropin stimulation test demonstrates a peak cortisol response above 18 micrograms per dL, confirming HPA axis recovery. Recovery typically requires 6 to 18 months; during this period, the patient must carry a steroid emergency card and know to double the dose during febrile illness or physiological stress.

Complications of Adrenalectomy and Postoperative Surveillance

Complications of laparoscopic adrenalectomy include hemorrhage (the most feared complication — particularly right adrenal vein avulsion, with conversion rates for bleeding of 2 to 5%), injury to adjacent organs (splenic injury during left adrenalectomy requiring splenectomy in 1 to 2%, pancreatic tail injury producing postoperative pancreatic fistula, diaphragmatic injury producing pneumothorax), port-site hernia (0.5 to 2%, more common with 12 mm trocar sites), and wound infection. Specific complications of open adrenalectomy for large tumors include higher rates of blood loss and transfusion, incisional hernia (particularly with subcostal or thoracoabdominal incisions), prolonged ileus, and — for ACC resections involving nephrectomy or IVC thrombectomy — renal insufficiency and thromboembolic events. Postoperative surveillance after adrenalectomy depends on the pathology: for pheochromocytoma, annual plasma free metanephrines are recommended lifelong (recurrence risk is 5 to 15% overall and higher in hereditary syndromes); for ACC, cross-sectional imaging every 3 months for the first 2 years, then every

6 months for years 3 to 5, then annually (local recurrence and distant metastasis rates are high even after R0 resection, with 50 to 80% of patients experiencing recurrence within 2 years); for aldosteronoma, follow-up assessment of blood pressure and potassium at 1 to 3 months (persistent hypertension may require continued antihypertensive therapy); and for cortisol-producing adenoma, serial cosyntropin stimulation testing every 3 to 6 months until HPA axis recovery is confirmed.

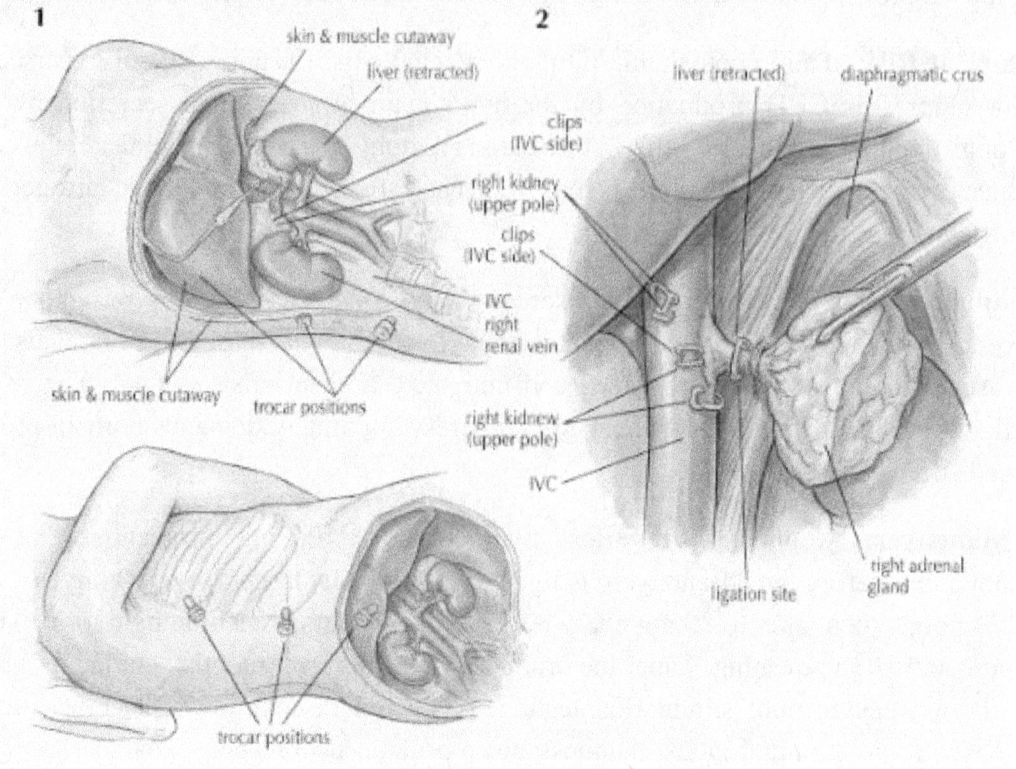

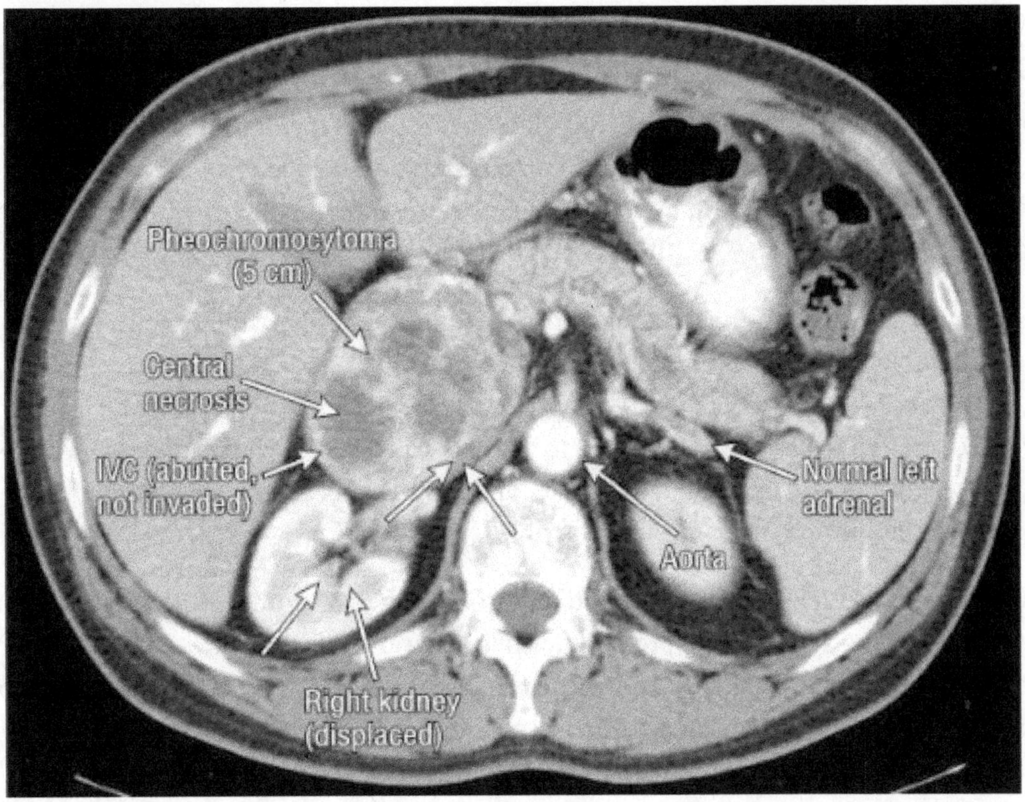

Clinical Case — Pheochromocytoma With Intraoperative Hypertensive Crisis

A 38-year-old woman is referred for evaluation of a 4 cm right adrenal mass discovered incidentally on CT for renal colic. She reports episodic headaches, palpitations, and diaphoresis. Plasma free metanephrines are markedly elevated (normetanephrine 12.4 nmol/L, metanephrine 3.8 nmol/L — both more than three times the upper limit of normal), confirming a biochemical diagnosis of pheochromocytoma. She is started on phenoxybenzamine 10 mg twice daily, titrated over 2 weeks to 30 mg twice daily until seated blood pressure is below 130/80 mmHg with orthostatic hypotension. High-sodium diet and liberal fluids are prescribed. Propranolol 20 mg three times daily is added after 1 week of alpha-blockade for reflex tachycardia. At surgery, a right laparoscopic transabdominal adrenalectomy is performed in the lateral decubitus position. The right adrenal vein is identified on the posterolateral IVC and clip-ligated as the first step. During subsequent gland mobilization, a brief catecholamine surge produces systolic blood pressure of 220 mmHg — the anesthesiologist administers intravenous phentolamine 2 mg bolus and a nicardipine infusion, controlling the blood pressure within 3 minutes. After complete gland removal, the blood pressure drops to 90/60 mmHg (rebound hypotension from catecholamine withdrawal) — this is managed with intravenous fluids and a brief phenylephrine infusion. The specimen is extracted intact in a retrieval bag. Pathology confirms a 4.2 cm pheochromocytoma with PASS score of 3 (low risk of malignancy). Postoperatively, all antihypertensive medications are discontinued, and the patient is normotensive at 6-week follow-up.

Right Adrenal Vein Avulsion from the Inferior Vena Cava: The right adrenal vein is only 2 to 5 mm long — any lateral traction on the right adrenal gland before vein ligation transmits force directly to the IVC wall, risking caval avulsion and torrential venous hemorrhage. **Safe maneuver:** identify and clip-ligate the right adrenal vein as the first operative step before applying any traction to the gland; place at least two clips on the IVC side.

Catecholamine Crisis During Pheochromocytoma Resection: Manipulation of a pheochromocytoma releases catecholamines that can produce lethal hypertensive crisis, tachyarrhythmias, myocardial infarction, or stroke — historically carrying mortality exceeding 30% without preparation. **Safe maneuver:** preoperative alpha-blockade for 10 to 14 days with phenoxybenzamine or doxazosin, volume expansion, beta-blockade ONLY after adequate alpha-blockade; ligate the adrenal vein first; have intravenous phentolamine and nitroprusside available.

Adrenal Cortical Insufficiency After Cortisol-Producing Adenoma Resection: Chronic cortisol excess from a functioning adenoma suppresses the contralateral adrenal gland — unilateral adrenalectomy removes the only functioning adrenal tissue, producing adrenal crisis if stress-dose steroids are not provided. **Safe maneuver:** administer hydrocortisone 100 mg IV at induction and taper over 48 to 72 hours; maintain oral replacement for 6 to 18 months until HPA axis recovery is confirmed by cosyntropin stimulation testing.

Tumor Capsule Rupture During Adrenocortical Carcinoma Resection: Morcellation or capsule rupture during resection of an adrenocortical carcinoma converts a potentially curable localized cancer into disseminated peritoneal disease — dramatically worsening prognosis. **Safe maneuver:** perform en bloc resection with intact tumor capsule; use a specimen retrieval bag; if the tumor is adherent to adjacent structures, resect them en bloc rather than dissecting the tumor off their surface.

Summary and Key Concepts

The right adrenal vein is only 2 to 5 mm long and drains directly into the posterolateral IVC — it must be identified and clip-ligated before the adrenal gland is mobilized to prevent caval avulsion.

Early venous control is paramount in pheochromocytoma surgery — ligating the adrenal vein as the first operative step minimizes catecholamine release during subsequent gland manipulation.

Preoperative alpha-blockade for pheochromocytoma (phenoxybenzamine or doxazosin for 10 to 14 days with volume expansion) is one of the most critical perioperative protocols in endocrine surgery — inadequate preparation carries a mortality risk exceeding the technical risks of the operation.

Beta-blockade must NEVER be initiated before adequate alpha-blockade in pheochromocytoma — unopposed alpha-mediated vasoconstriction from beta-blockade alone worsens hypertension and may precipitate hypertensive crisis.

Open adrenalectomy with en bloc resection and intact tumor capsule is the standard for adrenocortical carcinoma — capsule rupture or morcellation converts localized disease to peritoneal dissemination.

Cortisol-producing adenomas require perioperative stress-dose glucocorticoids because the suppressed contralateral adrenal cannot mount a cortisol response — HPA axis recovery takes 6 to 18 months.

Posterior retroperitoneoscopic adrenalectomy offers direct access to the adrenal gland without entering the peritoneal cavity and allows bilateral adrenalectomy without repositioning — ideal for patients with prior abdominal surgery or bilateral disease.

CHAPTER 17: OPERATIONS OF THE ARTERIES

Learning Objectives

1. Describe the surgical anatomy of the major arterial systems, including the carotid bifurcation, the abdominal aorta and its branches, the iliac system, and the lower extremity arterial tree from the common femoral artery to the pedal vessels.
2. Perform a carotid endarterectomy with appropriate shunt placement, arteriotomy technique, plaque removal, and patch angioplasty closure to prevent perioperative stroke.
3. Select the appropriate operative strategy (open repair versus endovascular) for abdominal and thoracoabdominal aortic aneurysms based on patient anatomy, comorbidities, and aneurysm morphology.
4. Apply the principles of infrainguinal arterial bypass, including conduit selection, anastomotic technique, and assessment of distal runoff.
5. Execute a balloon catheter embolectomy for acute arterial occlusion and apply damage-control principles to peripheral arterial trauma, including temporary vascular shunts and reversed saphenous vein interposition grafts.

Surgical Anatomy of the Major Arteries

The Carotid System

The common carotid artery (CCA) arises from the brachiocephalic artery on the right and directly from the aortic arch on the left. Both ascend within the carotid sheath (alongside the internal jugular vein laterally and the vagus nerve posteriorly) and bifurcate at the upper border of the thyroid cartilage (approximately C3-C4) into the internal carotid artery (ICA) and external carotid artery (ECA). The carotid bulb — the dilated ICA origin — is the most common site of atherosclerotic plaque and the target of carotid endarterectomy. The ICA has no branches in the neck and enters the skull through the carotid canal to supply the anterior and middle cerebral circulation. The ECA gives off multiple branches (superior thyroid, ascending pharyngeal, lingual, facial, occipital, posterior auricular, maxillary, and superficial temporal arteries). The surgical landmark distinguishing the ICA from the ECA is that the ECA has branches while the ICA does not.

The Aorta and Its Branches

The thoracic aorta is divided into the ascending aorta (from the aortic root to the brachiocephalic artery origin), the aortic arch (from which the brachiocephalic, left common carotid, and left subclavian arteries arise), and the descending thoracic aorta (from the left subclavian origin to the diaphragmatic hiatus at approximately the T12 vertebral level). The abdominal aorta extends from the aortic hiatus to the bifurcation into the common iliac arteries at approximately the L4 vertebral level (the level of the umbilicus). The major visceral branches of the abdominal aorta are the celiac trunk (left gastric, common hepatic, splenic arteries — at T12/L1), the superior mesenteric artery (SMA — at L1, supplying the midgut from the ligament of Treitz to the splenic flexure), the renal arteries (at L1-L2, arising laterally), the inferior mesenteric artery (IMA — at L3, supplying the hindgut from the splenic flexure to the upper rectum), and the gonadal arteries. The infrarenal abdominal aorta (below the renal arteries) is the most common site of abdominal aortic aneurysm (AAA), and the surgical exposure for open AAA repair requires retraction of the transverse colon superiorly, evisceration of the small bowel to the right, and incision of the posterior peritoneum over the aorta.

The Lower Extremity Arterial Tree

The common iliac artery bifurcates into the external iliac artery (which becomes the common femoral artery below the inguinal ligament) and the internal iliac (hypogastric) artery (supplying the pelvis and gluteal region). The common femoral artery (CFA) is the primary arterial access point for all endovascular procedures and the inflow site for infrainguinal bypasses — it lies in the femoral triangle, midway between the anterior superior iliac spine and the pubic symphysis, lateral to the femoral vein. The CFA bifurcates approximately 4 cm below the inguinal ligament into the superficial femoral artery (SFA — which traverses the adductor canal and becomes the popliteal artery at the adductor hiatus) and the profunda femoris (deep femoral artery — the most important collateral pathway in femoral-popliteal occlusive disease). The popliteal artery passes through the popliteal fossa and trifurcates below the knee into the anterior tibial artery, the posterior tibial artery, and the peroneal (fibular) artery. The anterior tibial artery becomes the dorsalis pedis artery on the dorsum of the foot; the posterior tibial artery passes behind the medial malleolus into the plantar arch.

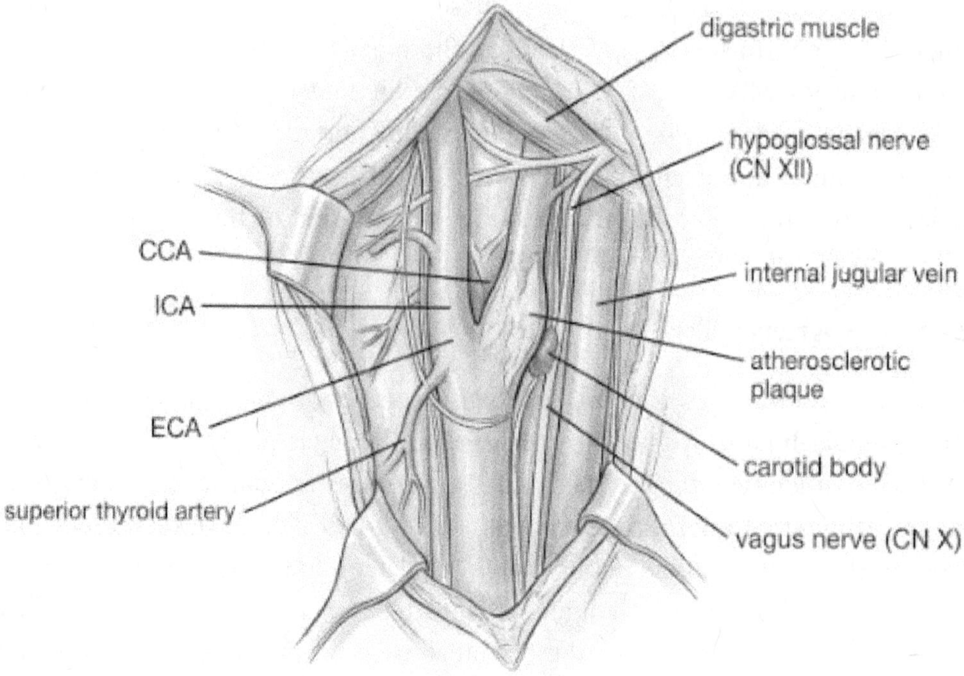

Carotid Endarterectomy

Indications and Patient Selection

Carotid endarterectomy (CEA) is indicated for symptomatic carotid stenosis of 50% or greater (by NASCET criteria — symptoms include ipsilateral transient ischemic attack, amaurosis fugax, or nondisabling stroke within the preceding 6 months) and for asymptomatic carotid stenosis of 60 to 70% or greater with a perioperative stroke/death rate below 3% (established by the ACAS and ACST trials). The benefit of CEA is greatest in symptomatic patients with 70 to 99% stenosis (absolute risk reduction of approximately 16% at 2 years versus medical therapy alone in the NASCET trial) and diminishes for moderate stenosis (50 to 69%). Timing of CEA after a neurological event is important — early surgery (within 14 days of the index event) maximizes stroke prevention benefit because the risk of recurrent stroke is highest in the first 2 weeks; however, surgery should be deferred for 4 to 6 weeks after a major disabling stroke to allow cerebral edema to resolve and avoid hemorrhagic conversion. Contraindications to CEA include complete (100%) carotid occlusion (no benefit to endarterectomy once the vessel is fully thrombosed), prior radical neck dissection with scarring at the carotid bifurcation, radiation-induced carotid stenosis (restenosis rates are high — transfemoral carotid artery stenting may be preferred), and contralateral vocal cord paralysis (because CEA risks injury to the ipsilateral vagus or recurrent laryngeal nerve, and bilateral vocal cord paralysis produces airway compromise).

Operative Technique

The patient is positioned supine with the head turned away from the operative side. A longitudinal incision along the anterior border of the sternocleidomastoid exposes the CCA, ICA, and ECA within the carotid sheath. The vagus nerve (running posteriorly between the CCA and internal jugular vein), hypoglossal nerve (crossing superiorly over the ICA and ECA), and ansa cervicalis are identified and preserved. After systemic heparinization (80 to 100 units per kilogram), vascular clamps are applied to the ICA first (preventing distal embolization), then the CCA and ECA. A longitudinal arteriotomy extends from the CCA across the bulb into the diseased ICA. A carotid shunt is placed if selective shunting criteria are met (stump pressure below 40 mmHg, EEG changes, or cerebral oximetry changes). The plaque is removed in the endarterectomy plane between the outer media and the plaque, working from the CCA distally. The distal ICA endpoint must be clean and tacked down with 6-0 or 7-0 polypropylene sutures to prevent an intimal flap. The arteriotomy is closed with patch angioplasty (Dacron, bovine pericardium, or saphenous vein) rather than primary closure — patch closure significantly reduces perioperative stroke and long-term restenosis.

THE OPERATIVE DANGER ZONE ATLAS — Cranial Nerve Injury During Carotid Endarterectomy

---

The Zone: The carotid bifurcation and the superior extent of the dissection during carotid endarterectomy — the area where the hypoglossal nerve (CN XII) crosses over the ICA and ECA at the level of the digastric muscle, and where the vagus nerve (CN X) runs within the carotid sheath posterior to the common carotid artery. The marginal mandibular branch of the facial nerve (CN VII) is at risk if the incision or retraction extends above the angle of the mandible.

The Structure at Risk: The hypoglossal nerve (CN XII), the vagus nerve (CN X, including its recurrent laryngeal branch), and the marginal mandibular branch of the facial nerve (CN VII). The hypoglossal nerve crosses the distal ICA and ECA superiorly and must be mobilized to access the distal extent of the plaque. The vagus nerve lies within the carotid sheath — in an aberrant course (present in 1 to 5% of patients), it may run anterior to the CCA rather than posterior, placing it directly in the line of the incision.

The Consequence: Hypoglossal nerve injury causes ipsilateral tongue deviation toward the injured side, with dysarthria and difficulty with mastication and swallowing. Vagus nerve injury (or its recurrent laryngeal branch) causes ipsilateral vocal cord paralysis with hoarseness; if bilateral (as when contralateral vagus injury exists from a prior CEA), vocal cord paralysis produces airway obstruction requiring tracheostomy. Marginal mandibular nerve injury causes drooping of the ipsilateral corner of the mouth. These injuries occur in 5 to 8% of CEA cases overall, though most are neuropraxic and recover within weeks to months.

The Safe Maneuver: Identify the hypoglossal nerve before dividing any tissue crossing the ICA at the superior extent of the dissection — it crosses from lateral to medial, often with the ansa cervicalis descending from it. Mobilize it gently with a vessel loop rather than retracting it with a sharp instrument. Identify the vagus nerve within the carotid sheath before applying vascular clamps — if it courses anteriorly, mobilize it posteriorly with a vessel loop. Avoid extending the skin incision above the angle of the mandible to protect the marginal mandibular nerve. Before contralateral CEA, confirm ipsilateral vocal cord function with indirect laryngoscopy.

CLINICAL PEARL: Patch angioplasty closure of the carotid arteriotomy (using Dacron, bovine pericardium, or autologous saphenous vein) significantly reduces both perioperative stroke and long-term restenosis compared with primary closure. Routine patch closure is the current standard of care for CEA — primary closure should be reserved only for patients with a large-caliber ICA in whom the arteriotomy can be closed without narrowing.

Open Aortic Aneurysm Repair (Abdominal and Thoracoabdominal)

Indications and Preoperative Assessment

Open surgical repair of abdominal aortic aneurysm (AAA) is indicated for aneurysms measuring 5.5 cm or greater in men and 5.0 cm or greater in women (at these thresholds, the annual rupture risk exceeds the operative mortality risk), for aneurysms growing at a rate exceeding 1 cm per year regardless of absolute size, and for symptomatic aneurysms (back or abdominal pain attributable to the aneurysm) and ruptured aneurysms. Preoperative assessment includes CT angiography to define aneurysm anatomy (proximal neck length and angulation, renal artery involvement, iliac artery morphology), cardiac risk stratification (the majority of AAA patients have concomitant coronary artery disease — cardiac catheterization or stress testing is indicated for patients with active cardiac symptoms or poor functional capacity), and pulmonary function testing (thoracoabdominal repairs require single-lung ventilation). The decision between open repair and endovascular aneurysm repair (EVAR) is based on patient anatomy and fitness — open repair is preferred when the anatomy is unfavorable for EVAR (short infrarenal neck less than 15 mm, severely angulated neck greater than 60 degrees, small or diseased iliac arteries precluding device delivery), in younger patients (open repair has superior long-term durability with lower reintervention rates), and in patients who cannot comply with the lifelong surveillance required after EVAR.

Operative Technique for Infrarenal AAA Repair

Open infrarenal AAA repair is performed through a midline transperitoneal approach or a left retroperitoneal approach. The transperitoneal approach provides wide exposure and access to both iliac systems but requires small bowel evisceration; the retroperitoneal approach (through a left flank incision with medial rotation of the left kidney) provides direct access to the aorta without entering the peritoneal cavity and is preferred for hostile abdomens, juxtarenal aneurysms, and patients with prior abdominal surgery. After achieving proximal and distal vascular control, the aneurysm sac is opened longitudinally (inlay technique — the sac is not excised). Lumbar arteries bleeding back into the sac are suture-ligated from within. A Dacron or expanded polytetrafluoroethylene (ePTFE) tube graft is sewn to the proximal aortic neck with a running 3-0 or 4-0 polypropylene suture, and the distal anastomosis is constructed to the aortic bifurcation (tube graft) or to each common iliac artery (bifurcated graft — used when the aneurysm extends to the aortic bifurcation or when concomitant iliac aneurysms are present). Before completing the distal anastomosis, back-bleeding from the iliac arteries and forward-bleeding from the graft are confirmed to ensure the absence of thromboembolism. The aneurysm sac is closed over the graft to separate it from the overlying duodenum — failure to do so risks aortoenteric fistula, a catastrophic late complication.

THE OPERATIVE DANGER ZONE ATLAS — Left Renal Vein Injury During Infrarenal Aortic Cross-Clamping

The Zone: The infrarenal aortic neck during exposure for proximal aortic clamping — the left renal vein crosses the anterior surface of the aorta immediately below the renal arteries, running from left to right to enter the IVC. The proximal aortic clamp must be placed BELOW the renal arteries, in exactly the area where the left renal vein crosses.

The Structure at Risk: The left renal vein. It crosses the aorta anteriorly at the level of the left renal artery origin and is the first structure encountered when exposing the infrarenal aortic neck from an anterior (transperitoneal) approach. It receives the left gonadal vein inferiorly and the left adrenal vein superiorly. In approximately 3% of patients, a retroaortic left renal vein passes behind the aorta — this variant is at particular risk during posterior dissection of the aortic neck.

The Consequence: Inadvertent injury to the left renal vein produces brisk venous hemorrhage that obscures the operative field and delays aortic clamping — particularly dangerous in ruptured AAA repair where rapid proximal control is life-saving. If the left renal vein is ligated (deliberately or inadvertently), the left kidney maintains drainage through three collateral pathways (the left adrenal vein to the inferior phrenic vein, the left gonadal vein, and the left lumbar veins) — ligation is tolerated IF these collaterals are intact, but if the gonadal and adrenal branches have already been divided during dissection, ligation causes left renal venous hypertension, renal infarction, and renal failure.

The Safe Maneuver: Identify the left renal vein early during infrarenal aortic exposure — it is the landmark for the proximal neck. Retract it superiorly with a vein retractor to expose the aortic neck below. If the renal vein limits exposure of a juxtarenal aneurysm, it may be divided between ligatures, but ONLY after confirming the gonadal and adrenal branches are intact (they provide collateral drainage). In ruptured AAA with hemodynamic instability, supraceliac aortic clamping at the diaphragmatic hiatus provides immediate proximal control without the need to expose the infrarenal neck — the clamp is moved distally to the infrarenal position once the patient is stabilized and the anatomy is defined.

Endovascular Aneurysm Repair (EVAR and TEVAR)

Anatomical Requirements and Device Selection

Endovascular aneurysm repair (EVAR) deploys a covered stent graft within the aneurysm from a transfemoral approach, excluding the aneurysm sac from arterial pressure without requiring laparotomy or aortic clamping. Standard infrarenal EVAR requires specific anatomical criteria: an infrarenal aortic neck length of at least 15 mm (measured from the lowest renal artery to the start of the aneurysm), a neck diameter of 18 to 32 mm (depending on the device), a neck angulation of less than 60 degrees, and iliac arteries of adequate diameter (typically greater than 7 mm) and without severe tortuosity or calcification to allow device delivery. The graft lands proximally on the infrarenal neck and distally in the common iliac arteries (or the external iliac arteries with internal iliac embolization if the iliac arteries are aneurysmal). Fenestrated and branched endografts extend the indications to juxtarenal and suprarenal aneurysms by incorporating fenestrations or directional branches for the renal and visceral arteries — these are technically demanding procedures performed at high-volume centers.

Endoleaks and Surveillance

Endoleaks — persistent blood flow into the excluded aneurysm sac — are the principal limitation of EVAR and the reason patients require lifelong surveillance after endovascular repair. Type I endoleaks (flow around the proximal or distal seal zones — the graft is not sealed to the aortic wall) are high-pressure leaks that require immediate treatment (extension cuff, remodeling balloon, or open conversion) because they expose the aneurysm sac to systemic arterial pressure and confer a rupture risk equivalent to an untreated aneurysm. Type II endoleaks (flow into the sac from patent branch vessels — typically the IMA or lumbar arteries) are the most common type (20 to 30% incidence), are low-pressure, and the majority seal spontaneously; intervention (coil embolization or sac ligation) is indicated only if the aneurysm sac enlarges during surveillance. Type III endoleaks (flow through defects in the graft fabric or between modular graft components) are high-pressure and require relining or replacement. Type V endoleaks (endotension — sac enlargement without a demonstrable leak) are managed by open conversion if progressive enlargement is documented. Standard EVAR surveillance consists of CT angiography at 1 month, 6 months, and 12 months post-procedure, then annually. Ultrasound is an accepted alternative for long-term surveillance when sac size is stable.

Endoleak Type	Source	Pressure	Management
Type I	Proximal or distal seal zone failure	High (systemic)	Immediate repair — extension cuff, balloon, or open conversion
Type II	Patent branch vessels (IMA, lumbar arteries)	Low	Observe; intervene only if sac enlarges (coil embolization)
Type III	Graft fabric defect or modular disconnection	High (systemic)	Relining or component replacement
Type IV	Graft porosity (within 30 days)	Low	Self-limited; observe
Type V	Endotension (sac growth, no visible leak)	Unknown	Open conversion if progressive enlargement

Lower Extremity Arterial Bypass (Femoral-Popliteal and Femoral-Tibial)

Indications and Conduit Selection

Infrainguinal arterial bypass is performed for limb-threatening ischemia (Rutherford categories 4 to 6 — rest pain, non-healing ulcer, or gangrene) and for lifestyle-limiting claudication (Rutherford categories 2 to 3) that has failed medical therapy and exercise rehabilitation. The choice of bypass target depends on preoperative arterial imaging (CT angiography or conventional angiography) — the distal anastomosis is placed on the most proximal patent artery with continuous runoff to the foot (the above-knee popliteal artery if the SFA is occluded but the popliteal is patent; the below-knee popliteal artery if the above-knee popliteal is diseased; or a tibial artery — anterior tibial, posterior tibial, or peroneal — if the popliteal artery is occluded). The greater saphenous vein (GSV) is the conduit of choice for all infrainguinal bypasses — autologous vein has superior long-term patency compared with prosthetic grafts, particularly for below-knee targets (5-year primary patency rates of 60 to 80% for vein versus 30 to 50% for prosthetic below the knee). The GSV may be used in situ (left in its anatomical bed with the valves incised using a valvulotome and the side branches ligated) or as a reversed vein graft (harvested, reversed to render the valves incompetent, and tunneled anatomically). When the GSV is unavailable (previously harvested for coronary artery bypass, varicose, or inadequate diameter — less than 3 mm), alternative autologous conduits include the small saphenous vein, arm veins (cephalic or basilic), and composite sequential vein grafts. Prosthetic grafts (ePTFE or Dacron) are acceptable for above-knee femoral-popliteal bypass, where the patency difference between vein and prosthetic is smaller, but are inferior to vein for all below-knee reconstructions.

Anastomotic Technique and Graft Surveillance

The proximal anastomosis is constructed end-to-side on the common femoral artery using a running 5-0 or 6-0 polypropylene suture. The graft is tunneled anatomically (subfascial, along the course of the native SFA and popliteal artery) to the distal target. The distal anastomosis is constructed end-to-side on the target artery — the arteriotomy must be placed on a segment of artery with adequate inflow and outflow, away from heavily calcified segments that resist suturing and prevent the vessel wall from forming a compliant, hemostatic seal. A completion angiogram or duplex ultrasound is performed to confirm graft patency, exclude technical errors (intimal flaps, retained valve leaflets in in situ grafts, graft kinks, or anastomotic stenosis), and document the runoff. Postoperative graft surveillance with duplex ultrasound is performed at 1, 3, 6, and 12 months and then every 6 months to detect developing stenoses (particularly at the proximal and distal anastomoses and within the vein graft itself) before they progress to graft thrombosis — stenoses detected by surveillance can be treated with percutaneous transluminal angioplasty or surgical patch angioplasty, preserving graft function. A peak systolic velocity ratio greater than 3.5 across a stenosis or an absolute velocity greater than 300 cm per second indicates a hemodynamically significant lesion warranting intervention.

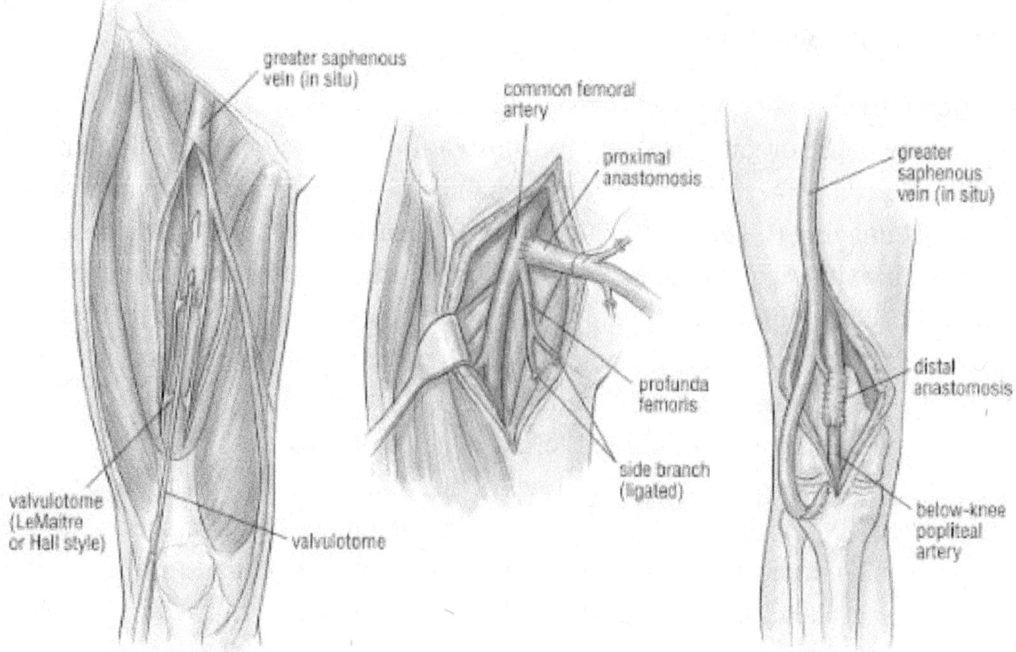

THE OPERATIVE DANGER ZONE ATLAS — Popliteal Vein Injury During Below-Knee Popliteal Artery Exposure

---

The Zone: The medial approach to the below-knee popliteal artery — the incision is made one fingerbreadth behind the posterior border of the tibia, the crural fascia is incised, and the popliteal artery is exposed by retracting the medial head of the gastrocnemius posteriorly. The popliteal vein lies immediately deep and posterior to the popliteal artery, directly in the path of dissection.

The Structure at Risk: The popliteal vein (a deep vein critical for lower extremity venous drainage) and the tibial nerve (which lies superficial and posterior to the popliteal vein). The intimate relationship between the popliteal artery and vein — they share a common adventitial sheath — means that circumferential dissection of the artery for distal anastomosis construction requires separating these two vessels, and injudicious posterior dissection risks entering the vein wall.

The Consequence: Popliteal vein injury produces significant venous hemorrhage in a confined space, obscuring the arterial target. More importantly, popliteal vein ligation or thrombosis (from repair-site narrowing) produces acute deep venous obstruction of the leg, causing limb swelling, venous hypertension, and potentially venous gangrene — a devastating complication that can lead to amputation of the leg the bypass was intended to save. Tibial nerve injury causes sensory loss in the sole of the foot and weakness of ankle plantar flexion.

The Safe Maneuver: Approach the below-knee popliteal artery from its anteromedial aspect — identify it by palpation or Doppler, then dissect directly onto the arterial wall using fine-tipped scissors and gentle spreading dissection. Dissect only the anterior and lateral circumference of the artery (enough to pass a vessel loop for control) — do not attempt to circumferentially mobilize the artery off the vein unless absolutely necessary. If the vein is inadvertently entered, repair it with a lateral 6-0 polypropylene suture rather than ligating it. Preserve the tibial nerve by staying anterior to it during the approach.

Embolectomy and Thrombectomy

Clinical Presentation and Diagnosis of Acute Arterial Occlusion

Acute arterial occlusion presents with the classic six Ps: pain (sudden onset, severe, distal), pallor, pulselessness, poikilothermia (cold limb), paresthesia, and paralysis — the last two (paresthesia and paralysis) are signs of advanced ischemia indicating tissue death if flow is not restored within hours. The two principal causes are embolism (a thrombus or atheromatous material from a proximal source — most commonly the left atrium in atrial fibrillation, a left ventricular mural thrombus after myocardial infarction, or an aortic or iliac plaque — lodging at an arterial bifurcation) and thrombosis (acute thrombosis of a pre-existing atherosclerotic stenosis or of a bypass graft). Distinguishing embolism from thrombosis guides management: embolic occlusion typically occurs in a patient with atrial fibrillation, is sudden in onset with no prior claudication history, affects the common femoral or popliteal bifurcation, and has no collateral development (the limb is profoundly ischemic); thrombotic occlusion occurs in a patient with known peripheral arterial disease, may have a stuttering onset with prior claudication, and often has better-developed collaterals (the limb is less acutely threatened). Acute limb ischemia is classified by the Rutherford system: category I (viable — no immediate threat, can tolerate further workup), category IIa (marginally threatened — salvageable if promptly treated), category IIb (immediately threatened — salvageable with immediate revascularization), and category III (irreversible — major tissue loss or permanent nerve damage, amputation indicated).

Balloon Catheter Embolectomy Technique

Balloon catheter (Fogarty catheter) embolectomy is performed through a transverse arteriotomy in the common femoral artery (the CFA is the preferred access point because it provides access to the entire lower extremity arterial tree and is easily exposed under local anesthesia). A 3-French or 4-French Fogarty embolectomy catheter is passed distally through the arteriotomy into the occluded vessel, advanced beyond the embolus, the balloon is inflated with saline (just enough to produce gentle apposition against the arterial wall — over-inflation causes intimal injury and vessel rupture), and the catheter is withdrawn, dragging the thrombus out through the arteriotomy. Multiple passes are made until no further thrombus is retrieved and brisk back-bleeding from the distal vasculature is established. Proximal embolectomy (into the iliac system and aorta) is performed with a larger (5-French or 6-French) Fogarty catheter passed retrograde through the same CFA arteriotomy. A completion angiogram is mandatory after embolectomy to confirm complete clot removal, exclude residual thrombus, and identify an underlying stenosis that may have caused the thrombosis. Intraoperative thrombolytic infusion (tissue plasminogen activator directly into the vessel through the embolectomy catheter) may be used as an adjunct for small-vessel thrombus that cannot be retrieved mechanically. Postoperatively, systemic anticoagulation with heparin is initiated immediately to prevent rethrombosis, followed by long-term oral anticoagulation (warfarin or a direct oral anticoagulant) if the embolic source is cardiac.

CAUTION: Reperfusion syndrome after revascularization of an acutely ischemic limb can produce a systemic inflammatory response with hyperkalemia (from release of intracellular potassium from ischemic muscle), myoglobinuria (from rhabdomyolysis, risking acute renal failure if myoglobin precipitates in the renal tubules), metabolic acidosis, and compartment syndrome. Monitor serum potassium, creatine kinase, and urine myoglobin closely after revascularization. Fasciotomy should be performed prophylactically if ischemia time exceeds 4 to 6 hours or if compartment pressures are elevated.

Operative Management of Peripheral Arterial Trauma

Principles of Vascular Trauma Management

Peripheral arterial injuries result from penetrating trauma (stab wounds, gunshot wounds — the most common mechanism in civilian practice), blunt trauma (fractures and dislocations — particularly supracondylar humeral fractures causing brachial artery injury in children, and knee dislocations causing popliteal artery injury in adults), and iatrogenic causes (catheterization, arterial lines). The clinical signs of arterial injury are divided into hard signs (active hemorrhage, expanding or pulsatile hematoma, palpable thrill or audible bruit, absent distal pulses with signs of ischemia — any hard sign mandates immediate operative exploration) and soft signs (history of hemorrhage now controlled, diminished but palpable distal pulses, proximity of the wound to a major vessel, peripheral nerve deficit — soft signs warrant further evaluation with CT angiography or duplex ultrasound). The ankle-brachial index (ABI) is a rapid screening tool — an ABI below 0.9 in an injured extremity is highly sensitive for arterial injury and warrants imaging.

Operative Repair Techniques

Operative repair follows a systematic approach: proximal and distal vascular control (clamps, vessel loops, or intraluminal balloon catheters — obtain control before exploring the hematoma), debridement to normal intima, Fogarty catheter thrombectomy proximally and distally, systemic heparinization (if the injury burden permits), and definitive repair. Options include lateral arteriorrhaphy (for small lacerations that can be repaired without reducing lumen diameter by more than 50%), end-to-end anastomosis (for less than 2 cm of arterial loss with tension-free mobilization), and interposition grafting (for greater than 2 cm segmental loss — reversed saphenous vein is the preferred conduit; prosthetic grafts are avoided in contaminated wounds). Temporary vascular shunts are used in damage-control settings when the patient is hemodynamically unstable — the shunt restores distal perfusion while the patient is resuscitated, with definitive repair at reoperation within 24 to 48 hours. Completion angiography confirms technical adequacy. Concomitant venous injuries are repaired when feasible to preserve venous outflow — ligation is reserved for damage control. Fasciotomy is performed liberally with prolonged ischemia (more than 4 to 6 hours), combined arteriovenous injury, or suspected compartment syndrome.

THE OPERATIVE DANGER ZONE ATLAS — Popliteal Artery Disruption in Posterior Knee Dislocation

The Zone: The popliteal fossa during posterior knee dislocation — the popliteal artery is tethered proximally at the adductor hiatus and distally at the soleal arch (where it passes beneath the tendinous arch of the soleus muscle). These two fixed points prevent the artery from accommodating the sudden posterior displacement of the tibia, placing maximum tensile and shearing force on the arterial segment between them.

The Structure at Risk: The popliteal artery. Popliteal artery injury occurs in approximately 20 to 40% of posterior knee dislocations — the injury ranges from intimal tears and thrombosis (which may present with initially palpable pulses that disappear over hours as the intimal flap propagates) to complete arterial transection. The popliteal vein and the common peroneal nerve (wrapping around the fibular neck) are frequently injured concurrently.

The Consequence: Missed popliteal artery injury after knee dislocation produces limb-threatening ischemia with an amputation rate of 80 to 90% if the ischemia time exceeds 6 to 8 hours. The popliteal artery has limited collateral pathways (the geniculate arteries), and acute occlusion — particularly when combined with popliteal vein injury — produces a profoundly ischemic limb that rapidly progresses to irreversible tissue death. Even reperfused limbs carry a 10 to 15% amputation rate from compartment syndrome and reperfusion injury.

The Safe Maneuver: All posterior knee dislocations require vascular assessment regardless of palpable pulses — perform serial ABI measurements (ABI less than 0.9 mandates CT angiography or immediate exploration) or obtain CT angiography on all patients. If arterial injury is confirmed, urgent exploration and repair (reversed saphenous vein interposition graft from the contralateral leg is the standard conduit) within 6 hours of injury is critical. In the damage-control setting, a temporary intraluminal vascular shunt restores perfusion immediately while the orthopedic injury is stabilized with an external fixator. Four-compartment fasciotomy of the leg is performed prophylactically in all patients with popliteal artery repair after knee dislocation.

Clinical Case — Acute Lower Extremity Ischemia From Femoral Artery Embolism

A 72-year-old man with atrial fibrillation (not anticoagulated) presents with sudden right leg pain and numbness of 3 hours duration. The right leg is pale and cool from mid-thigh distally with absent pulses below the groin. Sensation is diminished in the foot, but motor function is preserved (weakened dorsiflexion and plantar flexion) — Rutherford category IIb (immediately threatened). Urgent right CFA exploration under local anesthesia reveals a saddle embolus at the femoral bifurcation. A 4-French Fogarty catheter retrieves organized thrombus from the SFA and each tibial vessel; a 5-French catheter clears the iliac system proximally. Completion angiography confirms patent pedal flow with no residual thrombus. The arteriotomy is closed with patch angioplasty. Intravenous heparin is initiated immediately, transitioned to warfarin for long-term anticoagulation. At 24 hours, compartment pressures are normal —

the short ischemia time (3 hours) obviated fasciotomy. At 2-week follow-up, pedal pulses are palpable with full neurologic recovery.

THE OPERATIVE DANGER ZONE ATLAS — Arterial Surgery Dangers

Cranial Nerve Injury During Carotid Endarterectomy: The hypoglossal nerve (CN XII) crosses over the ICA and ECA at the superior extent of the dissection, and the vagus nerve (CN X) runs within the carotid sheath — injury during CEA causes tongue deviation, vocal cord paralysis, or airway compromise. **Safe maneuver:** identify CN XII before dividing any crossing tissue; locate CN X within the sheath before clamping; mobilize nerves with vessel loops, never sharp retraction.

Left Renal Vein Injury During Infrarenal Aortic Cross-Clamping: The left renal vein crosses the anterior aorta at the infrarenal neck — the exact site where the proximal aortic clamp must be placed. Injury produces brisk hemorrhage; ligation without intact collaterals (gonadal, adrenal, lumbar veins) causes renal failure. **Safe maneuver:** identify the left renal vein as the landmark for the infrarenal neck; retract it superiorly; if division is needed, confirm collateral branches are intact first.

Popliteal Vein Injury During Below-Knee Popliteal Artery Exposure: The popliteal vein lies immediately deep and posterior to the popliteal artery, sharing a common adventitial sheath — circumferential dissection of the artery for distal bypass anastomosis risks entering the vein. **Safe maneuver:** dissect only the anterior and lateral arterial surface; do not mobilize the artery off the vein unless necessary; repair any vein injury with lateral venorrhaphy rather than ligation.

Popliteal Artery Disruption in Posterior Knee Dislocation: The popliteal artery is tethered at the adductor hiatus and soleal arch — posterior knee dislocation tears or thromboses the artery in 20 to 40% of cases, with amputation rates exceeding 80% if ischemia time exceeds 6 to 8 hours. **Safe maneuver:** assess vascular status in all knee dislocations regardless of palpable pulses; obtain CT angiography or serial ABI; repair within 6 hours with reversed saphenous vein graft; perform prophylactic four-compartment fasciotomy.

Summary and Key Concepts

The carotid bulb (ICA origin) is the most common site of extracranial atherosclerotic disease — carotid endarterectomy is indicated for symptomatic stenosis of 50% or greater and asymptomatic stenosis of 60 to 70% or greater.

Patch angioplasty closure of the carotid arteriotomy is the standard of care — it significantly reduces perioperative stroke and long-term restenosis compared with primary closure.

Open infrarenal AAA repair uses the inlay technique — the aneurysm sac is opened but not excised, and the prosthetic graft is sewn within the sac, which is then closed over the graft to prevent aortoenteric fistula.

Endovascular aneurysm repair (EVAR) requires lifelong surveillance for endoleaks — Type I and III endoleaks are high-pressure leaks requiring immediate intervention, while Type II endoleaks are low-pressure and are observed unless the sac enlarges.

The greater saphenous vein is the conduit of choice for all infrainguinal arterial bypasses — it has superior long-term patency compared with prosthetic grafts, particularly for below-knee targets.

Acute arterial embolism is treated with Fogarty balloon catheter embolectomy through the common femoral artery — completion angiography is mandatory to confirm complete clot removal.

All posterior knee dislocations require vascular assessment regardless of palpable pulses — popliteal artery injury occurs in 20 to 40% of cases and carries an amputation rate exceeding 80% if ischemia time exceeds 6 to 8 hours.

CHAPTER 18: OPERATIONS OF THE VEINS AND LYMPHATICS

Learning Objectives

1. Describe the surgical anatomy of the superficial and deep venous systems of the lower extremity, including the saphenofemoral and saphenopopliteal junctions, the perforator veins, and the relationship between venous valvular incompetence and chronic venous insufficiency.
2. Perform venous thrombectomy for iliofemoral deep vein thrombosis and understand the indications for inferior vena cava filter placement.
3. Select the appropriate technique for varicose vein surgery (high ligation and stripping, endovenous thermal ablation, or ultrasound-guided foam sclerotherapy) based on anatomical pattern and clinical severity.
4. Apply the principles of lymph node biopsy, sentinel lymph node biopsy, and lymphovenous anastomosis for the management of lymphedema.

Surgical Anatomy of the Venous and Lymphatic Systems

Superficial and Deep Venous Systems of the Lower Extremity

The lower extremity venous system is divided into the superficial system (within the subcutaneous tissue, above the deep fascia), the deep system (within and deep to the muscular compartments), and the perforating veins (connecting the superficial to the deep system through the deep fascia). The great saphenous vein (GSV) is the principal superficial vein — it originates from the dorsal venous arch of the foot, ascends anterior to the medial malleolus, courses along the medial leg and thigh, and joins the common femoral vein at the saphenofemoral junction (SFJ) in the groin, approximately 4 cm below and lateral to the pubic tubercle. The SFJ is the critical surgical landmark in saphenous surgery — at this junction, the GSV passes through the saphenous opening (fossa ovalis) in the fascia lata to join the femoral vein. Several tributaries converge at the SFJ (the superficial epigastric, superficial circumflex iliac, and external pudendal veins — the so-called flush ligation requires division of all tributaries at the junction to prevent neovascularization and recurrence). The small saphenous vein (SSV) originates behind the lateral malleolus, ascends along the posterior calf, and typically joins the popliteal vein at the saphenopopliteal junction (SPJ) in the popliteal fossa — the level of the SPJ is variable (between 2 and 7 cm above the knee crease) and must be mapped with duplex ultrasound before surgery.

Deep Venous Anatomy and Perforators

The deep venous system of the lower extremity follows the arterial anatomy: paired tibial veins coalesce into the popliteal vein, which becomes the femoral vein (formerly called the superficial femoral vein — a misnomer that caused clinical errors, because ligation of this 'superficial' femoral vein actually ligates a deep vein, producing severe venous insufficiency), which joins the profunda femoris vein to form the common femoral vein below the inguinal ligament, continuing as the external iliac vein. Perforator veins connect the superficial to the deep system at predictable locations: the Cockett (posterior tibial) perforators along the medial lower leg, the Boyd perforator below the knee, and the Hunterian (mid-thigh) and Dodd (distal thigh) perforators along the medial thigh. Normal perforator valves direct flow from superficial to deep — when these valves become incompetent, blood refluxes from the deep system into the superficial veins during calf muscle contraction, producing ambulatory venous hypertension that drives the clinical syndrome of chronic venous insufficiency (skin changes, pigmentation, lipodermatosclerosis, and venous ulceration). The inferior vena cava (IVC) receives the common iliac veins at the L5 vertebral level and ascends to the right of the aorta to enter the right atrium through the diaphragm at the T8 level.

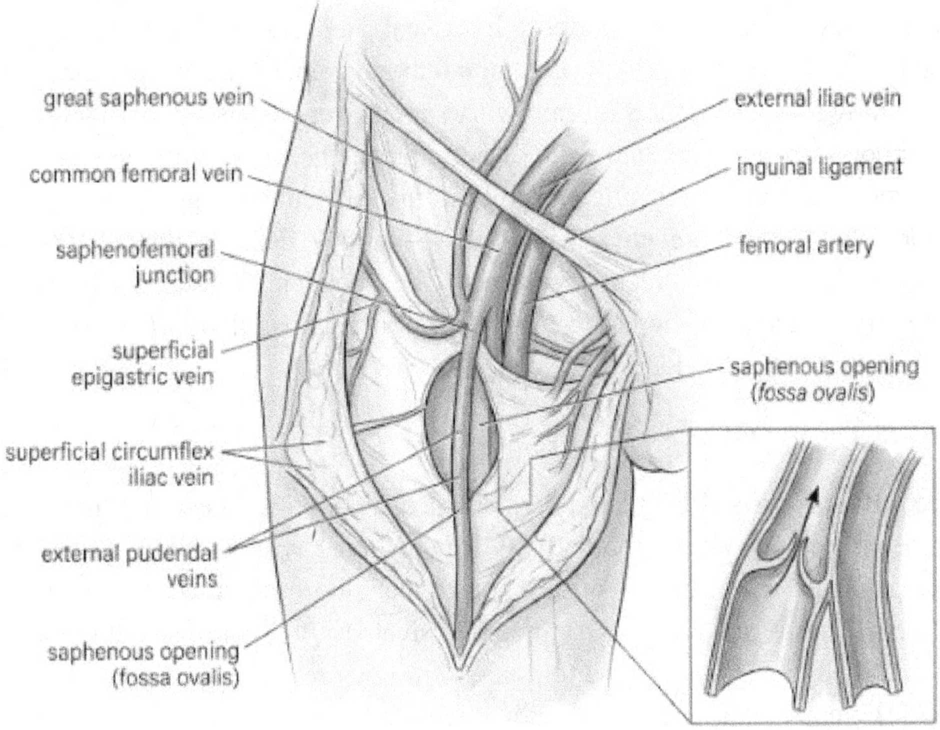

The Lymphatic System

The lymphatic system parallels the venous system and is responsible for interstitial fluid absorption, immune surveillance, and lipid transport. Lymph from the lower extremity drains through superficial lymphatics (following the GSV to the inguinal lymph nodes) and deep lymphatics (following the deep veins to the pelvic lymph nodes). The inguinal lymph nodes are divided into superficial (above the fascia lata, draining the skin of the lower extremity, perineum, and lower abdominal wall) and deep (within the femoral canal, medial to the femoral vein — the node of Cloquet or Rosenmuller is the most superior deep inguinal node). The thoracic duct is the largest lymphatic vessel, draining the entire body below the diaphragm and the left upper body — it ascends through the posterior mediastinum and arches over the left subclavian artery to drain into the junction of the left internal jugular and subclavian veins (the left venous angle). The right lymphatic duct drains the right upper body into the right venous angle. Surgical disruption of lymphatic channels (during groin dissection, axillary dissection, or pelvic lymphadenectomy) is the most common cause of secondary lymphedema.

Venous Thrombectomy and IVC Filter Placement

Indications for Surgical Venous Thrombectomy

Surgical venous thrombectomy is indicated for acute iliofemoral deep vein thrombosis (DVT) causing phlegmasia cerulea dolens (massive venous obstruction producing a cyanotic, swollen, painful limb with impending venous gangrene) or phlegmasia alba dolens (white, painful, swollen limb from extensive iliofemoral DVT) when pharmacomechanical catheter-directed thrombolysis is not available or has failed. The goal of thrombectomy is to restore venous outflow and prevent limb loss — a Fogarty venous thrombectomy catheter (a large-bore, balloon-tipped catheter designed for the low-pressure venous system) is passed through a venotomy in the common femoral vein, advanced into the iliac veins and IVC, inflated, and withdrawn to extract the thrombus. An arteriovenous fistula (a side-to-side anastomosis between the common femoral artery and vein, or a branch of the SFA to the femoral vein using a short saphenous vein loop) is constructed after thrombectomy to maintain high-velocity flow through the cleared iliofemoral segment and prevent rethrombosis — the AV fistula is ligated at 6 to 12 weeks when endothelialization of the venous lumen is complete. The patient is systemically anticoagulated with heparin intraoperatively and transitioned to long-term oral anticoagulation (minimum 6 months, often lifelong for unprovoked iliofemoral DVT).

Catheter-Directed Thrombolysis

Catheter-directed thrombolysis (CDT) and pharmacomechanical thrombectomy have largely supplanted open surgical thrombectomy for iliofemoral DVT in patients without phlegmasia. A multi-sidehole infusion catheter is placed directly into the thrombus under fluoroscopic guidance (via popliteal vein or posterior tibial vein access), and tissue plasminogen activator (tPA) is infused at 0.5 to 1.0 mg per hour for 12 to 24 hours, with serial venograms to assess thrombus resolution. Pharmacomechanical devices (AngioJet, EKOS) combine mechanical disruption with thrombolytic infusion to accelerate clot resolution and reduce the total lytic dose. The ATTRACT trial demonstrated that CDT reduces the severity of post-thrombotic syndrome (PTS) at 6 months in patients with proximal DVT, although the 24-month primary endpoint did not reach statistical significance — patient selection (younger patients, acute iliofemoral DVT with severe symptoms) is critical for identifying those most likely to benefit. After clot resolution, underlying iliac vein stenosis (particularly May-Thurner syndrome — compression of the left common iliac vein by the right common iliac artery) is identified by intravascular ultrasound (IVUS) and treated with venous stenting, which significantly reduces DVT recurrence.

Inferior Vena Cava Filter Placement

Inferior vena cava (IVC) filters are indicated for patients with acute proximal DVT or pulmonary embolism (PE) who have an absolute contraindication to therapeutic anticoagulation (active hemorrhage, recent intracranial surgery, hemorrhagic stroke), who have recurrent PE despite adequate anticoagulation, or who have massive PE with hemodynamic compromise where any additional embolic burden would be fatal. Retrievable IVC filters are preferred over permanent filters when the contraindication to anticoagulation is expected to resolve — the filter is placed via the femoral or internal jugular vein under fluoroscopic guidance and positioned in the infrarenal IVC below the renal veins (suprarenal placement is used when the thrombus extends above the renal veins or in pregnant patients to avoid compression by the gravid uterus). The filter is deployed at the L2-L3 level, and its position is confirmed fluoroscopically. Retrievable filters should be removed once the patient can be safely anticoagulated — prolonged filter dwell times increase the risk of IVC thrombosis (occurring in 5 to 30% of patients with permanent filters), filter migration, IVC perforation, filter fracture with embolization of strut fragments, and post-thrombotic syndrome from chronic IVC obstruction. Current guidelines emphasize that IVC filter placement does not substitute for anticoagulation — it prevents PE but does not treat DVT, and anticoagulation should be initiated as soon as the contraindication resolves.

THE OPERATIVE DANGER ZONE ATLAS — Iliac Vein Perforation During Venous Thrombectomy

The Zone: The common and external iliac veins during retrograde passage of a Fogarty venous thrombectomy catheter from the common femoral venotomy. The iliac veins are thin-walled, non-muscular vessels that lie on the pelvic brim — the catheter must navigate the confluence of the internal and external iliac veins and the junction with the IVC, areas where the vein wall is adherent to the periosteum and where chronic inflammation from organized thrombus further weakens the wall.

The Structure at Risk: The iliac vein wall. Unlike arterial walls, venous walls lack a robust muscular media and are easily perforated by excessive balloon inflation, forceful catheter advancement against organized or adherent thrombus, or misdirection of the catheter tip into a branch or through a weakened wall segment. The left common iliac vein is particularly vulnerable at the site of May-Thurner compression, where chronic pulsatile compression by the overlying right common iliac artery produces intimal hypertrophy (venous spur) and wall thinning.

The Consequence: Perforation of the iliac vein produces retroperitoneal hemorrhage — bleeding into the pelvis that is difficult to detect initially (the venotomy access is in the groin, so the surgeon does not directly visualize the pelvic veins) and difficult to control once identified. Retroperitoneal hemorrhage from a venous source is low-pressure but high-volume, producing hemodynamic instability if not recognized promptly. Open pelvic exploration to repair an iliac vein perforation is a major undertaking that significantly increases morbidity.

The Safe Maneuver: Inflate the thrombectomy balloon gently — use just enough saline to produce contact with the vein wall without overdistending it. Never force the catheter past resistance — if the catheter does not advance freely, organized thrombus may be adherent and requires catheter-directed thrombolysis rather than mechanical extraction. Use intraoperative fluoroscopy to confirm catheter position within the iliac vein before inflating the balloon. If the thrombus does not retrieve cleanly with gentle passes, convert to catheter-directed thrombolysis rather than escalating mechanical force. Monitor hemodynamic parameters continuously during thrombectomy — unexplained tachycardia or hypotension may indicate concealed retroperitoneal bleeding.

Varicose Vein Surgery and Endovenous Ablation

Classification and Clinical Assessment

Varicose veins are classified by the CEAP system — Clinical severity (C0 to C6: C0, no visible disease; C1, telangiectasias or reticular veins; C2, varicose veins; C3, edema; C4a, pigmentation or eczema; C4b, lipodermatosclerosis or atrophie blanche; C5, healed venous ulcer; C6, active venous ulcer), Etiology (congenital, primary, secondary), Anatomy (superficial, deep, perforator), and Pathophysiology (reflux, obstruction, both). Treatment is indicated for symptomatic varicose veins (C2 with symptoms — pain, heaviness, itching, night cramps), chronic venous insufficiency (C3 to C6), and for cosmetic concerns in C1 to C2 when conservative measures (compression stockings, exercise, elevation) have failed. Preoperative duplex ultrasound mapping is mandatory to identify the source and pattern of venous reflux — the ultrasound must demonstrate the saphenofemoral and saphenopopliteal junctions, the extent of GSV and SSV reflux, the status of the deep venous system (to exclude deep vein obstruction, which would make superficial ablation harmful), and incompetent perforator veins.

Endovenous Thermal Ablation

Endovenous thermal ablation (radiofrequency ablation [RFA] or endovenous laser ablation [EVLA]) has replaced open surgical stripping as the first-line treatment for GSV and SSV reflux. Under ultrasound guidance, the ablation catheter (radiofrequency: ClosureFast; laser: 1470 nm diode fiber) is introduced percutaneously through the GSV at or below the knee, advanced to within 2 cm of the SFJ (for the GSV) or 2 cm of the SPJ (for the SSV), and energy is delivered to produce thermal destruction of the vein wall, causing fibrosis and permanent occlusion. Tumescent anesthesia (dilute lidocaine with epinephrine in normal saline) is injected under ultrasound guidance around the entire length of the treated vein — the tumescent fluid serves three purposes: analgesia, compression of the vein wall around the catheter to maximize thermal contact, and a heat sink that protects the surrounding skin and saphenous nerve from thermal injury. The catheter tip must be positioned at least 2 cm from the SFJ to prevent thermal extension into the common femoral vein, which could produce deep vein thrombosis. Endovenous thermal ablation produces occlusion rates exceeding 95% at 5 years, with significantly less postoperative pain, faster return to normal activity, and equivalent long-term clinical outcomes compared with surgical stripping.

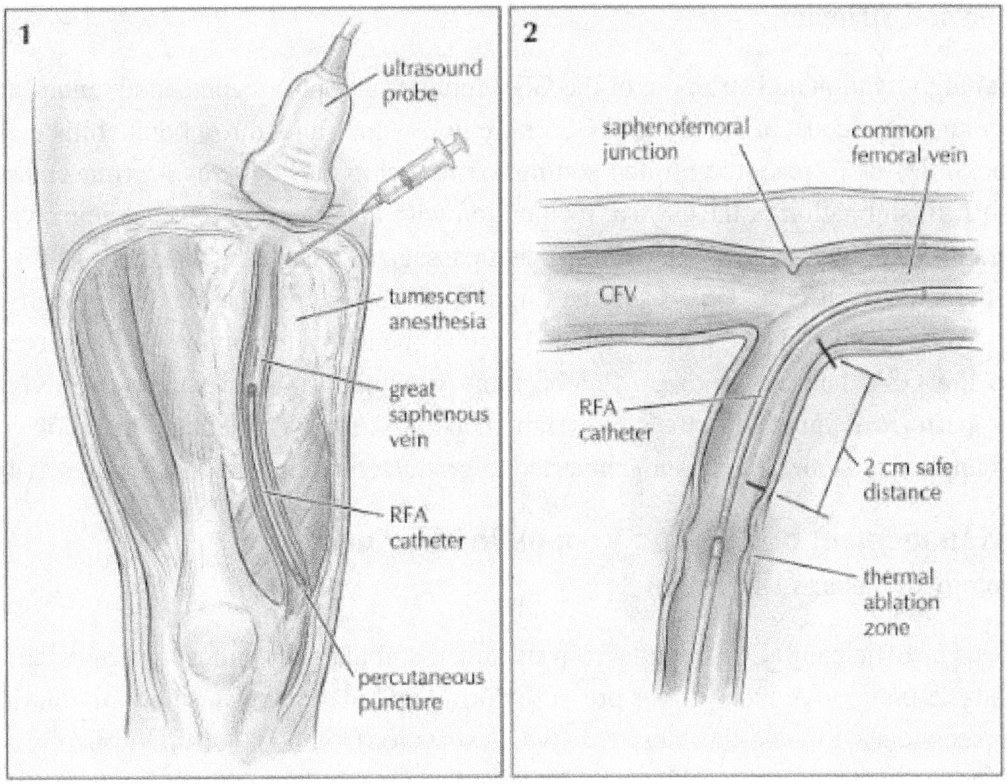

Complications of Endovenous Ablation

Complications of endovenous thermal ablation include endovenous heat-induced thrombosis (EHIT — extension of thrombus from the treated GSV into the common femoral vein, classified by extent: class 1, thrombus at the SFJ not extending into the CFV; class 2, thrombus extending less than 50% across the CFV lumen; class 3, thrombus extending more than 50% across the CFV; class 4, complete CFV occlusion). EHIT class 1 is observed with serial duplex ultrasound; class 2 and above are treated with therapeutic anticoagulation. The incidence of EHIT is approximately 1 to 3% and is minimized by positioning the catheter tip at least 2 cm from the SFJ and ensuring the GSV is compressed around the catheter by adequate tumescent anesthesia. Other complications include ecchymosis and induration along the treated vein (common, self-limited), skin burns (from inadequate tumescent insulation — more common with laser than radiofrequency), paresthesia from saphenous nerve thermal injury (2 to 5%, more common when below-knee GSV segments are treated), and phlebitis of untreated varicose tributaries (which may require secondary treatment with sclerotherapy or phlebectomy 4 to 6 weeks after the truncal ablation).

High Ligation and Stripping

Open surgical high ligation and stripping of the GSV remains an option when endovenous ablation is not feasible (very large, tortuous, or aneurysmal GSV; previous superficial thrombophlebitis making catheter passage impossible) or in resource-limited settings. The technique involves a groin crease incision to expose the SFJ, flush ligation of the GSV at its junction with the common femoral vein (with division of all SFJ tributaries to prevent neovascularization), and passage of a Babcock stripper or PIN stripper from the groin to the knee to strip the GSV from the thigh. The GSV below the knee is typically not stripped (to preserve it as a potential bypass conduit and to avoid saphenous nerve injury — the nerve runs in close proximity to the GSV below the knee). Phlebectomy (ambulatory stab avulsion) of visible varicose tributaries is performed through 2 to 3 mm stab incisions using a phlebectomy hook. Compression bandaging is applied postoperatively and converted to graduated compression stockings at 48 hours.

Surgical Management of Chronic Venous Insufficiency

Pathophysiology of Venous Ulceration

Chronic venous insufficiency (CVI) results from sustained ambulatory venous hypertension — the failure of the calf muscle pump to reduce venous pressure during ambulation because of valvular incompetence (primary or secondary to post-thrombotic valve destruction), venous obstruction, or both. Normal ambulatory venous pressure in the ankle drops from approximately 80 to 90 mmHg (standing hydrostatic pressure) to 20 to 30 mmHg during calf muscle contraction; in CVI, the pressure remains elevated at 60 to 80 mmHg because reflux through incompetent valves rapidly refills the venous system between contractions. This sustained venous hypertension is transmitted to the capillary bed, producing transcapillary fibrinogen leakage, pericapillary fibrin cuff deposition (the fibrin cuff hypothesis), white blood cell trapping and activation, release of inflammatory mediators, and ultimately tissue hypoxia, lipodermatosclerosis, and ulceration. Venous ulcers characteristically occur in the gaiter zone (above the medial malleolus), are shallow with irregular borders and a granulating base, and are associated with surrounding pigmentation (hemosiderin deposition), lipodermatosclerosis (woody induration), and dermatitis.

Surgical Interventions for Venous Ulceration

The cornerstone of venous ulcer management is compression therapy (multi-layer compression bandaging achieving 30 to 40 mmHg at the ankle), which reduces ambulatory venous hypertension and heals approximately 70% of venous ulcers within 6 months. Surgical interventions are added when compression alone fails or when correctable venous pathology is identified on duplex ultrasound. Superficial venous ablation (endovenous ablation or stripping of the incompetent GSV) is the most effective surgical intervention for venous ulcers — the EVRA trial demonstrated that early endovenous ablation combined with compression healed venous ulcers faster and reduced ulcer recurrence at 12 months compared with compression alone (hazard ratio 0.81 for time to healing). Subfascial endoscopic perforator surgery (SEPS) interrupts incompetent perforator veins beneath the deep fascia using an endoscopic approach through a small incision away from the ulcer bed — this is indicated when large incompetent perforators (greater than 3.5 mm) are identified on duplex ultrasound feeding the ulcer area, particularly when superficial reflux has already been treated. Deep venous reconstruction (valve repair, valve transposition, or venous stenting for iliac obstruction) is reserved for severe CVI refractory to superficial ablation and perforator interruption — deep venous surgery is technically demanding and performed at specialized centers.

THE OPERATIVE DANGER ZONE ATLAS — Common Femoral Vein Injury During Saphenofemoral Junction Ligation

The Zone: The saphenofemoral junction during high ligation of the great saphenous vein — the GSV joins the common femoral vein (CFV) through the saphenous opening in the fascia lata. The dissection to identify, isolate, and flush-ligate the GSV at its junction with the CFV occurs within centimeters of the femoral vein, femoral artery, and femoral nerve.

The Structure at Risk: The common femoral vein. The junction is a thin-walled, low-pressure vessel, and the tributary veins (superficial epigastric, superficial circumflex iliac, external pudendal) converge in a cluster around the SFJ that must be individually identified and divided. In redo groin surgery (for recurrent varicose veins), scarring from the previous operation obliterates the normal tissue planes and makes the CFV difficult to distinguish from the GSV stump, increasing the risk of inadvertent CFV ligation or lateral wall injury.

The Consequence: Inadvertent ligation of the common femoral vein produces acute deep venous obstruction of the entire lower extremity — massive limb swelling, venous hypertension, and risk of venous gangrene if collateral outflow through the profunda system is insufficient. Lateral injury to the CFV produces hemorrhage that is difficult to control in the confined groin dissection field. In redo surgery, CFV injury rates increase severalfold because the junction anatomy is distorted by scarring and neovascularization.

The Safe Maneuver: Identify the common femoral vein definitively before ligating any vessel at the SFJ — trace the GSV from the thigh into the junction rather than starting the dissection at the junction itself. Confirm the CFV by visualizing it above and below the SFJ (it continues as the external iliac vein above and receives the profunda femoris vein below). In redo surgery, use intraoperative duplex ultrasound to locate and mark the CFV before making the skin incision. Never ligate a vessel at the SFJ until you are certain it is the GSV and not the CFV — if uncertain, open the vessel and inspect for venous tributaries versus deep venous flow.

Lymph Node Biopsy and Lymphatic Surgery

Excisional and Sentinel Lymph Node Biopsy

Excisional lymph node biopsy is performed for diagnosis when fine-needle aspiration or core biopsy is inadequate — typically for suspected lymphoma (where architectural assessment of the entire node is essential for classification), granulomatous disease (sarcoidosis, tuberculosis), or reactive lymphadenopathy that fails to resolve. The node is excised intact (not incised or morcellated, which destroys architecture) through a small incision directly over the palpable node. The surgeon must orient the specimen for the pathologist and handle it gently (do not crush with forceps). For cervical lymph node biopsy, the spinal accessory nerve (CN XI), the phrenic nerve, and the internal jugular vein are at risk depending on the node's location within the posterior or anterior triangle. For inguinal lymph node biopsy, the saphenous vein and its tributaries, the femoral vessels, and the femoral nerve are at risk — the dissection should remain superficial to the fascia lata unless a deep inguinal node is specifically targeted.

Sentinel lymph node biopsy (SLNB) identifies the first node in the lymphatic drainage basin of a primary tumor — a negative sentinel node predicts that the remaining nodes in the basin are also negative, sparing the patient a complete lymphadenectomy. SLNB is the standard of care for clinically node-negative melanoma (Breslow thickness greater than 0.8 mm or with ulceration) and for clinically node-negative invasive breast cancer. The sentinel node is identified by preoperative lymphoscintigraphy (technetium-99m sulfur colloid injection around the primary tumor), intraoperative injection of a vital blue dye (isosulfan blue or methylene blue), or both — the sentinel node is the first node that is blue, hot (detected by the gamma probe), or both. Indocyanine green (ICG) fluorescence-guided SLNB using a near-infrared camera is an emerging alternative. The sentinel node is excised and examined by the pathologist (touch-prep cytology for intraoperative assessment, followed by permanent sectioning with immunohistochemistry for cytokeratin if initial sections are negative). False-negative rates for SLNB are approximately 5 to 10% and are minimized by dual-tracer technique, excising all blue and hot nodes, and ensuring the surgeon achieves a learning curve of at least 20 to 30 cases.

THE OPERATIVE DANGER ZONE ATLAS — Thoracic Duct Injury During Left Cervical Lymph Node Biopsy

---

The Zone: The left supraclavicular fossa and the confluence of the left internal jugular and subclavian veins (the left venous angle) — this is where the thoracic duct arches over the subclavian artery and drains into the venous system. Any surgical dissection in the left lower posterior triangle or supraclavicular region risks encountering the thoracic duct.

The Structure at Risk: The thoracic duct. It is the largest lymphatic vessel in the body, draining lymph and chyle (intestinal fat absorbed into the lacteals) from the entire body below the diaphragm and the left upper body. The duct is a thin, translucent, easily overlooked structure that is difficult to identify visually — lymphatic fluid is clear or milky (if the patient has recently eaten), and the duct lacks the obvious color and pulsatility of blood vessels.

The Consequence: Thoracic duct injury produces a chyle leak (chylous fistula) — persistent drainage of milky, lipid-rich lymphatic fluid through the wound or into the chest (chylothorax if the duct is injured during thoracic surgery). High-output chyle leaks (more than 500 mL per day) produce significant nutritional depletion (loss of protein, fat, fat-soluble vitamins, lymphocytes, and immunoglobulins), dehydration, and immunosuppression. A chyle leak that does not respond to conservative management (low-fat or medium-chain triglyceride diet, octreotide, total parenteral nutrition) requires surgical ligation of the thoracic duct — a technically challenging reoperation.

The Safe Maneuver: When performing lymph node biopsy in the left supraclavicular region, dissect superficially and avoid the deep triangle behind the clavicle where the thoracic duct enters the venous angle. If clear or milky fluid is encountered during dissection, immediately clip or ligate the leaking lymphatic — small lymphatic leaks that are ligated at the time of initial surgery rarely develop into clinically significant chyle fistulae. Ask the anesthesiologist to have the patient perform a Valsalva maneuver at the end of the dissection to increase thoracic duct pressure and reveal any occult leak before wound closure.

Lymphovenous Anastomosis and Vascularized Lymph Node Transfer

Surgical treatment of lymphedema has evolved from purely ablative procedures (debulking, liposuction) to physiological procedures that restore lymphatic drainage. Lymphovenous anastomosis (LVA) is a microsurgical technique that creates direct connections between functioning lymphatic channels and adjacent subdermal venules (0.3 to 0.8 mm diameter anastomoses) using supermicrosurgery (operating under 20 to 40 times magnification with 11-0 or 12-0 nylon sutures). LVA is most effective in early-stage lymphedema (ISL stage I to early stage II) when functioning lymphatic channels are still present — it is less effective in advanced fibrotic disease (late stage II to stage III) where lymphatic channels have been replaced by scar. Indocyanine green lymphangiography is used preoperatively and intraoperatively to identify patent lymphatic channels and map potential LVA sites. Vascularized lymph node transfer (VLNT) transplants a lymph node flap from an unaffected donor site (typically the lateral thoracic, submental, or supraclavicular nodes with their vascular pedicle) to the affected extremity — the transplanted nodes act as a lymphatic pump, absorbing interstitial fluid and draining it into the venous system through the flap's venous pedicle. VLNT is indicated for more advanced lymphedema and can be combined with LVA for optimal results.

KEY POINT: The EVRA trial demonstrated that early endovenous ablation of superficial venous reflux combined with compression heals venous ulcers faster and reduces ulcer recurrence at 12 months compared with compression therapy alone — establishing early intervention on the superficial venous system as the standard of care for venous ulceration in patients with confirmed superficial reflux.

Clinical Case — Phlegmasia Cerulea Dolens Requiring Venous Thrombectomy

A 54-year-old woman with recently diagnosed ovarian cancer presents with sudden onset of massive left leg swelling, cyanotic discoloration from the groin to the foot, and severe pain of 6 hours duration. The left leg is tense, dusky, and cool with absent pedal pulses (arterial compromise from venous congestion).

Duplex ultrasound confirms complete thrombosis of the left common femoral, external iliac, and common iliac veins. CT venography demonstrates extension into the IVC. The diagnosis is phlegmasia cerulea dolens — a surgical emergency. Intravenous heparin is started immediately. The patient is taken to the operating room for left common femoral venotomy and iliofemoral venous thrombectomy. A large-bore Fogarty venous catheter retrieves massive organized thrombus from the iliac veins and IVC under fluoroscopic guidance. After thrombectomy, a temporary arteriovenous fistula is constructed between a branch of the SFA and the femoral vein to maintain flow velocity and prevent rethrombosis. Completion venography demonstrates restored iliofemoral venous outflow. A prophylactic four-compartment below-knee fasciotomy is performed for the prolonged ischemia. Postoperatively, the leg color and temperature normalize within hours. The patient is maintained on therapeutic anticoagulation and transitions to long-term low-molecular-weight heparin (preferred in malignancy-associated VTE). The AV fistula is ligated at 8 weeks. At 3-month follow-up, the leg circumference is 2 cm larger than the contralateral side, with mild post-thrombotic edema managed with compression stockings.

THE OPERATIVE DANGER ZONE ATLAS — Venous and Lymphatic Surgery Dangers

Iliac Vein Perforation During Venous Thrombectomy: The iliac veins are thin-walled vessels that lie on the pelvic brim — aggressive catheter passage or balloon overinflation during thrombectomy risks perforation, producing retroperitoneal hemorrhage that is difficult to detect and control. **Safe maneuver:** inflate the balloon gently, never force past resistance, use fluoroscopic guidance, and convert to catheter-directed thrombolysis if organized thrombus does not retrieve cleanly.

Common Femoral Vein Injury During Saphenofemoral Junction Ligation: The CFV lies immediately deep to the SFJ — inadvertent ligation produces acute deep venous obstruction with massive limb swelling and risk of venous gangrene. Risk is highest in redo groin surgery where scarring distorts the anatomy. **Safe maneuver:** trace the GSV from the thigh into the junction; confirm the CFV above and below the SFJ; use intraoperative duplex in redo cases; never ligate until the vessel identity is certain.

Thoracic Duct Injury During Left Cervical Lymph Node Biopsy: The thoracic duct arches through the left supraclavicular fossa to drain into the left venous angle — dissection in this area risks duct injury, producing a chyle leak with nutritional depletion and immunosuppression. **Safe maneuver:** dissect superficially in the left supraclavicular region; clip any clear or milky lymphatic immediately; perform a Valsalva maneuver at the end of dissection to reveal occult leaks.

Saphenous Nerve Thermal Injury During Endovenous Ablation Below the Knee: The saphenous nerve runs in close proximity to the GSV below the knee, within the same fascial compartment — thermal ablation of the below-knee GSV risks nerve injury producing medial leg and foot numbness. **Safe maneuver:** limit thermal ablation to the above-knee GSV (the below-knee segment is treated with foam sclerotherapy or phlebectomy instead); ensure adequate tumescent anesthesia as a heat sink around the treated segment.

Summary and Key Concepts

The great saphenous vein joins the common femoral vein at the saphenofemoral junction approximately 4 cm below and lateral to the pubic tubercle — flush ligation of all SFJ tributaries is essential to prevent neovascularization and varicose vein recurrence.

Endovenous thermal ablation (radiofrequency or laser) has replaced open stripping as the first-line treatment for saphenous vein reflux, with occlusion rates exceeding 95% at 5 years and significantly less postoperative morbidity.

The EVRA trial established that early endovenous ablation combined with compression heals venous ulcers faster and reduces recurrence compared with compression alone.

Phlegmasia cerulea dolens (massive iliofemoral DVT with limb-threatening venous congestion) is a surgical emergency requiring venous thrombectomy or catheter-directed thrombolysis to prevent venous gangrene and limb loss.

Sentinel lymph node biopsy identifies the first draining node of a primary tumor — a negative sentinel node predicts negative regional nodes, sparing the patient complete lymphadenectomy.

The thoracic duct drains into the left venous angle (junction of the left internal jugular and subclavian veins) — surgical dissection in the left supraclavicular region risks thoracic duct injury producing a chyle leak.

Lymphovenous anastomosis is a microsurgical physiological procedure for early-stage lymphedema — it creates direct connections between functioning lymphatic channels and subdermal venules to bypass obstructed lymphatic pathways.

CHAPTER 19: OPERATIONS OF THE CHEST

Learning Objectives

1. Describe the surgical anatomy of the thorax, including the intercostal neurovascular bundle, the pulmonary hilum, the mediastinal compartments, and the course of the recurrent laryngeal nerves.
2. Perform a thoracotomy and a video-assisted thoracoscopic (VATS) approach with appropriate port placement, single-lung ventilation, and safe entry into the pleural space.
3. Execute the key steps of anatomic pulmonary resection (lobectomy, segmentectomy, pneumonectomy), including individual ligation of the hilar structures and bronchial stump management.
4. Manage empyema and trapped lung through decortication, and place and manage a chest tube using the triangle of safety.

Surgical Anatomy of the Thorax

The Chest Wall and Intercostal Neurovascular Bundle

The chest wall consists of 12 pairs of ribs, the sternum, and the thoracic vertebrae, covered by layers of muscle (external intercostal, internal intercostal, and innermost intercostal muscles). The intercostal neurovascular bundle (vein, artery, nerve — VAN, from superior to inferior) runs in the costal groove along the inferior border of each rib, between the internal intercostal and innermost intercostal muscles. This anatomical relationship dictates that all chest wall procedures (thoracotomy, chest tube insertion, intercostal nerve block) must enter the pleural space or the intercostal space by passing over the superior border of the rib below, not along the inferior border where the neurovascular bundle lies. The internal thoracic (internal mammary) arteries descend 1 to 2 cm lateral to the sternal border, supplying the anterior chest wall and giving rise to the superior epigastric artery — they are at risk during parasternal incisions, anterior chest wall resections, and during internal mammary lymph node dissection for breast cancer staging.

Pulmonary Hilum and Fissures

The pulmonary hilum contains the pulmonary artery, two pulmonary veins (superior and inferior), the bronchus, bronchial arteries, lymph nodes, and the pulmonary ligament. On the right, the anatomy from anterior to posterior is: superior pulmonary vein, pulmonary artery (the right main pulmonary artery passes anterior to the right main bronchus), and bronchus (eparterial — the right upper lobe bronchus arises above the pulmonary artery, which is unique to the right side). On the left, the pulmonary artery arches over the left main bronchus (the artery is superior and the bronchus is posterior and inferior) — the left main bronchus is longer than the right, and the left recurrent laryngeal nerve loops beneath the aortic arch at the level of the ligamentum arteriosum before ascending between the trachea and esophagus to innervate the left vocal cord. The oblique fissure separates the upper from the lower lobe on both sides; the horizontal (minor) fissure on the right separates the upper from the middle lobe. Incomplete fissures (occurring in 30 to 50% of patients) complicate anatomic lobectomy because the parenchymal bridge between lobes must be divided with a stapler, increasing the risk of air leak.

The Mediastinum

The mediastinum is divided into anterior (between the sternum and the pericardium — containing the thymus, fat, lymph nodes, and internal mammary vessels), middle (containing the heart, pericardium, great vessels, trachea, main bronchi, and phrenic nerves), and posterior (between the pericardium and the vertebral bodies — containing the esophagus, descending aorta, thoracic duct, vagus nerves, sympathetic chains, and azygos venous system) compartments. Each compartment has a characteristic differential diagnosis for masses: anterior mediastinum — thymoma, lymphoma, teratoma, thyroid goiter (the 4 Ts, with thyroid replacing the older 'terrible lymphoma'); middle mediastinum — bronchogenic cyst, lymphadenopathy, pericardial cyst; posterior mediastinum — neurogenic tumors (schwannoma, neurofibroma, ganglioneuroma), esophageal duplication cyst, meningocele.

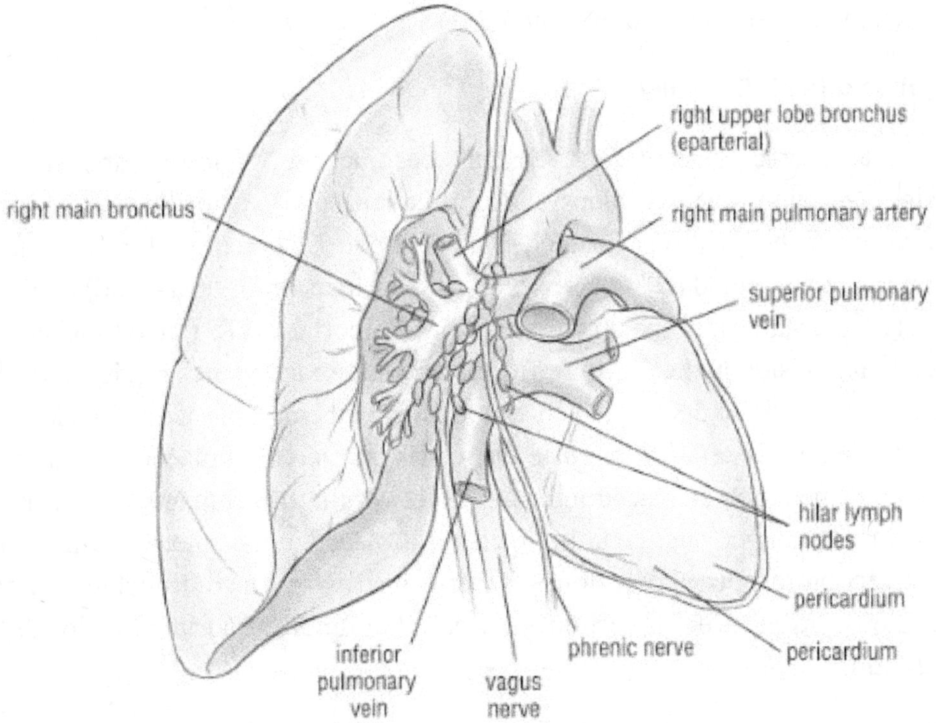

Thoracotomy and Video-Assisted Thoracoscopic Surgery (VATS)

Posterolateral Thoracotomy

Posterolateral thoracotomy provides the widest exposure to the hemithorax and remains the standard approach for complex pulmonary resections, esophageal surgery, and thoracic emergencies. The patient is placed in the lateral decubitus position with the operative side up. The incision extends from the anterior axillary line posteriorly and inferiorly around the tip of the scapula, curving superiorly between the scapula and the spine. The latissimus dorsi and serratus anterior muscles are divided (or the serratus is spared by retracting it anteriorly in muscle-sparing modifications). The pleural space is entered through the fifth intercostal space (for upper lobe surgery) or sixth intercostal space (for lower lobe surgery) by incising the intercostal muscles along the superior border of the rib below. A rib spreader (Finochietto retractor) is placed and opened gradually to avoid rib fracture. At closure, pericostal sutures are placed around the ribs above and below (not through the ribs, which fracture easily) to approximate the intercostal space, and the muscles are closed in layers. An intercostal nerve block with bupivacaine or placement of an epidural catheter provides postoperative analgesia — inadequate pain control after thoracotomy produces splinting, hypoventilation, retained secretions, and pneumonia.

VATS Technique and Port Placement

Video-assisted thoracoscopic surgery (VATS) has become the preferred approach for anatomic lobectomy, wedge resection, pleural biopsy, decortication, and sympathectomy, offering reduced postoperative pain, shorter hospital stays, and equivalent oncologic outcomes for early-stage lung cancer compared with thoracotomy. Standard VATS uses 2 to 4 port incisions (5 to 12 mm) and a utility incision (3 to 5 cm, without rib spreading) for specimen extraction. Uniportal VATS (single-incision thoracoscopy) uses a single 3 to 4 cm incision in the fourth or fifth intercostal space in the anterior axillary line. Single-lung ventilation (achieved with a double-lumen endotracheal tube or a bronchial blocker) is essential for VATS — the operative lung is deflated to create the working space. Port placement follows the principle of triangulation: the camera port is placed inferiorly, the working instruments are placed through ports that triangulate toward the target, and the utility incision is placed in the anterior axillary line at the level of the hilum. Conversion to open thoracotomy is performed when uncontrollable hemorrhage occurs, when dense adhesions prevent safe dissection, or when the tumor is too large or locally advanced for thoracoscopic resection.

Pulmonary Resection (Lobectomy, Segmentectomy, Pneumonectomy)

Preoperative Pulmonary Assessment for Lung Resection

Every candidate for anatomic lung resection requires preoperative assessment of pulmonary reserve to determine whether the patient can tolerate the planned resection without postoperative respiratory failure. The initial assessment is spirometry: predicted postoperative (ppo) FEV1 and ppoDLCO are calculated by multiplying the preoperative value by the fraction of functioning lung segments that will remain after resection (the segment-counting method or quantitative perfusion scanning). If both ppoFEV1 and ppoDLCO are greater than 60% predicted, the patient is considered low-risk and no further testing is needed. If either is between 30% and 60% predicted, cardiopulmonary exercise testing (CPET) with measurement of peak oxygen consumption (VO2max) is performed — a VO2max greater than 20 mL/kg/min indicates low risk, 10 to 20 mL/kg/min indicates moderate risk, and less than 10 mL/kg/min indicates high risk (lobectomy may still be considered in high-risk patients using sublobar resection or after preoperative pulmonary rehabilitation, but pneumonectomy is generally contraindicated). Stair climbing is a simple surrogate: a patient who can climb five flights of stairs without stopping has adequate reserve for lobectomy. Smoking cessation for at least 4 weeks before surgery reduces postoperative pulmonary complications by approximately 50%.

Anatomic Lobectomy

Anatomic lobectomy with systematic mediastinal lymph node dissection is the standard surgical treatment for early-stage non-small cell lung cancer (NSCLC) in patients with adequate pulmonary reserve. The operation involves individual identification, ligation, and division of the lobar pulmonary artery branches, the lobar pulmonary vein (or veins), and the lobar bronchus — these three hilar structures are stapled or ligated individually (not en masse, which prevents accurate pathological staging and increases the risk of bronchopleural fistula). The fissure is completed with an endoscopic stapler where incomplete. The sequence of hilar dissection varies by lobe: for right upper lobectomy, the truncus anterior branch of the pulmonary artery is divided first, followed by the superior pulmonary vein, then the right upper lobe bronchus, and finally the posterior ascending artery; for right lower lobectomy, the inferior pulmonary vein is divided first, then the basilar artery trunk, the superior segmental artery, and the lower lobe bronchus. Mediastinal lymph node dissection (stations 2R, 4R, 7, 8, 9 on the right; stations 5, 6, 7, 8, 9 on the left) is performed for staging and has been shown to improve staging accuracy and may improve survival compared with lymph node sampling alone.

Sublobar Resection — Segmentectomy and Wedge Resection

Anatomic segmentectomy has emerged as an oncologically acceptable alternative to lobectomy for small (2 cm or less) peripheral NSCLC based on the JCOG0802 and CALGB 140503 trials, which demonstrated equivalent overall survival and lower rates of pulmonary function loss compared with lobectomy. Segmentectomy requires identification and division of the segmental artery, segmental vein, and segmental bronchus, followed by division of the intersegmental plane (identified by inflation-deflation demarcation or indocyanine green fluorescence). Adequate surgical margins (at least 2 cm or greater than the tumor diameter, whichever is larger) are mandatory. Wedge resection (non-anatomic stapled excision of the lung parenchyma containing the tumor) is reserved for patients with insufficient pulmonary reserve for lobectomy or segmentectomy, for diagnostic biopsies of indeterminate pulmonary nodules, and for metastasectomy — wedge resection has higher local recurrence rates than anatomic resection for primary lung cancer.

THE OPERATIVE DANGER ZONE ATLAS — Pulmonary Artery Injury During Hilar Dissection for Lobectomy

The Zone: The pulmonary hilum during individual ligation of the lobar pulmonary artery branches — particularly the posterior ascending artery of the right upper lobe (which arises from the interlobar portion of the pulmonary artery within the fissure), the superior segmental artery of the lower lobe (which must be identified separately from the basilar trunk), and the left upper lobe artery branches (which lie in close proximity to the left main pulmonary artery).

The Structure at Risk: The main pulmonary artery and its major branches. The pulmonary artery is a thin-walled, high-flow vessel that operates at low pressure (systolic 25 mmHg) — its wall is significantly thinner and more fragile than systemic arteries of comparable caliber. Traction on a lobar branch during dissection can tear the branch at its origin from the main pulmonary artery, converting a controlled lobectomy into an uncontrolled hemorrhage from the main pulmonary artery.

The Consequence: Pulmonary artery injury during lobectomy produces rapid, high-volume hemorrhage that fills the operative field and can be fatal within minutes. In VATS lobectomy, the confined working space makes hemorrhage control particularly challenging — blood obscures the camera, and the surgeon must decide rapidly between attempting VATS repair and converting to thoracotomy. The mortality rate of intraoperative pulmonary artery injury during lobectomy is 1 to 2%.

The Safe Maneuver: Dissect each pulmonary artery branch individually with meticulous technique — encircle each branch with a vessel loop before stapling or ligating. Avoid excessive traction on artery branches, which can avulse them at their origin. When working in an incomplete fissure, divide the parenchymal bridge with a stapler BEFORE dissecting the artery in the fissure — the stapler creates a controlled division plane and avoids blind dissection near the artery. If hemorrhage occurs during VATS, apply direct pressure with a sponge stick, maintain single-lung ventilation, and convert to thoracotomy immediately — do not persist with VATS repair of a major pulmonary artery injury.

Pneumonectomy

Pneumonectomy (removal of the entire lung) is indicated when the tumor involves the main bronchus, extends across the fissure to involve multiple lobes, or involves the main pulmonary artery at its origin in a way that precludes individual lobar vessel division. Pneumonectomy carries significantly higher morbidity and mortality than lobectomy (operative mortality 5 to 8% versus 1 to 3% for lobectomy), and right pneumonectomy carries higher mortality than left pneumonectomy because the right lung contributes approximately 55% of total lung function. The hilar structures are divided individually: the main pulmonary artery is doubly ligated and divided, the superior and inferior pulmonary veins are stapled individually, and the main bronchus is divided with a bronchial stapler as close to the carina as possible (a long bronchial stump is at higher risk for bronchopleural fistula because it lacks the blood supply to heal). The bronchial stump is reinforced with a pedicled intercostal muscle flap, pericardial fat pad, or pleural flap — particularly after right pneumonectomy and after induction chemoradiation, which impairs bronchial stump healing. The pneumonectomy space fills with serous fluid over weeks and eventually obliterates. A balanced chest tube (if placed) is maintained on water seal only — NEVER on suction, because suction shifts the mediastinum toward the pneumonectomy side, compressing the remaining lung and producing cardiovascular compromise.

Complications of Pulmonary Resection

The major complications of pulmonary resection include air leak (the most common complication, occurring in 10 to 15% of lobectomies — most seal spontaneously within 5 to 7 days; persistent air leak beyond 7 days may require pleurodesis, autologous blood patch, or reoperation), bronchopleural fistula (BPF — a communication between the bronchial stump and the pleural space, occurring in 1 to 4% of pneumonectomies and less than 0.5% of lobectomies, presenting with sudden massive air leak, subcutaneous emphysema, and empyema; BPF is a surgical emergency requiring chest tube drainage of the empyema and stump revision with muscle flap reinforcement), postoperative pneumonia (5 to 10%, higher in patients with poor preoperative pulmonary function and inadequate pain control), atrial fibrillation (10 to 20% after lobectomy, up to 40% after pneumonectomy — the most common cardiac complication, managed with rate control and cardioversion), and post-pneumonectomy pulmonary edema (a poorly understood form of acute lung injury affecting the remaining lung after pneumonectomy, with a mortality rate exceeding 50% — minimized by restricting intraoperative and postoperative intravenous fluids to less than 2 liters in the first 24 hours).

Chest Wall Resection and Reconstruction

Indications and Oncologic Principles

Chest wall resection is indicated for primary chest wall tumors (chondrosarcoma — the most common primary malignant chest wall tumor, Ewing sarcoma, osteosarcoma, soft tissue sarcomas), for locally invasive lung cancers directly extending into the chest wall (T3 NSCLC — en bloc chest wall resection with lobectomy is standard for these tumors), and for radiation-induced chest wall necrosis. The oncologic principle is wide local excision with at least 4 cm margins for primary malignancies (or an uninvolved rib above and below the tumor), with en bloc resection of the involved lung parenchyma if the tumor extends into the lung. Reconstruction depends on the size and location of the defect: defects less than 5 cm or those covered by the scapula may not require prosthetic reconstruction; larger defects require a rigid prosthetic patch (polypropylene mesh, Gore-Tex, or methylmethacrylate sandwich — two layers of mesh with methylmethacrylate cement between them for chest wall rigidity) to prevent paradoxical chest wall motion and respiratory compromise, covered by a soft tissue flap (latissimus dorsi, pectoralis major, rectus abdominis, or omentum) for wound coverage and obliteration of dead space.

THE OPERATIVE DANGER ZONE ATLAS — Intercostal Artery Hemorrhage During Chest Wall Resection

The Zone: The posterior intercostal space during chest wall resection — the posterior intercostal arteries arise directly from the descending thoracic aorta (intercostal spaces 3 through 11) and are high-pressure vessels with substantial diameter (3 to 5 mm) that retract into the paravertebral musculature when transected, making hemostasis difficult.

The Structure at Risk: The posterior intercostal arteries. Unlike the anterior intercostal arteries (which arise from the internal thoracic artery and are small, easily controlled), the posterior intercostal arteries are direct aortic branches operating at systemic arterial pressure. They run along the costal groove beneath the intercostal vein and nerve, and their posterior segments are deep to the erector spinae muscles, where retraction after transection makes them inaccessible to direct clamping.

The Consequence: Transection of a posterior intercostal artery without prior control produces brisk arterial hemorrhage that can be difficult to identify and control — the artery retracts posteriorly into the paravertebral muscles, and blind clamping in this area risks injury to the thoracic spinal cord (the artery of Adamkiewicz, the major anterior spinal cord feeder, arises from a posterior intercostal artery, most commonly on the left between T9 and T12).

The Safe Maneuver: Ligate or clip posterior intercostal arteries BEFORE dividing the rib or intercostal space — identify each artery in the costal groove by palpation or direct visualization as the rib is exposed, and place clips or suture ligatures on both sides of the planned transection point. When performing wide chest wall resections, control the intercostal vessels at the posterior extent of the resection first (working from posterior to anterior). If a retracted intercostal artery bleeds from within the paravertebral muscles, identify the bleeding point with gentle muscle separation and place a figure-of-eight absorbable suture — do not blindly clamp deeply, because the spinal canal is immediately medial.

Decortication and Empyema Management

Staging and Operative Management of Empyema

Empyema (infection within the pleural space) progresses through three stages: stage 1 (exudative — free-flowing parapneumonic effusion with thin fluid and low WBC count, managed by chest tube drainage and antibiotics), stage 2 (fibrinopurulent — loculated fluid with fibrin strands and septations dividing the pleural space into pockets that impede drainage, requiring either intrapleural fibrinolytic therapy with tPA and DNase or VATS debridement and washout), and stage 3 (organizing — a thick, inelastic fibrous peel (cortex) encases the lung, preventing re-expansion even after fluid evacuation, requiring formal decortication). Decortication is the surgical removal of the fibrous peel from the visceral pleural surface to allow the trapped lung to re-expand and fill the hemithorax. It is performed via VATS (for early stage 3 with a relatively thin peel) or thoracotomy (for established stage 3 with a thick, leathery cortex). The peel is incised and peeled off the visceral pleura using a combination of blunt and sharp dissection, working from the apex toward the diaphragm — the dissection plane is between the peel and the visceral pleura, which must be preserved to prevent massive air leak from the lung surface. Complete decortication allows the lung to expand fully, obliterating the empyema cavity and restoring ventilatory mechanics.

Open Window Thoracostomy and Muscle Flap Closure

Open window thoracostomy (Eloesser flap or Clagett procedure) is reserved for patients who are too debilitated for formal decortication, who have a chronic empyema cavity that cannot be obliterated by lung re-expansion, or who have a bronchopleural fistula with ongoing contamination. One to three rib segments are resected overlying the empyema cavity, and the skin edges are marsupialized to the parietal pleura to create a permanent open window into the pleural space — this allows the empyema cavity to drain freely, be packed with damp dressings, and gradually fill with granulation tissue. Once the cavity is clean and granulating (typically weeks to months), it may be closed in a staged fashion using a muscle flap (latissimus dorsi, serratus anterior, or pectoralis major rotated into the cavity to obliterate the dead space) with or without an omental flap. The Clagett procedure (open drainage followed by filling the cavity with antibiotic solution and primary wound closure) is an alternative for selected patients with a clean, well-granulated cavity and no bronchopleural fistula.

Mediastinal Surgery

Mediastinoscopy and Mediastinal Lymph Node Assessment

Cervical mediastinoscopy is the gold-standard procedure for pathological staging of mediastinal lymph nodes in lung cancer. A 3 cm transverse incision is made in the suprasternal notch, and the pretracheal fascia is entered with blunt finger dissection. A mediastinoscope is advanced along the anterior surface of the trachea into the superior and middle mediastinum, allowing biopsy of paratracheal (stations 2R, 2L, 4R, 4L), subcarinal (station 7), and tracheobronchial lymph nodes. The principal hazard is hemorrhage from inadvertent biopsy of a mediastinal vessel — the innominate artery crosses anterior to the trachea at the level of the sternal notch and must be identified by palpation before the mediastinoscope is advanced. The left recurrent laryngeal nerve runs in the tracheoesophageal groove and is at risk during left paratracheal node biopsy. Endobronchial ultrasound-guided transbronchial needle aspiration (EBUS-TBNA) has largely replaced mediastinoscopy as the initial mediastinal staging procedure because it is less invasive and can access the same stations plus hilar nodes, but mediastinoscopy remains indicated when EBUS results are negative in patients with high clinical suspicion of N2 disease (where a false-negative EBUS would alter the treatment plan).

Thymectomy

Thymectomy is performed for thymoma (the most common anterior mediastinal tumor in adults — all thymomas require resection regardless of size because even small, encapsulated thymomas carry a risk of local invasion and recurrence) and for myasthenia gravis (MG — thymectomy produces clinical improvement or complete stable remission in approximately 60 to 70% of patients with non-thymomatous generalized MG, as demonstrated by the MGTX trial). The operative approaches include transcervical thymectomy (less invasive but limited exposure), partial sternotomy, full median sternotomy (the traditional approach for complete thymectomy, providing the widest exposure for resection of invasive thymoma), and robotic-assisted or VATS thymectomy (increasingly the standard for non-invasive thymoma and for MG without thymoma). Complete resection includes removal of all thymic tissue and the surrounding anterior mediastinal fat, because ectopic thymic tissue may harbor the pathology driving myasthenia. For invasive thymoma (Masaoka stage III or IV), en bloc resection of invaded structures (pericardium, lung, phrenic nerve, great vessels) is performed.

THE OPERATIVE DANGER ZONE ATLAS — Innominate Artery Injury During Cervical Mediastinoscopy

The Zone: The pretracheal space at the level of the thoracic inlet during cervical mediastinoscopy — the innominate (brachiocephalic) artery crosses the anterior surface of the trachea from left to right at approximately the level of the sternal notch, directly in the path of the advancing mediastinoscope.

The Structure at Risk: The innominate artery (the first branch of the aortic arch). It crosses the trachea at a level where the mediastinoscope is being advanced blindly through the pretracheal fascia — the artery pulsates and can be identified by palpation, but in the confined, blood-stained pretracheal space, it may be mistaken for a lymph node and biopsied. The superior vena cava, the azygos vein, and the main pulmonary artery are also at risk from deep biopsy in the subcarinal and right paratracheal stations.

The Consequence: Biopsy of the innominate artery produces life-threatening mediastinal hemorrhage — high-pressure arterial bleeding in the confined pretracheal space that is extremely difficult to control through the mediastinoscopy incision. Emergency sternotomy is required to achieve vascular control and repair the arterial injury. The mortality rate of major vascular injury during mediastinoscopy is approximately 5 to 10%.

The Safe Maneuver: Palpate the innominate artery with the index finger in the pretracheal space BEFORE inserting the mediastinoscope — it is a firm, pulsatile structure crossing the trachea at the level of the sternal notch. Never biopsy a pulsatile structure. Use the mediastinoscope to gently displace tissue and identify lymph nodes by their firm, non-pulsatile character before taking a biopsy. Use needle aspiration of suspicious nodes before excisional biopsy — aspiration of bright red blood confirms a vascular structure. Keep an emergency sternotomy tray available in the operating room during every mediastinoscopy.

Chest Tube Insertion and Management

Indications, Technique, and the Triangle of Safety

Chest tube (intercostal drain) insertion is indicated for pneumothorax (traumatic, spontaneous, or tension), hemothorax, pleural effusion requiring drainage, empyema, and postoperatively after thoracotomy or VATS. The standard insertion site is the triangle of safety — bordered anteriorly by the lateral border of the pectoralis major, posteriorly by the lateral border of the latissimus dorsi, inferiorly by a horizontal line at the level of the nipple (fifth intercostal space), and superiorly by the axilla. Insertion within this triangle avoids injury to the internal thoracic vessels (too anterior), the long thoracic nerve (too posterior), and the diaphragm and abdominal organs (too inferior). The technique involves a 2 to 3 cm incision over the rib below the target intercostal space, blunt dissection through the subcutaneous tissue and intercostal muscles using a curved clamp (entering over the superior border of the rib to avoid the intercostal neurovascular bundle below), digital exploration of the pleural space to confirm entry and sweep away adhesions, and insertion of the chest tube (28 to 32 French for hemothorax or empyema; 20 to 24 French for pneumothorax or simple effusion) directed apically for pneumothorax or basally for fluid. The tube is connected to an underwater seal drain (three-chamber system) with 20 cm H2O suction. The tube is secured with a suture and an occlusive dressing.

Management and Removal

Chest tube output is monitored for volume, character (blood, serous fluid, chyle, air), and trend. Criteria for chest tube removal include resolution of the indication (lung fully expanded on chest radiograph for pneumothorax; air leak ceased for more than 24 hours; fluid output less than 200 mL per 24 hours for effusion or hemothorax), absence of air leak on coughing or Valsalva, and clinical stability. The tube is removed at end-expiration (or during a Valsalva maneuver) to minimize the risk of air entry during removal. A retained hemothorax (more than 300 to 500 mL on imaging after initial tube drainage) requires early VATS evacuation — delayed intervention allows organization of the clot, producing fibrothorax and trapped lung that may ultimately require decortication. Massive hemothorax (initial output greater than 1,500 mL or ongoing output greater than 200 mL per hour for 2 to 4 hours) indicates a major vascular or parenchymal injury requiring urgent thoracotomy for hemorrhage control.

CLINICAL PEARL: The triangle of safety for chest tube insertion (anterior border of latissimus dorsi, lateral border of pectoralis major, fifth intercostal space at nipple level) avoids the most common sites of insertion-related injury. Chest tubes placed too anteriorly risk internal mammary vessel injury; too posteriorly risk the long thoracic nerve (producing winged scapula); too inferiorly risk transdiaphragmatic placement into the liver (right) or spleen (left).

Clinical Case — VATS Lobectomy for Early-Stage Lung Cancer

A 63-year-old woman with a 40-pack-year smoking history is found to have a 2.5 cm spiculated nodule in the right upper lobe on a low-dose CT lung cancer screening study. PET-CT demonstrates FDG avidity (SUVmax 8.2) in the nodule with no mediastinal lymph node uptake. EBUS-TBNA of stations 4R and 7 is negative for malignancy. Pulmonary function testing shows FEV1 of 2.1 L (85% predicted) with adequate DLCO. CT-guided percutaneous biopsy confirms adenocarcinoma. The patient undergoes VATS right upper lobectomy with systematic mediastinal lymph node dissection. Under single-lung ventilation, three port incisions and a 4 cm utility incision are placed. The truncus anterior branch of the pulmonary artery is identified, encircled, and divided with an endoscopic vascular stapler. The superior pulmonary vein is divided. The right upper lobe bronchus is divided with a bronchial stapler, and the posterior ascending artery is divided. The fissure is completed with a thick-tissue stapler. The specimen is extracted in a bag through the utility incision. Mediastinal lymph node dissection of stations 2R, 4R, 7, 8, and 9 yields 18 nodes, all negative for metastasis. Final pathology: pT1cN0M0 stage IA3 adenocarcinoma with negative margins. The patient is discharged on postoperative day 3 with the chest tube removed on day 2.

THE OPERATIVE DANGER ZONE ATLAS — Thoracic Surgery Dangers

Pulmonary Artery Injury During Hilar Dissection for Lobectomy: The pulmonary artery is thin-walled and fragile — traction on a lobar branch during dissection can avulse it from the main pulmonary artery, producing rapid, life-threatening hemorrhage. **Safe maneuver:** encircle each artery branch with a vessel loop before stapling; divide incomplete fissures with a stapler before dissecting arteries within them; convert VATS to thoracotomy immediately if major PA hemorrhage occurs.

Intercostal Artery Hemorrhage During Chest Wall Resection: Posterior intercostal arteries are direct aortic branches — transection without prior control produces arterial hemorrhage that retracts into the paravertebral muscles near the spinal canal. **Safe maneuver:** ligate posterior intercostal arteries before rib division; work from posterior to anterior; if a retracted artery bleeds, use gentle muscle separation and a figure-of-eight suture rather than blind deep clamping.

Innominate Artery Injury During Cervical Mediastinoscopy: The innominate artery crosses the anterior trachea at the sternal notch — directly in the mediastinoscope's path and easily mistaken for a lymph node. **Safe maneuver:** palpate for a pulsatile structure before inserting the mediastinoscope; never biopsy anything pulsatile; use needle aspiration before excisional biopsy; keep a sternotomy tray available.

Transdiaphragmatic Chest Tube Placement into the Abdomen: Chest tube insertion below the fifth intercostal space risks transdiaphragmatic placement into the liver (right) or spleen (left) — the diaphragm rises to the fourth intercostal space during full expiration. **Safe maneuver:** always insert within the triangle of safety; confirm the level of the fifth intercostal space at the nipple line; use digital exploration after entering the pleural space to confirm intrapleural position before inserting the tube.

Summary and Key Concepts

The intercostal neurovascular bundle runs along the inferior border of each rib (VAN — vein, artery, nerve from superior to inferior) — all chest procedures enter over the superior border of the rib below to avoid these structures.

VATS has become the preferred approach for anatomic lobectomy, offering reduced pain, shorter hospital stays, and equivalent oncologic outcomes for early-stage NSCLC compared with thoracotomy.

Anatomic lobectomy requires individual ligation of lobar pulmonary artery branches, pulmonary vein, and bronchus — en masse ligation is unacceptable because it prevents accurate staging and increases bronchopleural fistula risk.

Segmentectomy is an oncologically acceptable alternative to lobectomy for tumors 2 cm or less, with equivalent overall survival and better preservation of pulmonary function (JCOG0802 and CALGB 140503 trials).

Empyema progresses through three stages — exudative (chest tube drainage), fibrinopurulent (fibrinolysis or VATS), and organizing (decortication to remove the fibrous peel trapping the lung).

The triangle of safety (lateral border of pectoralis major, anterior border of latissimus dorsi, fifth intercostal space) is the standard insertion site for chest tubes, avoiding the internal mammary vessels, long thoracic nerve, and diaphragm.

Cervical mediastinoscopy provides access to paratracheal and subcarinal lymph node stations for lung cancer staging — the innominate artery crossing the trachea at the sternal notch is the principal hazard.

CHAPTER 20: OPERATIVE TRAUMA SURGERY

Learning Objectives

1. Apply the principles of damage control surgery, including abbreviated laparotomy with temporary abdominal closure, resuscitation in the intensive care unit, and planned return to the operating room for definitive repair.
2. Perform an exploratory laparotomy for abdominal trauma with systematic four-quadrant exploration, hemorrhage control using packing, and definitive repair of organ and vascular injuries.
3. Select the appropriate operative management for solid organ injuries (liver, spleen, kidney) and hollow viscus injuries based on injury grade, hemodynamic status, and the physiological reserve of the patient.
4. Execute an emergency department resuscitative thoracotomy, a neck exploration for penetrating trauma, and vascular repair of extremity arterial injuries using damage-control principles.

Principles of Damage Control Surgery

The Lethal Triad and the Damage Control Sequence

Damage control surgery (DCS) is a staged operative strategy for the severely injured patient who is in or approaching the lethal triad of hypothermia (core temperature below 35 degrees Celsius), metabolic acidosis (pH below 7.2, base deficit greater than 8 mEq/L), and coagulopathy (INR greater than 1.5, fibrinogen below 100 mg/dL). The triad is self-reinforcing: hypothermia impairs coagulation factor function and platelet aggregation, coagulopathy produces ongoing hemorrhage that drives acidosis, and acidosis worsens both hypothermia and coagulopathy — once established, this cycle cannot be reversed in the operating room regardless of technical surgical skill. The damage control sequence consists of three phases: phase 1, abbreviated operation (hemorrhage control and contamination control only — packing, ligation, stapled resection without anastomosis, temporary abdominal closure); phase 2, intensive care unit resuscitation (rewarming, correction of acidosis and coagulopathy with blood products, optimization of hemodynamics — typically 24 to 48 hours); and phase 3, planned return to the operating room for definitive repair (formal organ repair, intestinal anastomosis, fascial closure when the abdomen is compliant).

Indications for Damage Control

Damage control is indicated when the patient's physiology cannot tolerate a prolonged definitive operation — the decision to abbreviate is made early (within the first 30 to 60 minutes of laparotomy), based on physiological parameters rather than anatomic injury pattern. Specific indications include hemodynamic instability despite resuscitation (systolic pressure below 90 mmHg with transfusion requirement exceeding 10 units in the first 4 hours), two or more elements of the lethal triad, inability to achieve hemostasis due to coagulopathy (diffuse non-surgical bleeding from all raw surfaces), multiple cavitary injuries requiring prolonged operative time, and abdominal compartment syndrome (intra-abdominal pressure above 20 mmHg with new organ dysfunction). The damage control philosophy extends beyond the abdomen: damage control resuscitation (DCR — permissive hypotension with a target systolic of 80 to 90 mmHg until hemorrhage is controlled, balanced 1:1:1 blood product ratio, limited crystalloid, early tranexamic acid) is initiated simultaneously in the trauma bay.

Complications of Damage Control Surgery and Open Abdomen Management

The damage control sequence carries its own morbidity. The open abdomen (OA) — maintained with negative-pressure wound therapy between phase 1 and phase 3 — produces significant fluid losses (1 to 3 liters per day), enteroatmospheric fistula (5 to 15% of patients, particularly when bowel is exposed and desiccated), loss of abdominal domain (lateral retraction of the fascial edges makes delayed fascial closure increasingly difficult after 7 to 10 days), and intra-abdominal abscess (20 to 25%, requiring percutaneous or operative drainage). Fascial closure rates decrease from over 80% when achieved within 7 days to less than 30% when delayed beyond 14 days — sequential closure using NPWT with medial traction on the fascial edges maximizes the likelihood of primary closure. Patients who cannot achieve fascial closure require planned ventral hernia repair 6 to 12 months later. Abdominal compartment syndrome (ACS) is both an indication for and a complication of damage control — intra-abdominal pressure monitoring is mandatory, with decompressive laparotomy for sustained pressure above 20 mmHg with new organ dysfunction.

Massive Transfusion Protocol and Hemostatic Resuscitation

Massive transfusion is defined as the administration of 10 or more units of packed red blood cells (PRBCs) within 24 hours, or 4 or more units within 1 hour with anticipated ongoing need. Institutional massive transfusion protocols (MTPs) are activated early to ensure a continuous supply of blood products without crossmatching delays. The balanced ratio of 1:1:1 (PRBCs to fresh frozen plasma to platelets) is the current standard, based on the PROPPR trial demonstrating reduced mortality compared with lower ratios. Adjuncts include tranexamic acid (1 gram bolus followed by 1 gram over 8 hours, most effective within 3 hours of injury — the CRASH-2 trial demonstrated a 1.5% absolute mortality reduction), cryoprecipitate for fibrinogen below 150 mg/dL (target above 200 mg/dL), and calcium chloride replacement (citrate in banked blood chelates ionized calcium, producing hypocalcemia that worsens coagulopathy — maintain ionized calcium above 1.0 mmol/L). Viscoelastic hemostatic assays (thromboelastography or rotational thromboelastometry) provide real-time assessment of clot formation and lysis, enabling goal-directed therapy.

Exploratory Laparotomy for Abdominal Trauma

Indications and Initial Steps

Exploratory laparotomy for abdominal trauma is indicated for hemodynamic instability with a positive FAST or diagnostic peritoneal aspirate, peritonitis on examination, evisceration, diaphragmatic rupture on imaging, free intraperitoneal air, gunshot wounds traversing the peritoneal cavity, and stab wounds with peritoneal violation and deterioration. The operation begins with a generous midline laparotomy from xiphoid to pubis. Upon entering the abdomen, blood and clot are evacuated (manual scooping is faster than suction for large volumes), and four-quadrant packing is performed immediately (laparotomy pads in the right upper quadrant, left upper quadrant, pelvis, and paracolic gutters) to achieve temporary hemorrhage control by tamponade. After packing, the surgeon reassesses: if hemostasis is achieved, the operation proceeds systematically to identify all injuries; if hemorrhage continues, the source is addressed directly (usually a major vascular injury requiring exposure and repair).

Systematic Exploration

After initial hemorrhage control, the abdominal cavity is explored systematically. Packs are removed one quadrant at a time, starting with the least bloody quadrant: right upper quadrant (liver, right kidney, hepatic flexure, duodenum — the Kocher maneuver mobilizes the duodenum and head of pancreas to inspect the posterior duodenum, IVC, and right renal hilum), left upper quadrant (spleen, left kidney, splenic flexure, tail of pancreas, stomach), pelvis (bladder, rectum, iliac vessels, uterus and adnexa in women), and the entire small bowel (run from the ligament of Treitz to the ileocecal valve, inspecting both sides of the mesentery for hematoma and serosal injuries). The retroperitoneum is evaluated for expanding or pulsatile hematomas: central zone 1 hematomas (aorta, IVC, mesenteric vessels) are explored regardless of mechanism; lateral zone 2 hematomas (kidney, renal pedicle) are explored for penetrating trauma but may be observed for blunt trauma if the kidney is not actively bleeding and CT staging has been performed; pelvic zone 3 hematomas are NOT explored for blunt trauma (pelvic fracture — exploration releases tamponade and worsens hemorrhage) but ARE explored for penetrating trauma (iliac vessel injury).

THE OPERATIVE DANGER ZONE ATLAS — Pelvic Hematoma Exploration in Blunt Trauma

The Zone: The presacral and retroperitoneal pelvic space (zone 3) — the retroperitoneal compartment bounded by the pelvic brim superiorly, the sacrum posteriorly, and the pelvic sidewalls laterally. In blunt pelvic fracture, this space fills with blood from the disrupted presacral venous plexus (Batson plexus), fractured cancellous bone surfaces, and branches of the internal iliac artery.

The Structure at Risk: The presacral venous plexus — a valveless, thin-walled network of veins that drains the sacrum, rectum, and pelvic organs. These veins are not surgically controllable: they lack defined walls for suture repair, retract into the sacral foramina when divided, and bleed diffusely from innumerable small branches. The internal iliac artery branches (superior gluteal, obturator, lateral sacral) also contribute arterial hemorrhage in severe pelvic fractures.

The Consequence: Surgical exploration of a pelvic hematoma in blunt trauma releases the tamponade effect of the intact retroperitoneum — the contained hematoma decompresses into the free peritoneal cavity, and hemorrhage from the presacral plexus and fractured bone surfaces becomes uncontrollable. Blood loss accelerates from a tamponaded trickle to an exsanguinating torrent. This is one of the most lethal iatrogenic errors in trauma surgery — mortality from explored pelvic hematomas in blunt trauma approaches 75 to 100%.

The Safe Maneuver: Do NOT open the retroperitoneum over a pelvic hematoma in blunt trauma. Manage pelvic hemorrhage with a multimodal non-exploratory protocol: pelvic binder or external fixation to reduce fracture volume and tamponade venous bleeding, preperitoneal pelvic packing (through a lower midline or Pfannenstiel incision, placing three laparotomy pads directly against the pelvic brim and bladder without entering the retroperitoneum), and angioembolization of arterial bleeding sources identified on CT angiography. In penetrating trauma, zone 3 hematomas ARE explored because the mechanism (direct vessel laceration) requires surgical repair.

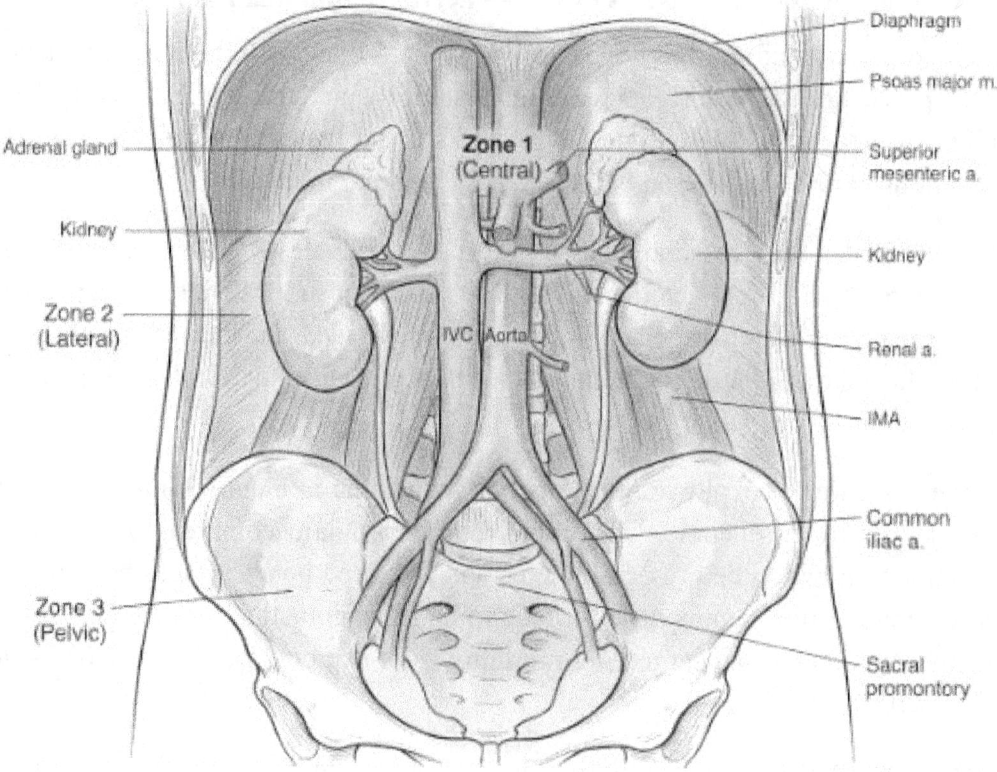

Operative Management of Solid Organ Injuries (Liver, Spleen, Kidney)

Liver Injury Management

The liver is the most commonly injured solid organ in penetrating abdominal trauma and the second most common in blunt trauma. The AAST grades liver injury from I (subcapsular hematoma less than 10% surface area) to VI (hepatic avulsion). The majority of grades I to III injuries are managed non-operatively in hemodynamically stable patients. Operative management is required for hemodynamic instability, grade IV to V injuries with active hemorrhage, and failure of non-operative management. Operative techniques include: perihepatic packing (the most important initial maneuver — laparotomy pads tamponade venous and parenchymal bleeding, effective for 60 to 80% of operative liver injuries), direct suture hepatorrhaphy (mattress sutures with omental pledgets placed across the laceration), hepatotomy with selective vascular ligation (finger fracture technique to expose and ligate individual bleeding vessels within the wound), and the Pringle maneuver (temporary clamping of the portal triad to reduce hepatic inflow; if bleeding stops, the source is parenchymal or portal venous; if bleeding continues, the source is retrohepatic IVC or hepatic vein — requiring atriocaval shunting or direct caval repair).

Grade	Hematoma	Laceration	Vascular
I	Subcapsular, less than 10% surface area	Capsular tear, less than 1 cm parenchymal depth	—
II	Subcapsular, 10 to 50% surface area; intraparenchymal less than 10 cm diameter	1 to 3 cm parenchymal depth, less than 10 cm length	—
III	Subcapsular, greater than 50% or expanding; ruptured subcapsular or parenchymal hematoma; intraparenchymal greater than 10 cm	Greater than 3 cm parenchymal depth	—
IV	—	Parenchymal disruption involving 25 to 75% of a hepatic lobe or 1 to 3 Couinaud segments	—
V	—	Parenchymal disruption involving greater than 75% of a hepatic lobe or greater than 3 Couinaud segments	Juxtahepatic venous injury (retrohepatic IVC or central major hepatic veins)
VI	—	—	Hepatic avulsion

THE OPERATIVE DANGER ZONE ATLAS — Retrohepatic Inferior Vena Cava Injury in Major Hepatic Trauma

The Zone: The retrohepatic space — the segment of the IVC behind the liver, from the confluence of the hepatic veins to the suprarenal IVC. This segment receives the three major hepatic veins (right, middle, left) and is surrounded by hepatic parenchyma, making surgical access extremely difficult. Grade V and VI liver injuries (deep lacerations extending to the hepatic veins or IVC, or hepatic avulsion) involve this zone.

The Structure at Risk: The retrohepatic inferior vena cava and the hepatic veins. These are large-caliber, thin-walled, valveless veins carrying the entire venous return from the lower body and the liver. They are fixed to the diaphragm and the liver parenchyma, making mobilization dangerous — any attempt to mobilize the liver off the IVC in the setting of retrohepatic venous injury risks converting a partially tamponaded injury into an uncontrolled exsanguinating hemorrhage.

The Consequence: Retrohepatic IVC or hepatic vein injury produces massive, high-volume venous hemorrhage that fills the operative field faster than it can be suctioned. The mortality rate for retrohepatic caval injuries exceeds 80%. Hemorrhage from this location does not respond to the Pringle maneuver (because the bleeding source is outflow, not inflow), and direct surgical repair requires either total hepatic vascular isolation (clamping the suprahepatic IVC, infrarenal IVC, portal triad, and aorta simultaneously — producing profound hemodynamic compromise) or atriocaval shunting.

The Safe Maneuver: If perihepatic packing controls the hemorrhage — leave the packs in place and close or temporarily close the abdomen (damage control). Packing is the safest maneuver for retrohepatic venous injuries because it preserves the natural tamponade. Do NOT remove the packs to 'look at the injury' — this releases the tamponade and can produce lethal hemorrhage. If packing fails and bleeding continues despite the Pringle maneuver, the injury is retrohepatic venous — mobilize for total hepatic vascular isolation only if the patient's physiology permits and the surgical team has experience with this maneuver. Angioembolization by interventional radiology is an adjunct for arterial bleeding sources identified on CT angiography.

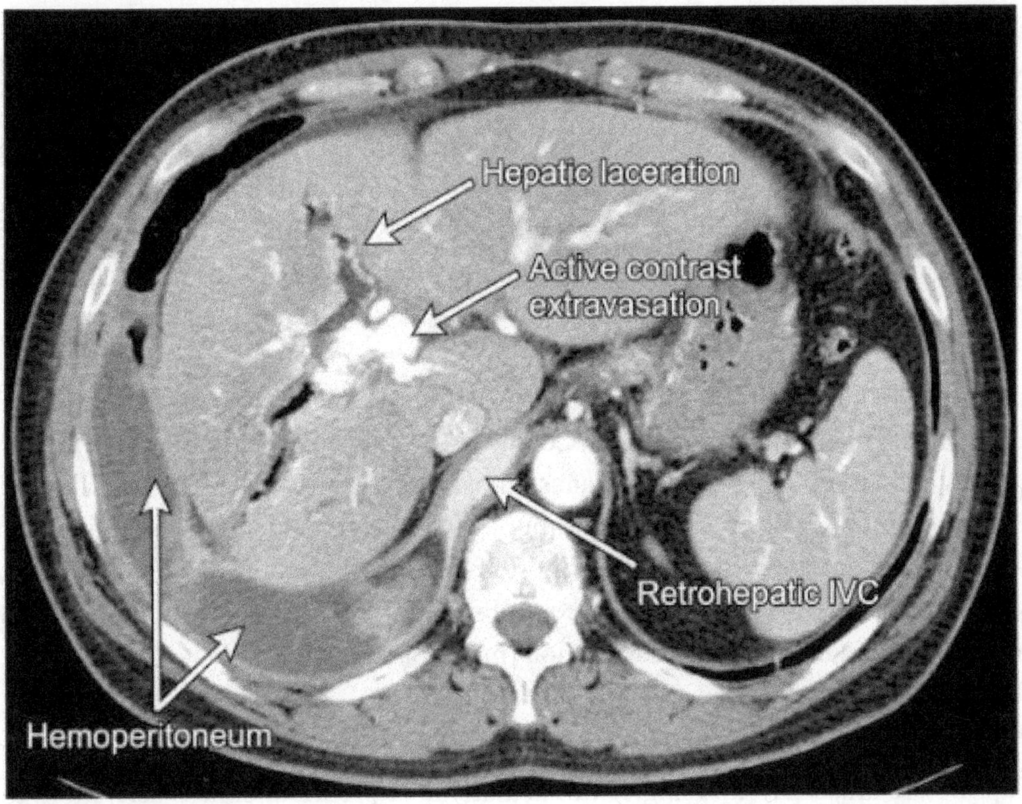

Spleen and Kidney Injury Management

The spleen is the most commonly injured organ in blunt abdominal trauma. Non-operative management (observation with serial imaging) is successful in 60 to 90% of hemodynamically stable patients with blunt splenic injury, including high-grade injuries, with angioembolization as an adjunct for AAST grade III or higher injuries with contrast blush on CT. Operative management (splenectomy or splenorrhaphy) is indicated for hemodynamic instability despite resuscitation, failure of non-operative management (dropping hemoglobin, increasing transfusion requirement), and associated injuries requiring laparotomy. Splenectomy is performed by ligating the short gastric vessels, mobilizing the spleen medially, and ligating the splenic artery and vein at the hilum individually (en masse hilar ligation is acceptable in the damage control setting). After splenectomy, patients require vaccination against encapsulated organisms (pneumococcus, meningococcus, Haemophilus influenzae type b) — ideally 14 days postoperatively. Renal injuries are managed non-operatively in the majority of cases (over 85% of blunt renal injuries), with operative exploration reserved for expanding or pulsatile perirenal hematomas, renal pedicle avulsion (grade V), and hemodynamic instability attributable to renal hemorrhage. Nephrectomy is the most common operative intervention for severe renal trauma — the contralateral kidney function must be confirmed (by preoperative CT or intraoperative palpation of the contralateral kidney) before performing nephrectomy.

Operative Management of Hollow Viscus Injuries

Small Bowel and Colon Injuries

Hollow viscus injuries are the third most common abdominal injury in penetrating trauma. Small bowel injuries are repaired primarily (two-layer closure with an inner running absorbable suture and outer interrupted seromuscular sutures) for lacerations involving less than 50% of the bowel circumference and without significant mesenteric injury. Injuries involving more than 50% of the circumference, multiple adjacent injuries, or injuries with devascularized segments require segmental resection with primary anastomosis — in the damage control setting, resection is performed with a stapler but the anastomosis is deferred (the stapled ends are left in discontinuity) until the patient is resuscitated and returned to the operating room for definitive reconstruction. Colon injuries are managed similarly: primary repair for small lacerations and resection with primary anastomosis for larger injuries — the traditional practice of mandatory colostomy for all destructive colon injuries has been abandoned based on evidence showing that primary repair and anastomosis are safe in most settings (even for left-sided injuries), with diversion (colostomy or ileostomy) reserved for damage control situations, massive fecal contamination, significant hemodynamic instability, and delayed presentation (more than 12 hours).

Duodenal and Pancreatic Injuries

Duodenal injuries are graded from I (single-wall hematoma or partial-thickness laceration) to V (massive disruption of the duodenopancreatic complex or devascularization). Grade I and II injuries are repaired primarily with a two-layer closure. Grade III injuries (disruption of 50 to 75% of the circumference or involving the ampulla) require repair with consideration of duodenal diversion (pyloric exclusion — the pylorus is stapled closed from inside the stomach through a gastrotomy, a gastrojejunostomy is constructed for gastric decompression, and the duodenal repair is protected from gastric secretions while it heals; the pyloric staple line opens spontaneously in 2 to 4 weeks). Grade IV and V injuries may require pancreaticoduodenectomy (trauma Whipple — a formidable operation performed in a damage control sequence). Pancreatic injuries are managed based on ductal integrity: injuries without main pancreatic duct disruption (grades I to II) are managed with drainage alone (closed-suction drains placed adjacent to the injury); injuries with main duct disruption (grade III and above) in the body or tail are managed with distal pancreatectomy (with or without splenectomy); injuries to the pancreatic head with duct disruption may require pancreaticoduodenectomy if the injury is not amenable to drainage and endoscopic stenting.

Gastric and Bladder Injuries

Gastric injuries occur in 5 to 15% of penetrating abdominal trauma cases and are uncommon in blunt trauma (less than 2%). The stomach is repaired primarily in two layers (inner running absorbable, outer interrupted seromuscular) for the majority of injuries. Complete transection or massive destruction of the stomach is rare but may require partial gastrectomy. Both the anterior and posterior walls must be inspected — posterior gastric wall injuries are identified by opening the gastrocolic omentum and entering the lesser sac. Bladder injuries are classified as extraperitoneal (managed non-operatively with catheter drainage for 10 to 14 days in most cases) or intraperitoneal (requiring operative repair — a two-layer closure with absorbable sutures, followed by catheter drainage). All repairs should be confirmed with a cystogram at 7 to 14 days before catheter removal. Bladder injuries are associated with pelvic fractures in up to 85% of cases — any patient with a pelvic fracture and gross hematuria should undergo CT cystography to evaluate for bladder rupture.

Diaphragm Injury Repair

Diagnosis and Operative Repair

Traumatic diaphragmatic injuries occur in 1 to 7% of patients with blunt abdominal trauma (from sudden increase in intra-abdominal pressure producing a radial tear, typically on the left — the liver protects the right hemidiaphragm from radial tears) and in 10 to 15% of patients with penetrating thoracoabdominal trauma. Left-sided injuries are more commonly diagnosed because herniation of abdominal contents (stomach, colon, omentum) into the left chest is visible on chest radiograph (elevated hemidiaphragm, bowel gas pattern in the chest, nasogastric tube curling into the chest). Right-sided injuries are often occult, because the liver plugs the defect and prevents herniation. Missed diaphragmatic injuries enlarge over time due to the persistent pressure gradient between the abdomen and thorax, eventually presenting years later as a diaphragmatic hernia with incarceration or strangulation of abdominal viscera in the chest — a surgical emergency. Repair is performed through a transabdominal approach during the acute phase (laparotomy or laparoscopy) using interrupted horizontal mattress sutures of non-absorbable material (1-0 polypropylene or polyester), closing the defect in a single layer without tension. Large defects may require a prosthetic mesh patch (polypropylene or dual-sided composite mesh). Late presentations with a large chronic hernia are repaired through a thoracotomy or thoracoscopy (the adhesions between the herniated viscera and the thoracic structures are best managed from above).

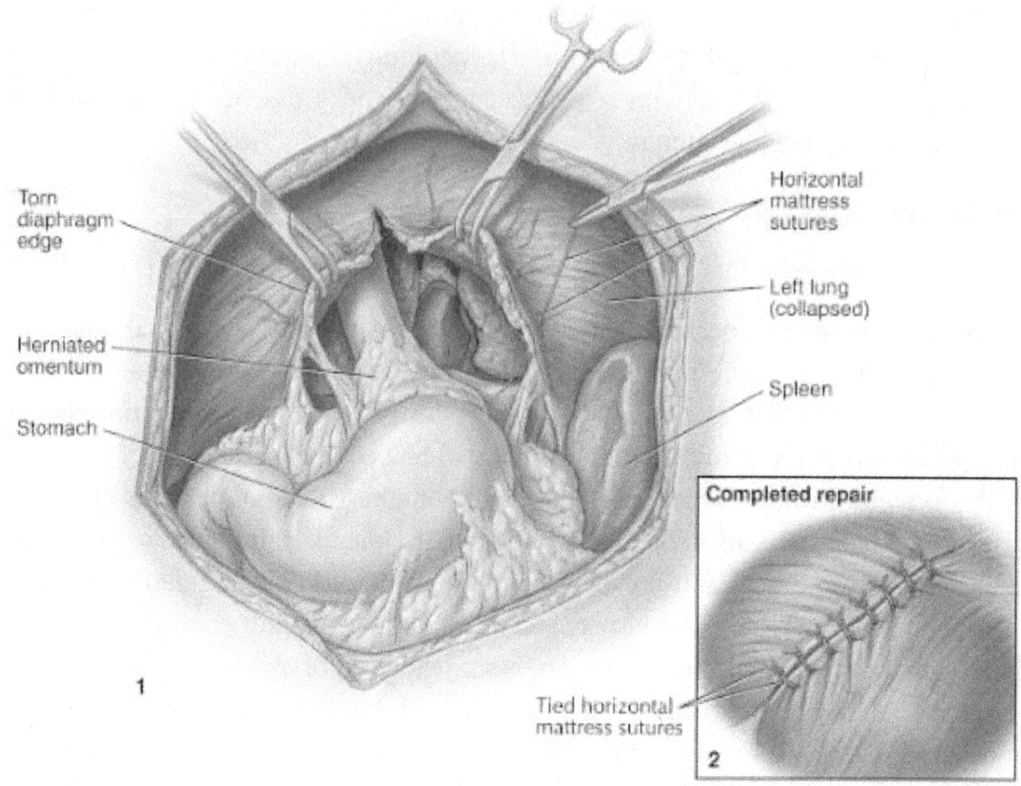

THE OPERATIVE DANGER ZONE ATLAS — Missed Diaphragmatic Injury Progressing to Strangulated Hernia

The Zone: The diaphragm — specifically the left posterolateral hemidiaphragm in blunt trauma (the most common location for radial tears) and any point of diaphragmatic penetration in thoracoabdominal stab or gunshot wounds. The danger zone is not only the moment of injury but the subsequent weeks to years during which an unrepaired defect silently enlarges.

The Structure at Risk: The abdominal organs that herniate through the defect — stomach, transverse colon, omentum, small bowel, and (in large left-sided defects) the spleen. Once herniated into the negative-pressure thoracic cavity, these organs become trapped by the rigid diaphragmatic ring, which acts as a constricting band around the herniated viscera.

The Consequence: A chronically unrepaired diaphragmatic defect inevitably enlarges and eventually produces incarceration (viscera trapped in the chest but viable) or strangulation (visceral blood supply compromised by the constricting defect, producing ischemia, necrosis, and perforation). A strangulated diaphragmatic hernia with gastric necrosis and perforation produces tension gastrothorax (gastric contents and air under pressure in the chest), mediastinal shift, cardiovascular collapse, and sepsis — with mortality rates of 30 to 60%.

The Safe Maneuver: Maintain a high index of suspicion for diaphragmatic injury in all thoracoabdominal penetrating trauma and in all blunt trauma with a mechanism capable of producing sudden intra-abdominal pressure spikes (high-speed motor vehicle collisions, falls from height). Inspect the entire diaphragm during every trauma laparotomy — both domes, from the esophageal hiatus to the central tendon. For left-sided penetrating trauma between the nipple line and the costal margin, diagnostic laparoscopy reliably identifies occult diaphragmatic injuries that are missed by CT scan. Repair all defects at the time of identification — even small puncture wounds — because the natural history of every unrepaired diaphragmatic defect is progressive enlargement.

Trauma Thoracotomy (Emergency Department and Operating Room)

Indications and Technique for Resuscitative Thoracotomy

Emergency department thoracotomy (EDT, resuscitative thoracotomy) is a last-resort intervention performed in patients in extremis or in cardiac arrest from traumatic injury. The indications with the highest survival rates are penetrating cardiac injuries (stab wounds to the cardiac box with witnessed cardiac arrest and less than 15 minutes of prehospital CPR — survival rate 10 to 35%) and cardiac tamponade with hemodynamic collapse. Indications with lower survival include penetrating thoracic injuries with witnessed arrest (less than 15 minutes CPR — survival 5 to 15%), blunt thoracic injuries with witnessed arrest (less than 10 minutes CPR — survival less than 2%), and abdominal exsanguination (EDT performed to cross-clamp the descending aorta for temporary hemorrhage control while the patient is transported to the operating room). EDT is futile and should not be performed for blunt trauma with no signs of life in the field, unwitnessed cardiac arrest, or prolonged CPR exceeding 15 minutes (penetrating) or 10 minutes (blunt).

The technique is a left anterolateral thoracotomy in the fifth intercostal space (inframammary crease), extending from the sternum to the posterior axillary line. The chest is entered rapidly with a scalpel and heavy scissors, the rib spreader is inserted, and the lung is retracted superiorly. The immediate objectives, performed in sequence, are: release of cardiac tamponade (the pericardium is opened longitudinally, anterior to the phrenic nerve, and blood clot is evacuated — if a cardiac wound is identified, it is controlled with digital pressure, a Foley catheter balloon, or a skin stapler until formal cardiorrhaphy can be performed), control of cardiac hemorrhage (direct suture repair of cardiac lacerations with pledgeted horizontal mattress sutures of 3-0 polypropylene), open cardiac massage (bimanual compression of the heart if in arrest), cross-clamping of the descending thoracic aorta (the aorta is palpated against the vertebral column posterior and medial to the esophagus and clamped with a DeBakey aortic clamp to redirect the limited cardiac output to the coronary and cerebral circulation and to reduce subdiaphragmatic hemorrhage), and hilar clamping or pulmonary tractotomy for massive pulmonary hemorrhage.

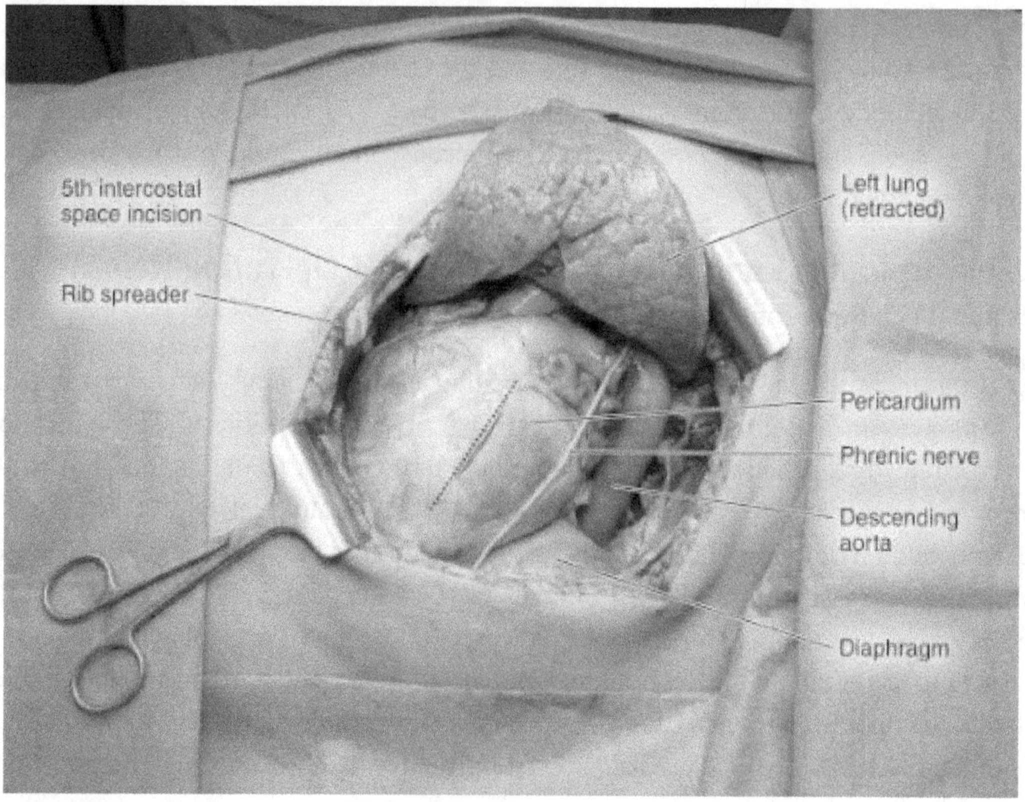

Neck Exploration for Penetrating Trauma

Anatomical Zones and Operative Approach

The neck is divided into three zones for penetrating trauma: zone I (from the clavicles/sternal notch to the cricoid cartilage — containing the thoracic outlet vessels, esophagus, trachea, thoracic duct, and lung apices), zone II (from the cricoid cartilage to the angle of the mandible — containing the carotid arteries, internal jugular veins, pharynx, larynx, esophagus, and cervical spine), and zone III (from the angle of the mandible to the base of the skull — containing the distal ICA, vertebral arteries, and cranial nerves as they exit the skull base). Zone II injuries are the most accessible surgically and are explored through an incision along the anterior border of the sternocleidomastoid. The traditional mandatory exploration policy for all zone II penetrating injuries has been replaced by selective management based on CT angiography — patients with hard signs of vascular injury (active hemorrhage, expanding hematoma, absent pulse, bruit or thrill) or aerodigestive injury (air bubbling through the wound, subcutaneous emphysema, hematemesis, dysphagia) undergo immediate operative exploration; patients without hard signs undergo CT angiography for anatomic assessment, followed by selective operative, endovascular, or non-operative management. Zone I and zone III injuries are more difficult to expose operatively and are more commonly managed with endovascular techniques (stent grafting, embolization).

THE OPERATIVE DANGER ZONE ATLAS — Esophageal Injury Missed During Neck Exploration

The Zone: The cervical esophagus, lying posterior to the trachea and anterior to the prevertebral fascia — a location that makes it the most commonly missed injury in penetrating neck trauma. The esophagus has no serosal layer, making small perforations difficult to identify visually, and its posterior position means the surgeon must actively rotate the trachea and esophagus to inspect the posterior wall.

The Structure at Risk: The cervical esophagus itself. Unlike vascular injuries (which bleed and declare themselves) and airway injuries (which leak air), esophageal perforations may be initially occult — a small perforation in the posterior esophageal wall can leak saliva and bacteria into the deep cervical fascial spaces without obvious external signs during the initial hours.

The Consequence: A missed cervical esophageal perforation produces deep neck space infection (retropharyngeal or prevertebral abscess), descending mediastinitis (infection tracks from the cervical fascial planes into the mediastinum along the prevertebral and visceral fascia), and sepsis. Mediastinitis from a missed esophageal perforation carries a mortality rate of 20 to 50% and requires aggressive surgical drainage (transcervical and often transthoracic) in addition to broad-spectrum antibiotics.

The Safe Maneuver: During every neck exploration for penetrating trauma, actively inspect the esophagus — retract the trachea medially and inspect the posterior esophageal wall directly, rotating the esophagus to visualize its full circumference. If a perforation is identified, repair it primarily in two layers (inner mucosa with absorbable sutures, outer muscular layer with interrupted silk or polypropylene) and drain the area widely. If the perforation is not visible but the trajectory crosses the esophageal axis, perform intraoperative flexible esophagoscopy or instill methylene blue through a nasogastric tube to detect an occult leak. A negative exploration of the esophagus at initial surgery does not exclude a delayed perforation — maintain a high index of suspicion postoperatively.

Operative Management of Extremity Vascular Trauma

Principles and Temporary Vascular Shunts

Extremity vascular trauma is managed according to the principles described in Chapter 17 (Operations of the Arteries). In the polytrauma patient, the damage control concept extends to extremity vascular injuries: temporary intraluminal vascular shunts (TIVS) restore distal perfusion immediately while the patient is resuscitated and stabilized for definitive repair. A shunt (Argyle, Sundt, or improvised from a segment of chest tube or nasogastric tube) is inserted into the proximal and distal ends of the transected artery and secured with vessel loops or silk ties. Shunts maintain patency for 24 to 48 hours without anticoagulation, providing a bridge to definitive repair. Definitive repair follows the same principles as elective arterial reconstruction: reversed saphenous vein interposition graft is the conduit of choice for all extremity arterial repairs in the trauma setting (prosthetic grafts are avoided in contaminated wounds). Four-compartment fasciotomy is performed prophylactically after all combined arterial and venous injuries, after ischemia time exceeding 4 to 6 hours, and after any reperfusion with clinical suspicion of compartment syndrome.

Compartment Syndrome After Reperfusion

Compartment syndrome is the most feared complication of extremity vascular injury. Ischemia-reperfusion injury produces massive edema within the closed fascial compartments, raising intracompartmental pressure above capillary perfusion pressure (compartment syndrome develops when pressure exceeds 30 mmHg or delta pressure falls below 30 mmHg). The classic presentation is pain out of proportion to injury, pain with passive stretch, and a tense swollen extremity — loss of pulses is a LATE finding indicating irreversible necrosis. Treatment is emergent fasciotomy: in the lower leg, four-compartment release through two incisions (medial for the superficial and deep posterior compartments, lateral for the anterior and lateral compartments); in the forearm, volar and dorsal fasciotomy. Incisions are left open and dressed with negative-pressure wound therapy, with delayed closure or grafting at 48 to 72 hours. Fasciotomy beyond 6 to 8 hours after onset results in muscle necrosis, rhabdomyolysis with myoglobinuric acute kidney injury, and a functionless extremity — delayed fasciotomy may be more harmful than amputation because of systemic reperfusion effects (hyperkalemia, renal failure, sepsis).

CAUTION: In blunt trauma, NEVER explore a pelvic (zone 3) hematoma — the hematoma is tamponading the hemorrhage from pelvic fracture venous plexus injury, and exploration releases the tamponade, converting a stable hematoma into an uncontrollable exsanguinating hemorrhage. Pelvic hemorrhage in blunt trauma is managed with external fixation, preperitoneal pelvic packing, and angioembolization — not surgical exploration.

Clinical Case — Damage Control Laparotomy for Gunshot Wound to the Abdomen

A 28-year-old man arrives with a gunshot wound to the left upper quadrant, systolic blood pressure 70 mmHg, heart rate 130, GCS 14, and positive FAST. He receives 2 units of uncrossmatched O-negative PRBCs and is taken to the operating room. At laparotomy, 2 liters of blood are evacuated and four-quadrant packing performed. The source is a through-and-through injury to the splenic flexure and a grade III splenic laceration with active hemorrhage. The spleen is removed rapidly. The colon injuries are resected with a GIA stapler without anastomosis — the stapled ends are left in discontinuity. At this point, the patient's temperature is 34.2 degrees Celsius, pH 7.18, INR 1.9 — he is in the lethal triad. The abdomen is temporarily closed with a negative-pressure dressing. Over 36 hours of ICU resuscitation, he is rewarmed, coagulopathy is corrected (total: 14 units PRBCs, 12 units FFP, 2 units platelets, 2 grams tranexamic acid), and acidosis resolves. He returns to the operating room at 48 hours: the colonic ends are trimmed and a hand-sewn anastomosis is performed, the abdomen is irrigated, and the fascia closed primarily. Discharge is on postoperative day 9.

Retrohepatic Inferior Vena Cava Injury in Major Hepatic Trauma: The retrohepatic IVC segment behind the liver is inaccessible and receives the hepatic veins — injury produces exsanguinating hemorrhage with mortality exceeding 80%. **Safe maneuver:** if perihepatic packing controls the hemorrhage, leave the packs and close (damage control); do NOT remove packs to inspect the injury; only attempt total hepatic vascular isolation if packing fails and the team has the expertise.

Missed Diaphragmatic Injury Progressing to Strangulated Hernia: Unrepaired diaphragmatic defects inevitably enlarge due to the abdominothoracic pressure gradient, producing incarceration and strangulation of herniated viscera with mortality of 30 to 60%. **Safe maneuver:** inspect both hemidiaphragms during every trauma laparotomy; use diagnostic laparoscopy for left thoracoabdominal penetrating trauma; repair all defects, even puncture wounds.

Esophageal Injury Missed During Neck Exploration: The cervical esophagus is the most commonly missed injury in penetrating neck trauma — occult perforation produces deep neck infection and descending mediastinitis with 20 to 50% mortality. **Safe maneuver:** actively inspect the full circumference of the esophagus during neck exploration; use intraoperative esophagoscopy or methylene blue if the trajectory is suspicious; repair in two layers and drain widely.

Pelvic Hematoma Exploration in Blunt Trauma: Opening a pelvic hematoma in blunt trauma releases the tamponade on venous plexus bleeding from pelvic fractures, converting a stable situation into uncontrollable hemorrhage. **Safe maneuver:** NEVER explore a zone 3 hematoma in blunt trauma; manage with external fixation, preperitoneal pelvic packing, and angioembolization.

Summary and Key Concepts

Damage control surgery is a staged operative strategy for patients in the lethal triad (hypothermia, acidosis, coagulopathy) — phase 1 abbreviates the operation to hemorrhage and contamination control only, with definitive repair deferred to phase 3 after ICU resuscitation.

Four-quadrant packing at the start of trauma laparotomy provides immediate hemorrhage control by tamponade — packs are then removed systematically one quadrant at a time during exploration.

Perihepatic packing is the most important initial maneuver for operative liver injuries — it controls hemorrhage in 60 to 80% of cases and is the safest approach for retrohepatic venous injuries (do not remove packs to inspect the injury).

The Pringle maneuver (portal triad clamping) differentiates hepatic parenchymal/portal bleeding (stops with Pringle) from retrohepatic caval/hepatic vein bleeding (continues despite Pringle).

Primary repair or resection with anastomosis has replaced mandatory colostomy for most destructive colon injuries — diversion is reserved for damage control, massive contamination, and delayed presentation.

Emergency department thoracotomy has the highest survival for penetrating cardiac injuries with witnessed arrest and less than 15 minutes of CPR — the immediate objectives are pericardiotomy, cardiac repair, open cardiac massage, and aortic cross-clamping.

Zone 3 (pelvic) hematomas in blunt trauma must NEVER be explored — exploration releases tamponade on pelvic venous plexus bleeding and causes uncontrollable hemorrhage.

CHAPTER 21: OPERATIONS OF THE SKIN AND SOFT TISSUE

Learning Objectives

1. Describe the layered anatomy of the skin and subcutaneous tissue, including the relationship of relaxed skin tension lines to incision planning and scar cosmesis.
2. Select the appropriate biopsy technique (shave, punch, incisional, excisional) for skin lesions of varying clinical suspicion, and perform an elliptical excision with a 3:1 length-to-width ratio along Langer lines.
3. Determine the correct excision margin for cutaneous melanoma based on Breslow depth, and describe the indications, technique, and significance of sentinel lymph node biopsy.
4. Apply the principles of oncological resection to soft tissue sarcomas, including the role of preoperative imaging, compartmental anatomy, and the margin requirements for limb-sparing surgery.
5. Differentiate between split-thickness and full-thickness skin grafts, design local flaps for wound reconstruction, assess burn depth and total body surface area, and perform escharotomy for circumferential burns.

Surgical Anatomy of the Skin and Subcutaneous Tissue

Layers of the Skin and Their Surgical Significance

The skin is the largest organ of the body, averaging 1.5 to 2.0 square meters in surface area, and consists of two principal layers with distinct surgical implications. The epidermis is the avascular outer layer composed of stratified squamous keratinized epithelium, organized from deep to superficial into the stratum basale (the germinative layer where epidermal stem cells reside), stratum spinosum, stratum granulosum, and stratum corneum. The dermis lies deep to the epidermis and is divided into the papillary dermis (loose connective tissue with capillary loops that supply the epidermis by diffusion) and the reticular dermis (dense irregular connective tissue containing collagen and elastin fibers, blood vessels, lymphatics, hair follicles, sebaceous glands, and nerve endings). The dermal-epidermal junction is critical surgically because the epidermal appendages — hair follicles and sweat glands — extend deep into the reticular dermis and even into the subcutaneous fat, and these appendages serve as the source of re-epithelialization for partial-thickness wounds and split-thickness skin graft donor sites.

Relaxed Skin Tension Lines and Incision Planning

Relaxed skin tension lines (RSTLs, Langer lines) represent the orientation of collagen fiber bundles in the reticular dermis and correspond to the natural skin creases visible on relaxed skin. Incisions placed parallel to RSTLs heal with narrower, flatter scars because the wound edges are not being pulled apart by the dominant collagen tension vectors — the wound closes under minimal tension, and the scar matures in alignment with the existing dermal architecture. Incisions placed perpendicular to RSTLs heal under constant lateral tension, which stimulates excessive collagen deposition and produces wide, raised, and hypertrophic scars. On the face, RSTLs generally follow the lines of facial expression (perpendicular to the underlying muscles of facial expression); on the trunk and extremities, they follow the skin creases that are visible when the tissue is relaxed. Every elective skin incision should be planned along RSTLs unless the anatomy of the lesion or the surgical approach requires a different orientation.

Vascular Supply and Lymphatic Drainage

The cutaneous blood supply is organized into two horizontal plexuses: the subdermal plexus at the dermal-subcutaneous junction and the subpapillary plexus at the junction of the papillary and reticular dermis. These plexuses receive perforating arterioles from the underlying named musculocutaneous or septocutaneous perforators — a principle that is the anatomical foundation of perforator flap design. Lymphatic drainage of the skin follows the superficial lymphatic channels in the subdermal plexus to regional lymph node basins, and the specific drainage pattern for any cutaneous site can be mapped preoperatively by lymphoscintigraphy — the basis of sentinel lymph node biopsy for melanoma and Merkel cell carcinoma.

Excision and Biopsy Techniques for Skin Lesions

Biopsy Techniques

The choice of biopsy technique depends on the clinical suspicion, the lesion location, and the information required for histopathological diagnosis. Shave biopsy removes the epidermis and superficial dermis tangentially with a blade or dermatome and is appropriate for superficial lesions where melanoma is not suspected — shave biopsy of a pigmented lesion suspected to be melanoma is contraindicated because it may transect the deep margin and prevent accurate Breslow depth measurement. Punch biopsy uses a cylindrical blade (2 to 8 mm diameter) to obtain a full-thickness specimen through epidermis, dermis, and subcutaneous fat, and is the technique of choice for inflammatory dermatoses, suspected deep dermal or subcutaneous pathology, and pigmented lesions requiring full-thickness histological assessment. Incisional biopsy removes a representative wedge of a large lesion (typically one that cannot be completely excised at the time of initial diagnosis) and is used for large soft tissue masses and extensive skin lesions where excisional biopsy would be mutilating before a definitive diagnosis is established.

Elliptical Excision Technique

Excisional biopsy with an elliptical incision is the standard technique for complete removal of skin lesions with a margin of normal tissue. The ellipse is designed with a length-to-width ratio of 3:1 to prevent standing cutaneous deformities (dog ears) at the wound apices. The long axis of the ellipse is oriented along the RSTLs whenever possible. The incision is made with a number 15 blade held perpendicular to the skin surface (beveling the edges inward produces a wedge-shaped wound that is difficult to close, while beveling outward produces everted wound edges that heal with a flat scar). The specimen is excised with a uniform depth through the subcutaneous fat, and the deep margin is the subcutaneous fat itself for benign lesions or the investing fascia for lesions suspicious for melanoma. Hemostasis is achieved with electrocautery (bipolar for facial lesions to minimize thermal spread), and the wound is closed in layers: deep dermal sutures of 4-0 polyglactin 910 to approximate the wound edges and eliminate dead space, followed by running subcuticular 5-0 poliglecaprone or interrupted nylon for the skin.

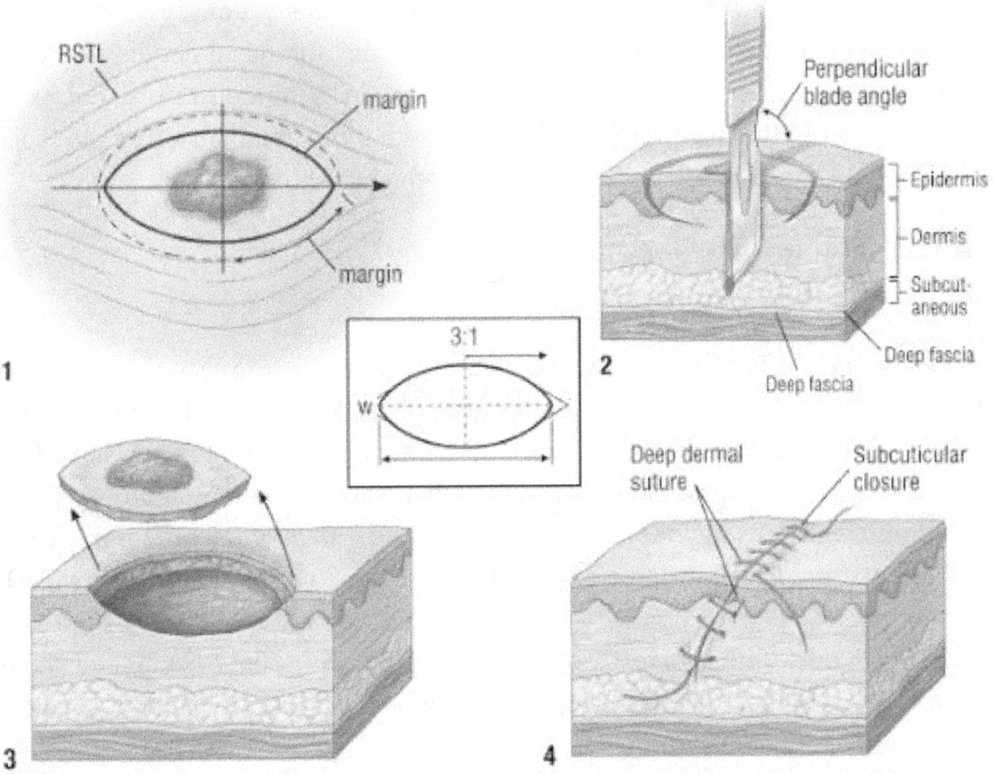

THE OPERATIVE DANGER ZONE ATLAS — Facial Nerve Branch Injury During Facial Skin Excision

---

The Zone: The lateral face and the area overlying the parotid gland, where the terminal branches of the facial nerve (CN VII) run superficially in the subcutaneous plane. The temporal branch crosses the zygomatic arch within the superficial temporal fascia, and the marginal mandibular branch runs along the inferior border of the mandible superficial to the facial artery and vein — both are at risk during excision of skin and subcutaneous lesions in these regions.

The Structure at Risk: The temporal branch of the facial nerve (responsible for frontalis muscle — forehead elevation and eyebrow raise) and the marginal mandibular branch (responsible for depressor anguli oris — lower lip depression and oral competence). Both branches become superficial as they exit the parotid gland and cross the zygomatic arch and mandible respectively, running within or just deep to the subcutaneous fat.

The Consequence: Division of the temporal branch produces ipsilateral inability to raise the eyebrow and wrinkle the forehead — a permanent and cosmetically significant deficit with no reliable surgical repair. Division of the marginal mandibular branch produces asymmetric smile and lower lip weakness with drooling and oral incompetence — the affected side cannot depress the lower lip, producing a visible asymmetry during speech and eating.

The Safe Maneuver: For excisions over the lateral face, keep the dissection superficial to the superficial musculoaponeurotic system (SMAS) — the SMAS is the fascial plane that separates the subcutaneous fat (safe plane) from the deeper parotid-masseteric layer containing the facial nerve branches. For excisions overlying the zygomatic arch, stay superficial to the superficial temporal fascia. For excisions near the mandibular border, identify the marginal mandibular branch by its relationship to the facial vessels — it crosses superficial to the facial artery at the mandibular angle.

Wide Local Excision for Melanoma

Excision Margins by Breslow Depth

Wide local excision (WLE) is the definitive surgical treatment for primary cutaneous melanoma. The excision margin — the distance of clinically normal skin excised circumferentially around the biopsy scar or residual lesion — is determined by the Breslow thickness (depth of invasion measured from the granular layer of the epidermis to the deepest melanoma cell) established on the initial biopsy. Current evidence-based margin recommendations are: melanoma in situ, 0.5 to 1.0 cm clinical margin; Breslow depth 1.0 mm or less, 1.0 cm margin; Breslow depth 1.01 to 2.0 mm, 1 to 2 cm margin; Breslow depth greater than 2.0 mm, 2 cm margin. The deep margin extends to the investing muscle fascia — the fascia is taken en bloc with the specimen only if it is clinically involved. These margins have been validated by randomized controlled trials demonstrating that wider margins do not improve melanoma-specific survival but narrower margins increase local recurrence rates.

Sentinel Lymph Node Biopsy

Sentinel lymph node biopsy (SLNB) identifies the first lymph node(s) draining the primary melanoma site and determines whether regional nodal metastasis is present. SLNB is indicated for melanomas with Breslow depth of 0.8 mm or greater, or for thinner melanomas with adverse features (ulceration, high mitotic rate, lymphovascular invasion). The technique involves preoperative lymphoscintigraphy (injection of technetium-99m sulfur colloid around the primary site, followed by gamma camera imaging to identify the draining nodal basin and the sentinel node within it), intraoperative injection of blue dye (isosulfan blue or methylene blue) at the primary site, and identification of the sentinel node by its blue coloration and radioactive signal using a handheld gamma probe. The sentinel node is excised and sent for permanent histopathological analysis with immunohistochemical staining (S-100, HMB-45, Melan-A). A positive sentinel node upstages the melanoma to stage III and informs decisions about completion lymph node dissection, adjuvant systemic therapy, and surveillance intensity.

CLINICAL PEARL: SLNB must be performed BEFORE or simultaneously with wide local excision — performing WLE first disrupts the lymphatic drainage pathways and can invalidate the sentinel node mapping. When re-excision is needed after an initial narrow-margin excision biopsy, SLNB is performed at the same operation as the WLE.

Management of Regional Nodal Disease

Completion lymph node dissection (CLND) after a positive SLNB has been the traditional approach, but the MSLT-II and DeCOG-SLT trials demonstrated that CLND does not improve melanoma-specific survival compared with active ultrasound surveillance of the nodal basin in patients with a positive sentinel node. Current practice reserves CLND for patients with clinically detected nodal disease (palpable lymphadenopathy confirmed by fine-needle aspiration), extracapsular extension on the sentinel node, or multiple positive sentinel nodes, and offers ultrasound surveillance as an alternative for patients with low-volume sentinel node metastasis.

Soft Tissue Sarcoma Resection

Principles of Oncological Resection

Soft tissue sarcomas are rare mesenchymal malignancies (approximately 13,000 new cases annually in the United States) arising in muscle, fat, connective tissue, and peripheral nerves. The majority (approximately 60%) occur in the extremities, with the remainder in the retroperitoneum (20%), trunk wall, and head and neck. The standard of care for localized extremity and trunk wall sarcomas is wide surgical resection with negative margins combined with radiation therapy. The goal of resection is an R0 margin — no tumor at the inked surgical margin on permanent histopathology. For extremity sarcomas, limb-sparing resection (wide excision with adjuvant radiation) achieves equivalent oncological outcomes to amputation and is the standard approach for the majority of tumors, with amputation reserved for tumors that encase the neurovascular bundle or involve the joint surface in a way that precludes functional limb preservation.

Preoperative Assessment and Compartmental Anatomy

Preoperative MRI with gadolinium contrast is mandatory for all extremity soft tissue sarcomas — it defines the tumor's relationship to the investing fascia, neurovascular structures, bone, and the anatomical compartment boundaries. The extremity is organized into anatomical compartments bounded by fascial septa: the thigh has three compartments (anterior, medial, posterior), the leg has four (anterior, lateral, superficial posterior, deep posterior), and the forearm has three (volar, dorsal, mobile wad). Intracompartmental sarcomas are confined within the fascial boundaries and are resected with a cuff of normal tissue including the overlying fascia. Extracompartmental sarcomas (extending through the investing fascia or along neurovascular bundles) require wider resection with careful attention to the tissue planes adjacent to critical structures. Core needle biopsy (14-gauge or larger) is the standard diagnostic technique — the biopsy tract must be placed in line with the planned resection incision so that it is excised en bloc with the specimen.

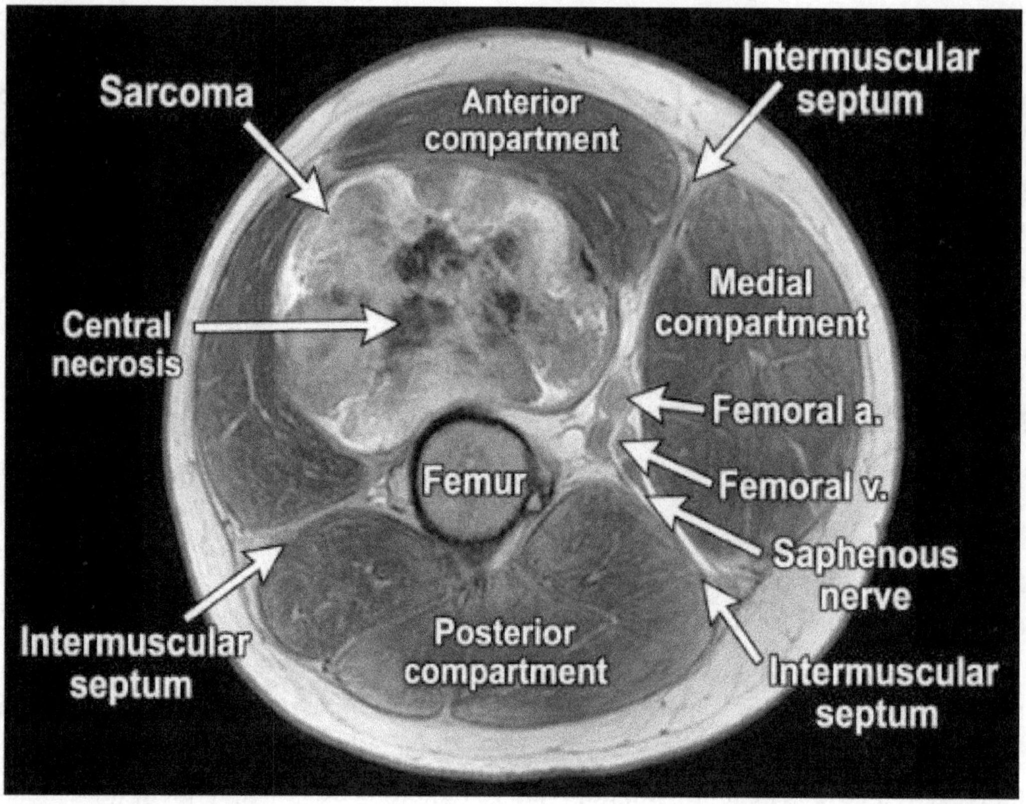

THE OPERATIVE DANGER ZONE ATLAS — Spinal Accessory Nerve Injury During Posterior Triangle Soft Tissue Resection

The Zone: The posterior triangle of the neck — bounded by the posterior border of the sternocleidomastoid anteriorly, the anterior border of the trapezius posteriorly, and the middle third of the clavicle inferiorly. The spinal accessory nerve (CN XI) crosses this triangle superficially, running on the levator scapulae muscle approximately 1 cm above Erb point (the intersection of the greater auricular nerve with the posterior border of the sternocleidomastoid), and is the most commonly injured nerve during posterior triangle surgery.

The Structure at Risk: The spinal accessory nerve (CN XI) — it exits the posterior border of the sternocleidomastoid at its midpoint and traverses the posterior triangle in the superficial investing fascia, running obliquely from superomedial to inferolateral to enter the anterior border of the trapezius at its junction with the middle and lower thirds. The nerve lies on the floor of the posterior triangle (on the levator scapulae and splenius capitis muscles) with only the investing cervical fascia and subcutaneous fat superficial to it.

The Consequence: Division or traction injury to the spinal accessory nerve produces trapezius muscle paralysis — the shoulder droops, the scapula rotates laterally and protrudes (scapular winging), and the patient cannot abduct the arm above 90 degrees. This produces chronic shoulder pain, weakness, and significant functional disability. Unlike facial nerve injuries, spinal accessory nerve injuries do not recover spontaneously in the majority of cases when the nerve is transected.

The Safe Maneuver: Before any dissection in the posterior triangle (for lymph node biopsy, soft tissue mass excision, or neck dissection), identify the spinal accessory nerve at its exit point from the posterior border of the sternocleidomastoid and trace it across the posterior triangle. Dissect superficial to the nerve for superficial lesions. Use nerve stimulation to confirm identification. Never excise a mass in the posterior triangle without first identifying and preserving CN XI, and never place a drain or suture that could entrap the nerve.

Skin Grafting and Local Flap Reconstruction

Split-Thickness and Full-Thickness Skin Grafts

Skin grafts are classified by the thickness of dermis included. Split-thickness skin grafts (STSGs) include the epidermis and a variable portion of the dermis (thin: 0.008 to 0.012 inches; intermediate: 0.012 to 0.018 inches; thick: 0.018 to 0.024 inches) and are harvested with a dermatome from the anterolateral thigh, buttock, or upper arm. Because the donor site retains the deep dermis with its epidermal appendages, it re-epithelializes by secondary intention in 10 to 21 days. STSGs are used for large defects, burn wound coverage, and wounds in areas where cosmesis is secondary to coverage. Full-thickness skin grafts (FTSGs) include the entire epidermis and dermis and are harvested by sharp excision from sites where the donor skin can be closed primarily (postauricular, supraclavicular, groin, antecubital fossa). FTSGs produce superior cosmetic results (less contraction, better color and texture match) but require a well-vascularized wound bed and are limited in size by the donor site.

Local Flap Design

Local flaps transfer adjacent tissue with its intact blood supply to reconstruct a wound defect, and are classified by the method of tissue movement. Advancement flaps move tissue in a single linear direction by undermining and advancing the flap edge into the defect (V-Y advancement, bipedicled advancement). Rotation flaps pivot a semicircular flap of skin and subcutaneous tissue around a pivot point into the defect, redistributing wound closure tension over a longer arc. Transposition flaps lift a rectangular or rhomboid flap of tissue over an intervening bridge of skin and place it into the adjacent defect (rhomboid flap, Z-plasty, bilobed flap). The choice of flap depends on the defect size, location, tissue laxity, and the availability of adjacent tissue — the principle of the reconstructive ladder guides the surgeon from the simplest closure (primary, secondary intention, STSG) upward to the most complex (free tissue transfer) only when simpler methods are inadequate.

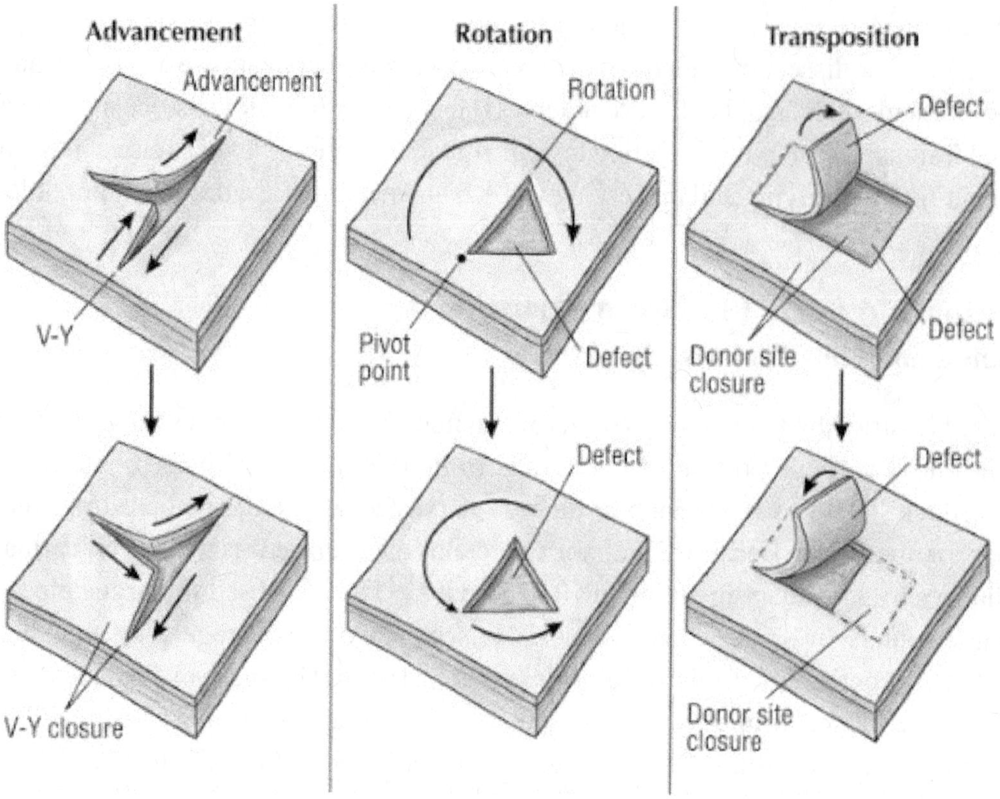

Graft Take and Complications

Skin graft survival depends on three sequential phases: imbibition (first 24 to 48 hours — the graft absorbs nutrients from the wound bed by passive diffusion, producing graft edema and a characteristic bluish discoloration), inosculation (days 2 to 4 — the graft capillaries align with recipient bed capillaries and establish direct vascular connections), and revascularization (days 4 to 7 — new capillary ingrowth from the wound bed penetrates the graft dermis). Graft failure occurs when any factor disrupts this sequence: hematoma or seroma beneath the graft (the most common cause of graft failure — lifts the graft off the wound bed, preventing imbibition and inosculation), infection (bacterial collagenase destroys the graft-bed interface), shear force (movement between the graft and bed disrupts the fragile neovascular connections), and an inadequate wound bed (avascular surfaces such as bare bone, tendon without paratenon, or irradiated tissue cannot support graft revascularization and require flap coverage instead).

THE OPERATIVE DANGER ZONE ATLAS — Saphenous Nerve Injury During Split-Thickness Skin Graft Harvest from the Thigh

The Zone: The medial thigh and the anteromedial leg — the standard donor sites for split-thickness skin graft harvest. The saphenous nerve, the longest sensory nerve in the body, runs in the subcutaneous tissue along the medial thigh and crosses from deep to superficial at the adductor canal (Hunter canal), emerging between the sartorius and gracilis muscles to lie in the subcutaneous fat of the medial leg alongside the great saphenous vein.

The Structure at Risk: The saphenous nerve (a pure sensory branch of the femoral nerve, carrying sensation from the medial leg and medial ankle). In the medial thigh, the nerve lies deep to the sartorius fascia and is relatively protected. However, in the distal medial thigh and medial leg, the nerve lies superficially in the subcutaneous fat — directly in the path of a dermatome harvesting a split-thickness graft from the anteromedial leg.

The Consequence: Dermatome transection of the saphenous nerve produces a permanent sensory deficit along the medial leg and medial ankle — a numb strip that is cosmetically minor but functionally significant in patients who rely on sensory feedback from the foot (diabetic patients, elderly patients with balance impairment). Neuroma formation at the transection site can produce chronic neuropathic pain at the donor site.

The Safe Maneuver: Harvest STSGs from the anterolateral thigh rather than the anteromedial thigh or medial leg — the lateral thigh has no major superficial sensory nerves in the standard harvest plane. Set the dermatome to the minimum thickness required for the clinical situation (thin grafts re-epithelialize faster and cause less donor site morbidity). If medial thigh harvest is required, harvest proximal to the knee (where the saphenous nerve is deeper) rather than distal.

Surgical Management of Burns and Complex Wounds

Assessment of Burn Depth and Total Body Surface Area

Burn depth is classified by the layers of skin destroyed. Superficial burns (first degree) involve the epidermis only, producing erythema and pain without blistering, and heal spontaneously in 3 to 5 days. Superficial partial-thickness burns (superficial second degree) destroy the epidermis and papillary dermis, producing blisters with a moist, pink, painful wound bed that blanches with pressure; these re-epithelialize from epidermal appendages in the retained reticular dermis within 10 to 14 days and rarely scar. Deep partial-thickness burns (deep second degree) destroy the epidermis and extend into the reticular dermis, producing a mottled pink-and-white wound bed with decreased sensation and sluggish capillary refill — these heal slowly (3 to 6 weeks) with significant scarring and often require excision and grafting. Full-thickness burns (third degree) destroy the entire epidermis and dermis, producing a dry, waxy, or leathery eschar that is insensate and does not blanch; these cannot re-epithelialize and require excision and grafting.

Burn Depth	Layers Destroyed	Clinical Appearance	Sensation	Healing Time	Treatment
Superficial (1st degree)	Epidermis only	Erythema, dry, no blisters	Painful	3–5 days	Topical moisturizer
Superficial partial (2nd degree)	Epidermis + papillary dermis	Blisters, moist, pink, blanches	Very painful	10–14 days	Topical antimicrobial, dressings
Deep partial (2nd degree)	Epidermis + reticular dermis	Mottled pink-white, sluggish refill	Decreased	3–6 weeks (scarring)	Excision and grafting often needed
Full thickness (3rd degree)	Entire skin (epidermis + dermis)	Waxy, leathery, dry eschar	Insensate	Cannot heal spontaneously	Excision and grafting required
4th degree	Skin + subcutaneous + deeper	Charred, visible fascia/muscle/bone	Insensate	Cannot heal spontaneously	Excision, flap, or amputation

Total body surface area (TBSA) burned is estimated using the rule of nines in adults (each arm 9%, each leg 18%, anterior trunk 18%, posterior trunk 18%, head 9%, perineum 1%) or the Lund-Browder chart (which adjusts for age-related body proportion differences and is more accurate in children). The patient's palm (including fingers) represents approximately 1% TBSA and is useful for estimating scattered or irregular burn patterns. Fluid resuscitation is guided by the Parkland formula: 4 mL of lactated Ringer solution per kilogram body weight per percent TBSA burned in the first 24 hours, with half administered in the first 8 hours from the time of injury and the remainder over the next 16 hours, titrated to a urine output of 0.5 to 1.0 mL/kg/hour.

Escharotomy and Fasciotomy

Circumferential full-thickness burns of the extremities, chest, or abdomen produce a rigid, inelastic eschar that acts as a constricting band. As underlying tissue edema develops during resuscitation, the unyielding eschar compresses the deep structures — in the extremities, this produces compartment syndrome with vascular compromise; in the chest, it restricts ventilation by limiting chest wall expansion. Escharotomy is performed at the bedside as an emergency procedure: the eschar is incised longitudinally along the medial and lateral aspects of the affected extremity (or along the anterior axillary lines for chest eschar) through the full thickness of the burned skin down to the subcutaneous fat. The incision should extend beyond the margins of the circumferential burn into normal tissue proximally and distally. The eschar edges separate immediately, releasing the constriction. Fasciotomy is performed in addition to escharotomy when clinical signs of compartment syndrome persist after escharotomy (absent distal pulses, tense compartments) or when electrical burns have caused deep tissue edema beneath intact fascia.

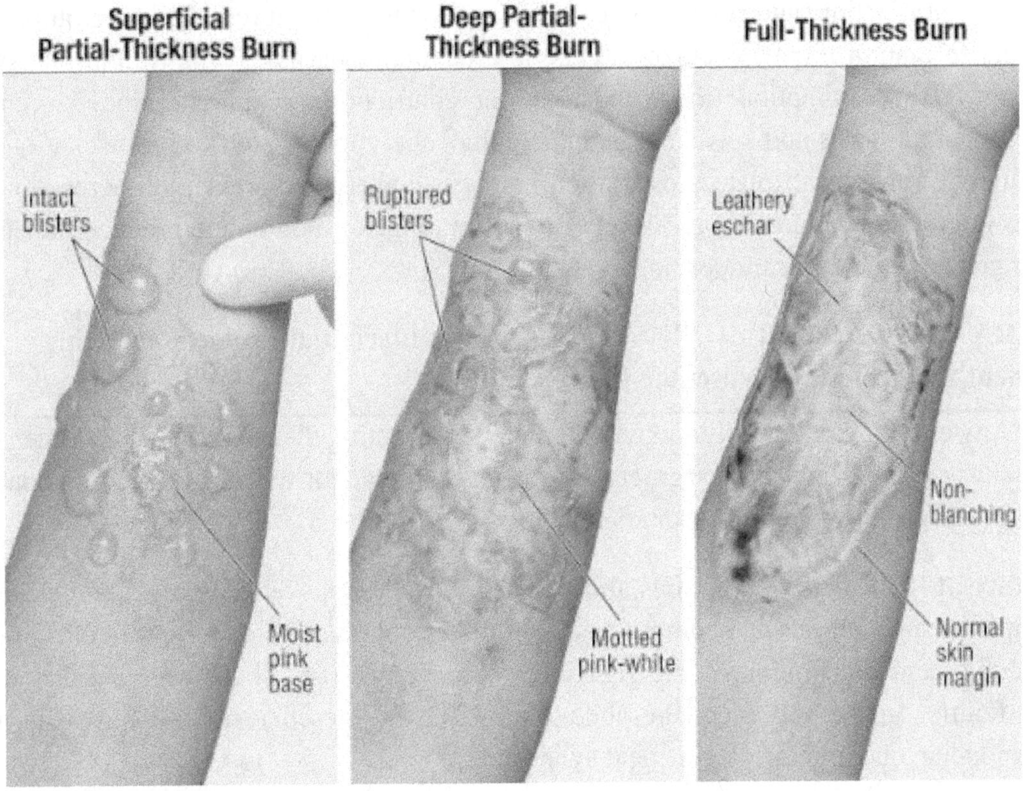

Burn Wound Excision and Grafting

Early tangential excision of deep partial-thickness and full-thickness burns with immediate split-thickness skin grafting is the standard of care — performed within the first 5 days of injury, early excision and grafting reduces hospital length of stay, decreases wound infection rates, and improves functional outcomes compared with serial debridement and delayed grafting. Tangential excision (using a Goulian or Watson knife) sequentially shaves the necrotic eschar in thin layers until a viable wound bed with punctate capillary bleeding is reached. The excised wound is then covered with STSG — meshed grafts (1.5:1 or 3:1 expansion ratio) are used for large burns to maximize coverage from limited donor sites, while sheet (unmeshed) grafts are used for cosmetically sensitive areas (face, hands, anterior neck). Temporary wound coverage with cadaveric allograft or synthetic biological dressings (Integra, Biobrane) is used when autograft donor sites are insufficient — these provide a biological barrier until donor sites re-epithelialize for re-harvest.

Complications and Special Populations in Burn Surgery

Major burn complications include burn wound sepsis (the leading cause of death in burn patients after the initial resuscitation period — diagnosed by quantitative wound biopsy showing more than 100,000 organisms per gram of tissue), inhalation injury (diagnosed by history of enclosed-space fire, soot in the oropharynx, hoarseness, and bronchoscopic findings of mucosal edema and carbonaceous deposits — managed with early intubation, pulmonary toilet, and bronchoscopy), hypertrophic scarring and contracture (occurring in up to 70% of deep partial and full-thickness burns, managed with pressure garments, silicone sheeting, and surgical release of functional contractures), and heterotopic ossification (ectopic bone formation in periarticular soft tissue after major burns). Pediatric burn surgery requires adjustment of TBSA estimation (the Lund-Browder chart, not the rule of nines — children have proportionally larger heads and smaller legs than adults), age-appropriate fluid resuscitation targets, and particular attention to growth plate preservation and scar contracture prevention across joints, because contractures in growing children progressively limit joint range of motion and produce skeletal deformity as the child grows while the scar does not.

THE OPERATIVE DANGER ZONE ATLAS — Circumferential Eschar Producing Compartment Syndrome and Vascular Compromise

The Zone: Any circumferential full-thickness burn of an extremity, the chest, or the abdomen — the rigid, inelastic eschar encircles the body segment completely and cannot expand to accommodate the tissue edema that develops during burn resuscitation.

The Structure at Risk: In the extremities: the arterial inflow, venous outflow, and the muscles within the fascial compartments — the eschar compresses all of these progressively as tissue edema increases. In the chest: the lungs and diaphragm — the rigid chest eschar prevents chest wall expansion, producing ventilatory failure. In the abdomen: the abdominal viscera — eschar rigidity raises intra-abdominal pressure, producing abdominal compartment syndrome.

The Consequence: Extremity compartment syndrome from circumferential eschar produces ischemic muscle necrosis within 4 to 6 hours if unrelieved — the limb is lost to myonecrosis, rhabdomyolysis, and potentially the patient to hyperkalemia and renal failure from myoglobin release. Chest eschar restriction produces progressive hypoxemia, hypercarbia, and respiratory arrest despite mechanical ventilation (because the ventilator cannot generate sufficient pressure to expand the rigid chest wall).

The Safe Maneuver: Monitor all circumferentially burned extremities with serial pulse checks (palpation and Doppler) and compartment pressure measurements during the resuscitation phase. Perform escharotomy immediately when distal pulses diminish or compartment pressures rise — the incision is placed along the medial and lateral mid-axial lines of the extremity, extending through the full-thickness eschar into subcutaneous fat, and carried beyond the burn margins into normal tissue. For chest burns, bilateral anterior axillary line escharotomies connected by a transverse subcostal incision release the constriction. Escharotomy is a bedside procedure that does not require anesthesia in full-thickness burns (the eschar is insensate).

Clinical Case — Wide Local Excision and Sentinel Lymph Node Biopsy for Melanoma

A 47-year-old woman presents with a 1.4 cm irregular pigmented lesion on her left upper back. Excisional biopsy reveals a 1.8 mm Breslow depth melanoma, Clark level IV, with ulceration and a mitotic rate of 4 per mm squared. Preoperative CT of the chest, abdomen, and pelvis is negative for distant metastasis. Lymphoscintigraphy demonstrates drainage to two sentinel nodes in the left axilla. At operation, the wide local excision is performed first with a 2 cm margin around the biopsy scar, taken down to the investing fascia of the latissimus dorsi, which is included in the specimen. The resulting defect is closed primarily after undermining. The sentinel lymph node biopsy is then performed through a separate axillary incision — the two sentinel nodes are identified by their blue discoloration and radioactivity, excised, and sent for permanent histopathology. Final pathology confirms negative peripheral and deep margins on the WLE specimen. One sentinel node is positive for a 0.4 mm micrometastasis detected on immunohistochemistry (HMB-45 positive). The patient is counseled on the results of the MSLT-II trial, and ultrasound surveillance of the left axilla every 4 months is chosen over completion axillary lymph node dissection. She is referred to medical oncology for consideration of adjuvant immunotherapy.

KEY POINT: For melanomas with Breslow depth greater than 2.0 mm, the recommended surgical margin is 2 cm. SLNB should be performed at the same operation as the WLE, with SLNB performed BEFORE or simultaneously with the wide excision to preserve lymphatic drainage pathways. Completion lymph node dissection for microscopic sentinel node metastasis does not improve survival and can be replaced by active ultrasound surveillance in appropriate patients.

THE OPERATIVE DANGER ZONE ATLAS — Skin and Soft Tissue Operative Dangers

Facial Nerve Branch Injury During Facial Skin Excision: The temporal and marginal mandibular branches of the facial nerve run superficially over the zygomatic arch and mandible, placing them at risk during excision of facial and parotid-region skin lesions. **Safe maneuver:** dissect superficial to the SMAS; identify the marginal mandibular branch by its relationship to the facial vessels at the mandibular angle.

Spinal Accessory Nerve Injury During Posterior Triangle Soft Tissue Resection: CN XI crosses the posterior triangle superficially from the sternocleidomastoid to the trapezius — transection produces permanent trapezius paralysis with shoulder droop and scapular winging. **Safe maneuver:** identify CN XI at its exit from the sternocleidomastoid before dissecting in the posterior triangle; use nerve stimulation to confirm.

Saphenous Nerve Injury During Split-Thickness Skin Graft Harvest from the Thigh: The saphenous nerve lies in the subcutaneous fat of the medial and anteromedial thigh and leg, directly in the path of a dermatome. **Safe maneuver:** harvest from the anterolateral thigh where no major superficial sensory nerves are present; if medial harvest is needed, stay proximal to the knee.

Circumferential Eschar Producing Compartment Syndrome and Vascular Compromise: Circumferential full-thickness burns create a rigid constricting band that compresses deep structures as resuscitation edema develops — producing extremity compartment syndrome or chest restriction. **Safe**

maneuver: monitor circumferentially burned extremities with serial Doppler pulse checks; perform escharotomy immediately along medial and lateral mid-axial lines when pulses diminish.

Summary and Key Concepts

Incisions planned along relaxed skin tension lines heal with narrower, flatter scars because the wound edges are not under lateral tension from the dominant collagen fiber orientation in the reticular dermis.

Shave biopsy of a pigmented lesion suspected of melanoma is contraindicated because transection of the deep margin prevents accurate Breslow depth measurement — punch biopsy or excisional biopsy with narrow margins is required for accurate staging.

Wide local excision margins for melanoma are determined by Breslow depth: in situ 0.5 to 1.0 cm, 1.0 mm or less gets 1.0 cm, 1.01 to 2.0 mm gets 1 to 2 cm, and greater than 2.0 mm gets 2 cm — sentinel lymph node biopsy is performed before or simultaneously with WLE.

Soft tissue sarcoma resection requires an R0 margin with a cuff of normal tissue; preoperative MRI defines compartmental anatomy, and the core needle biopsy tract must be placed in line with the planned resection incision for en bloc excision.

Split-thickness skin grafts include epidermis and variable dermis (donor site heals by re-epithelialization), while full-thickness grafts include entire dermis (donor site requires primary closure) — graft failure is most commonly caused by hematoma beneath the graft.

Burn depth determines treatment: superficial partial-thickness burns heal spontaneously in 10 to 14 days, while deep partial-thickness and full-thickness burns require tangential excision and split-thickness skin grafting, ideally within 5 days of injury.

Circumferential full-thickness burns require emergent escharotomy along medial and lateral mid-axial lines when distal pulses diminish or ventilation is compromised — the rigid eschar acts as a constricting band that cannot accommodate resuscitation edema.

CHAPTER 22 OPERATIONS OF THE SPLEEN

Surgical Anatomy of the Spleen and Splenic Hilum

Gross Anatomy and Peritoneal Relationships

The spleen occupies the left upper quadrant posterolaterally, nestled against the diaphragm between the ninth and eleventh ribs. Its diaphragmatic surface is smooth and convex, conforming to the curvature of the left hemidiaphragm, while the visceral surface bears the gastric, renal, and colic impressions that reflect its intimate contact with the stomach, left kidney, and splenic flexure of the colon. The organ is entirely intraperitoneal and suspended by a series of ligamentous attachments — the gastrosplenic, splenorenal, splenocolic, and splenophrenic ligaments — that together define the surgical planes the operator must divide to mobilize the spleen. The gastrosplenic ligament, extending from the greater curvature to the splenic hilum, contains the short gastric vessels and the left gastroepiploic artery; because these vessels traverse the ligament in its superior portion, division must proceed from inferior to superior with individual vessel ligation to avoid retraction and hemorrhage.

Splenic Hilum and Vascular Supply

The splenic artery, the largest branch of the celiac trunk, follows a characteristically tortuous course along the superior border of the pancreas before reaching the splenic hilum. At the hilum the artery divides into terminal branches in one of two principal patterns: a distributed type (70% of individuals), in which the artery gives off multiple long branches that enter the spleen over a broad hilum, and a compact or magistral type (30%), in which a short main trunk divides close to the splenic capsule. The distributed pattern elongates the hilar dissection but allows individual branch ligation, while the magistral pattern concentrates vessels in a narrow zone where mass ligation is technically simpler but carries greater risk of incorporating pancreatic tail tissue. The splenic vein forms behind the pancreatic tail and courses along the posterior surface of the pancreas to join the superior mesenteric vein, forming the portal vein. This intimate relationship between the splenic vein and the pancreatic tail is the anatomical basis for pancreatic injury during hilar dissection — the most consequential danger zone of splenic surgery.

Segmental Anatomy and Avascular Plane

The spleen lacks a true lobar architecture but demonstrates a segmental blood supply without interarterial anastomoses. Ligation of a segmental branch produces well-demarcated ischemia along the corresponding territory, which is the physiologic basis for partial splenectomy. The avascular plane between the upper and lower polar segments — identifiable by a color-change demarcation line after segmental vessel occlusion — guides capsular incision during parenchyma-sparing procedures. Understanding this segmental anatomy is essential for the surgeon contemplating splenic preservation in pediatric patients, those with hereditary spherocytosis, or patients with focal splenic pathology amenable to limited resection rather than total splenectomy.

Ligament	Contents	Surgical Significance
Gastrosplenic	Short gastric vessels, left gastroepiploic artery	Divided first in open splenectomy; superior vessels require individual ligation
Splenorenal	Splenic artery and vein, pancreatic tail	Contains the hilar vessels; careless dissection risks pancreatic tail injury
Splenocolic	Usually avascular or minor omental vessels	Divided to mobilize inferior pole; traction may tear splenic flexure serosa
Splenophrenic	Avascular or small diaphragmatic branches	Divided last during mobilization; bleeding from diaphragmatic surface is usually self-limited

Open Splenectomy

Indications and Preoperative Planning

Open splenectomy remains indicated when the spleen is massively enlarged (exceeding 20 cm in craniocaudal length or 1,000 g in estimated weight), when splenic trauma has produced hemodynamic instability that precludes laparoscopic positioning, or when concomitant procedures — such as distal pancreatectomy or left-sided portosystemic shunt construction — require an open field. Hematologic indications include immune thrombocytopenic purpura refractory to medical therapy, hereditary spherocytosis, hemolytic anemias unresponsive to corticosteroids, and staging or treatment of lymphoproliferative disorders. Preoperative preparation includes vaccination against encapsulated organisms (Streptococcus pneumoniae, Neisseria meningitidis, Haemophilus influenzae type b) administered at least two weeks before elective surgery, correction of thrombocytopenia or coagulopathy where feasible, and cross-matching of packed red blood cells.

Operative Technique

The patient is positioned supine with a bump under the left flank to elevate the left upper quadrant. A left subcostal or midline incision provides adequate exposure. The operation proceeds systematically: the splenocolic ligament is divided first to release the inferior pole, then the lateral peritoneal attachments and splenophrenic ligament are incised to allow medial rotation of the spleen into the wound. With the spleen delivered medially, the short gastric vessels in the gastrosplenic ligament are individually ligated and divided from inferior to superior — this sequence keeps tension off the uppermost and shortest vessels, which are most prone to avulsion. The splenic artery is then identified along the superior border of the pancreas and ligated in continuity before hilar dissection; early arterial ligation reduces splenic congestion and operative blood loss by up to 40%. The splenic hilum is divided between clamps with suture ligation of each pedicle, taking care to visualize the pancreatic tail and confirm it is not incorporated in any ligature. The splenic vein is ligated last. The splenic bed is inspected for hemostasis and pancreatic tail integrity; any capsular disruption of the pancreatic tail warrants closed suction drainage positioned near the injury.

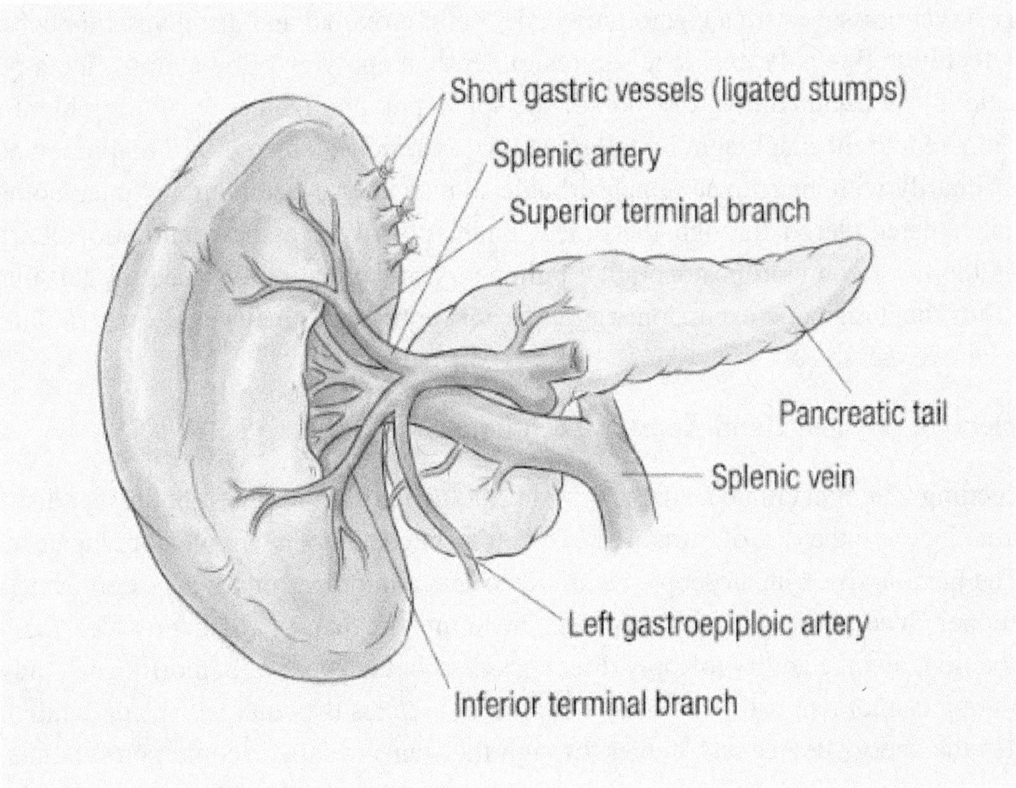

Search for Accessory Spleens

Accessory spleens are present in 10–30% of the population, most commonly located in the splenic hilum (56%), the gastrosplenic ligament (25%), and the splenocolic ligament. When splenectomy is performed for hematologic indications — particularly immune thrombocytopenic purpura — failure to identify and remove accessory spleens is the most common cause of operative failure and recurrent thrombocytopenia. A systematic search of the hilum, omentum, mesentery, pelvis, and left gonadal vessels is performed before closing. The greater omentum is examined by spreading it between the hands and palpating for discrete nodules; any suspicious tissue is excised and submitted for histopathologic confirmation.

CLINICAL PEARL: In immune thrombocytopenic purpura, the platelet count typically begins to rise within hours of splenic artery ligation — well before the spleen is fully mobilized and removed. A rapid intraoperative platelet rise confirms that the spleen is the primary site of platelet sequestration and destruction, reinforcing the appropriateness of the procedure.

Complications and Intraoperative Troubleshooting

The principal complications of open splenectomy include hemorrhage, pancreatic tail injury, diaphragmatic injury, and gastric wall perforation. Hemorrhage during hilar dissection most commonly arises from the splenic vein or its tributaries — the thin-walled venous system is more fragile than the arterial supply and tears readily under traction. If brisk venous hemorrhage is encountered, the surgeon should apply direct pressure with a laparotomy pad, obtain proximal and distal vascular control, and then repair the defect with fine polypropylene sutures rather than applying blind clamps into a pool of blood. Diaphragmatic injury occurs during division of the splenophrenic ligament or during blunt mobilization of a spleen adherent to the diaphragm by inflammatory adhesions; a recognized diaphragmatic laceration is repaired primarily with interrupted nonabsorbable sutures after evacuating any pneumothorax through a red rubber catheter placed through the defect under positive-pressure ventilation. Left lower lobe atelectasis is the most common postoperative pulmonary complication because the left upper quadrant incision inhibits diaphragmatic excursion; aggressive incentive spirometry and early ambulation are the primary preventive measures.

Massive Splenomegaly and Hand-Assisted Technique

Spleens exceeding 25 cm in craniocaudal length or 2,000 g in estimated weight present distinct technical challenges that increase the risk of intraoperative hemorrhage and conversion from laparoscopic to open approach. The hand-assisted laparoscopic technique offers a middle ground: a 7–8 cm hand port incision in the left upper quadrant admits the surgeon's nondominant hand, which provides tactile feedback, controlled traction, and the ability to apply direct pressure in the event of hemorrhage — advantages that pure laparoscopy cannot replicate. The hand elevates and rotates the enlarged spleen while the dominant hand operates the energy device and stapler through the standard laparoscopic ports. Studies comparing hand-assisted with pure laparoscopic splenectomy for spleens in the 20–30 cm range demonstrate lower conversion rates and reduced blood loss with the hand-assisted technique, without significant differences in postoperative pain, hospital stay, or wound complications. For spleens exceeding 30 cm, open splenectomy through a midline or left subcostal incision remains the safest approach.

THE OPERATIVE DANGER ZONE ATLAS — Pancreatic Tail Injury During Splenic Hilar Dissection

The Zone: The splenorenal ligament at the splenic hilum, where the terminal branches of the splenic artery and the origin of the splenic vein lie in direct contact with the pancreatic tail. In 30% of patients the pancreatic tail extends to within 1 cm of the splenic capsule, and in the compact (magistral) hilar pattern the vascular pedicle and pancreatic tissue overlap in a confined space that makes clean separation technically demanding.

The Structure at Risk: The pancreatic tail parenchyma and the main pancreatic duct. Incorporation of pancreatic tissue within a hilar vascular clamp or ligature causes crush injury and subsequent pancreatic fistula, while traction on the splenic vein during hilar mobilization can tear small pancreatic venous tributaries and produce hemorrhage that obscures the operative field and increases the likelihood of further pancreatic damage.

The Consequence: Pancreatic tail injury complicates 1–3% of splenectomies and produces a postoperative pancreatic fistula in up to 60% of recognized injuries. Unrecognized injuries present days to weeks later as peripancreatic fluid collections, abscess, or clinical pancreatitis. Pancreatic fistula prolongs hospitalization, necessitates percutaneous drainage, and occasionally requires reoperation for distal pancreatectomy.

The Safe Maneuver: Identify and palpate the pancreatic tail before placing any hilar clamps by sweeping a finger behind the hilum from lateral to medial. Ligate hilar vessels individually rather than using mass clamps. Maintain the plane of dissection anterior to the pancreatic tail. If the magistral hilar pattern is encountered and the pedicle is short, divide the splenic artery and vein as close to the splenic capsule as possible, accepting a slightly larger cuff of hilar fat rather than dissecting into the pancreatic tissue. Inspect the pancreatic tail after splenic removal; place a closed suction drain near the pancreatic tail if capsular disruption is identified or suspected.

Laparoscopic Splenectomy

Patient Selection and Positioning

Laparoscopic splenectomy has become the standard approach for elective splenectomy in spleens of normal to moderate size (up to approximately 20 cm). The procedure offers reduced postoperative pain, shorter hospital stay, fewer wound complications, and earlier return to activity compared with the open approach. The patient is positioned in the right lateral decubitus position at 45–60 degrees with the table flexed to open the space between the costal margin and the iliac crest. This positioning allows gravity to retract the colon and small bowel away from the left upper quadrant, providing exposure of the splenic hilum without mechanical retraction. Four ports are placed: a 12-mm camera port at the umbilicus, a 12-mm working port in the left midclavicular line, and two 5-mm accessory ports in the left anterior axillary line and subxiphoid position.

Operative Steps and Hilar Management

The operation begins with division of the splenocolic ligament using an energy device, which drops the splenic flexure inferiorly and exposes the inferior pole. The lateral peritoneal attachments and splenophrenic ligament are divided next, working from inferior to superior. The gastrosplenic ligament containing the short gastric vessels is divided with an ultrasonic or bipolar energy device — individual vessel sealing rather than clips is preferred because clips may dislodge during specimen manipulation. The splenic hilum is approached from the inferior pole after complete lateral and superior mobilization. The hilar vessels are divided using an endoscopic vascular stapler (2.5-mm staple height for vessels); a single or double firing across the hilum is usually sufficient. Before firing, the surgeon must confirm that the pancreatic tail is not within the stapler jaws by lifting the stapler and visualizing the posterior pancreatic tissue separately. The devascularized spleen is placed in a retrieval bag, morcellated, and extracted through an enlarged port site — intact retrieval is reserved for cases where histopathologic architecture must be preserved.

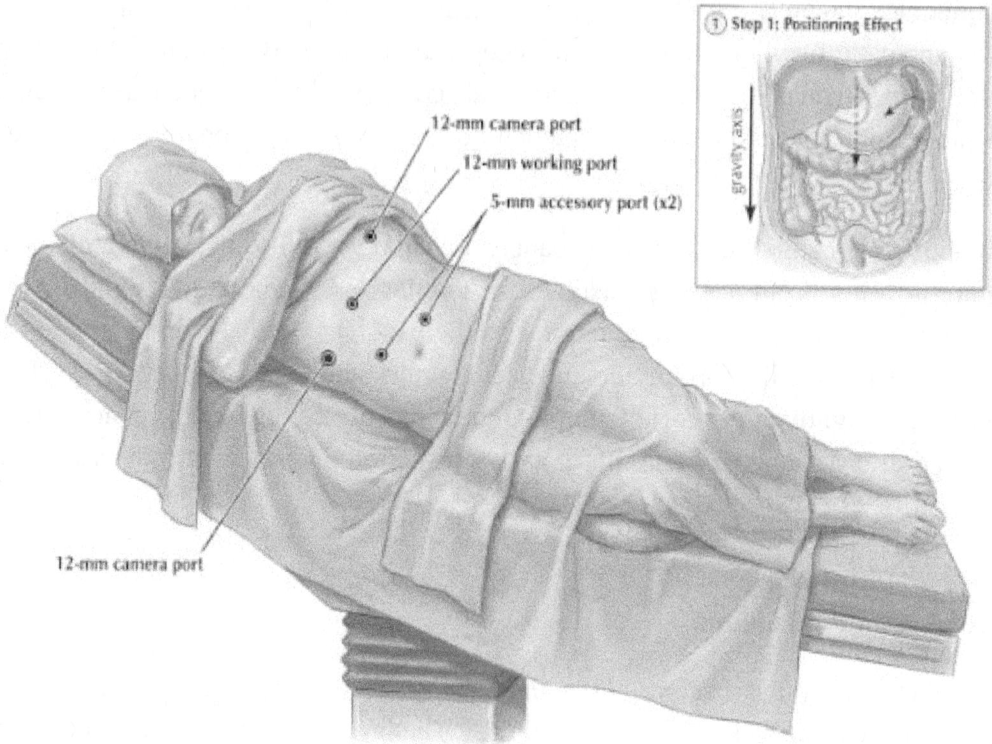

THE OPERATIVE DANGER ZONE ATLAS — Short Gastric Vessel Avulsion During Gastrosplenic Ligament Division

The Zone: The superior portion of the gastrosplenic ligament between the gastric fundus and the upper splenic pole, where the highest short gastric vessels are shortest (often less than 1 cm in length) and most tightly tethered. Excessive cephalad traction on the spleen during mobilization places these vessels under tension, converting them from identifiable structures into taut cords that avulse rather than divide cleanly.

The Structure at Risk: The short gastric vessels (vasa brevia) and the gastric fundal wall. Avulsion of a short gastric vessel produces brisk arterial hemorrhage from the retracted gastric stump that pools in the left upper quadrant and obscures the operative field. Aggressive attempts to control the bleeding with energy devices or graspers risk thermal or crush injury to the gastric fundus, producing a delayed gastric perforation or ischemic necrosis of the fundal wall.

The Consequence: Uncontrolled hemorrhage from short gastric avulsion is the most common reason for conversion from laparoscopic to open splenectomy, reported in 2–5% of laparoscopic cases. Iatrogenic gastric fundal injury produces a postoperative gastric leak that manifests as left upper quadrant sepsis, subphrenic abscess, or gastrocutaneous fistula — complications that carry substantial morbidity and require prolonged hospitalization.

The Safe Maneuver: Divide the gastrosplenic ligament from inferior to superior, handling the longest and most mobile vessels first and progressing to the shortest last. Minimize cephalad traction on the upper pole while dividing the superior short gastric vessels. Use an ultrasonic energy device that seals and divides simultaneously rather than clips, which may dislodge during subsequent manipulation. If the uppermost vessel is too short to isolate safely, consider leaving a small cuff of splenic tissue attached to the gastric wall rather than risking avulsion — this remnant can be cauterized flat or oversewn.

Partial Splenectomy and Splenic Preservation Techniques

Indications for Splenic Preservation

The immunologic consequences of total splenectomy — particularly the lifelong risk of overwhelming postsplenectomy infection — have driven increasing interest in parenchyma-sparing techniques whenever complete splenic removal is not oncologically or hematologically mandated. Partial splenectomy is best established in hereditary spherocytosis, where removing 80–85% of the splenic mass reduces hemolysis and transfusion requirements while preserving enough splenic tissue to maintain opsonization of encapsulated organisms. Other indications include benign splenic cysts, focal splenic tumors (hemangioma, hamartoma, lymphangioma), and selected cases of splenic trauma (AAST grades I–III) where the parenchymal injury is limited to one pole.

Technique of Partial Splenectomy

The operation depends on the segmental vascular anatomy described earlier. After full mobilization, the surgeon identifies the segmental artery supplying the territory to be resected and ligates it individually. A well-demarcated line of color change appears on the splenic capsule within minutes, marking the boundary between perfused and ischemic parenchyma. The capsule is scored 1 cm into the perfused side (to ensure a viable margin) and the parenchyma is divided using a combination of electrocautery, ultrasonic dissection, and topical hemostatic agents. Mattress sutures through the raw splenic surface buttressed with absorbable bolsters achieve capsular hemostasis. The remnant is confirmed to be well perfused by visual inspection — a dusky or mottled remnant suggests compromise of the remaining segmental supply and may require conversion to total splenectomy.

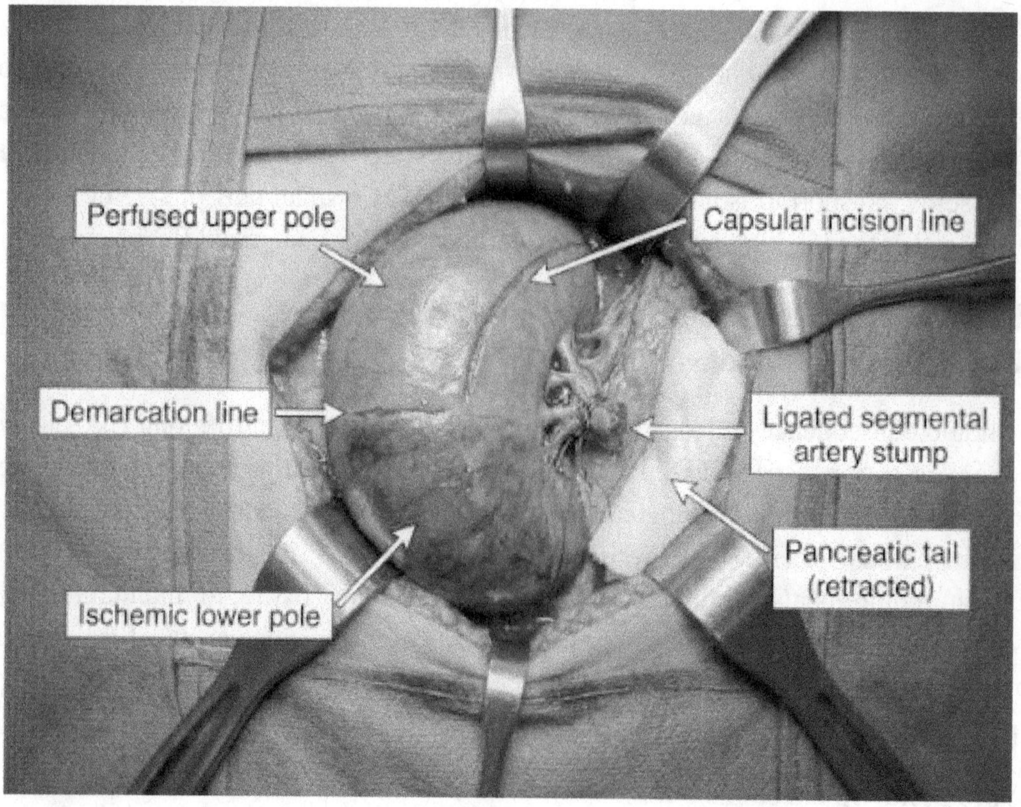

Pediatric Considerations in Splenic Preservation

Children are at substantially higher risk of OPSI than adults — the lifetime incidence of fatal postsplenectomy sepsis in children splenectomized before age 5 is estimated at 4–5%, compared with less than 1% in adults. This age-dependent risk has made partial splenectomy the preferred approach for hereditary spherocytosis in pediatric patients, where the operation is typically deferred until after age 5 when feasible. The standard pediatric partial splenectomy removes 80–85% of the splenic mass, retaining the upper pole on its preserved superior segmental artery. Postoperatively, the splenic remnant hypertrophies over 12–18 months, eventually providing measurable opsonin function as confirmed by the disappearance of Howell-Jolly bodies from the peripheral smear. Long-term studies demonstrate that children who undergo partial splenectomy maintain adequate pneumococcal antibody titers and do not require lifelong antibiotic prophylaxis, though they should still receive standard encapsulated organism vaccinations.

Splenic Salvage in Trauma

Nonoperative management is now the standard of care for hemodynamically stable patients with blunt splenic injury (AAST grades I–III), with success rates exceeding 90% when supported by serial clinical monitoring and CT surveillance. When operative intervention is required — because of hemodynamic instability, peritonitis, or failure of nonoperative management — splenic salvage techniques may still be considered if the injury is limited. Splenorrhaphy with absorbable mesh wrapping, topical hemostatic application, and argon beam coagulation can achieve hemostasis in selected grade II–III injuries. The decision to attempt salvage versus total splenectomy is made in the operating room based on the surgeon's assessment of injury severity, the patient's physiologic status, and the presence of other injuries requiring attention — a prolonged attempt at splenic salvage in a multiply injured patient with ongoing hemorrhage from other sources is not justified.

THE OPERATIVE DANGER ZONE ATLAS — Splenic Flexure Injury During Inferior Pole Mobilization

The Zone: The splenocolic ligament and the peritoneal reflection between the inferior pole of the spleen and the splenic flexure of the colon. In patients with a low-lying spleen or a redundant splenic flexure, the colon may be adherent to the inferior splenic capsule through inflammatory or congenital attachments that obscure the plane between the two organs. Blind inferior pole dissection in this configuration risks full-thickness colonic injury.

The Structure at Risk: The splenic flexure of the colon, specifically the antimesenteric wall that faces the splenic inferior pole. Serosal tears produce delayed adhesion-related complications, while full-thickness injuries cause fecal contamination of the left upper quadrant and postoperative abscess or peritonitis.

The Consequence: Iatrogenic colonic injury during splenectomy occurs in approximately 1–2% of cases and is more common with massive splenomegaly, where the enlarged spleen compresses and displaces the splenic flexure inferiorly and medially. Unrecognized full-thickness injury produces delayed peritonitis presenting 3–5 days postoperatively with fever, leukocytosis, and left upper quadrant tenderness — a clinical picture that may initially be attributed to subphrenic hematoma or postsplenectomy reactive thrombocytosis.

The Safe Maneuver: Identify the splenic flexure of the colon before beginning inferior pole dissection by following the transverse colon from its visible midline portion laterally into the left upper quadrant. Divide the splenocolic ligament under direct vision using sharp dissection rather than energy devices near the colonic wall. If inflammatory adhesions between the splenic capsule and the colonic wall are encountered, develop the plane from the colonic side — keeping the dissection immediately on the colonic serosa and leaving any adherent tissue on the splenic specimen. Inspect the splenic flexure circumferentially after mobilization; repair any serosal injuries with interrupted seromuscular sutures.

Postsplenectomy Considerations and Overwhelming Postsplenectomy Infection

Immunologic Consequences of Splenectomy

The spleen performs critical immunologic functions that are incompletely compensated by other reticuloendothelial organs after splenectomy. Its marginal zone B lymphocytes produce natural IgM antibodies against polysaccharide antigens on encapsulated bacteria — a function that other lymphoid tissues do not replicate. The splenic macrophages filter opsonized bacteria and immune complexes from the bloodstream with an efficiency that the hepatic Kupffer cells cannot match for poorly opsonized organisms. Loss of these functions produces a permanent state of increased susceptibility to invasive infection by encapsulated organisms, particularly Streptococcus pneumoniae (responsible for 50–70% of postsplenectomy sepsis), Neisseria meningitidis, and Haemophilus influenzae type b.

Pathophysiology and Clinical Course of Overwhelming Postsplenectomy Infection

Overwhelming postsplenectomy infection (OPSI) is a fulminant bacteremia that progresses from nonspecific prodromal symptoms — fever, malaise, rigors, vomiting — to septic shock, purpura fulminans, disseminated intravascular coagulation, and multiorgan failure within 12–24 hours. The mortality rate exceeds 50% even with aggressive critical care, and death may occur within hours of the first symptom. The lifetime risk of OPSI is estimated at 3–5%, with the highest incidence in the first two years after splenectomy, though cases have been reported decades later. The risk is greatest in children under five years of age and in patients splenectomized for hematologic malignancy. The hallmark pathophysiologic feature is an overwhelming bacterial load — blood cultures drawn at presentation often yield colony counts several orders of magnitude higher than those seen in bacteremia in immunocompetent patients, because the body lacks the splenic filter that normally clears low-grade bacteremia before it can amplify.

CAUTION: Every asplenic patient presenting with fever, regardless of how well they appear, must be treated as a potential OPSI case until proven otherwise. The window from mild symptoms to irreversible shock can be less than 12 hours. Empiric parenteral antibiotics covering Streptococcus pneumoniae (ceftriaxone 2 g IV) must be administered immediately — before blood culture results return and before any imaging workup is completed.

Prevention Strategies

Prevention of OPSI requires a multilayered approach combining vaccination, patient education, and in selected cases antibiotic prophylaxis. Vaccination is the cornerstone: pneumococcal conjugate vaccine (PCV15 or PCV20) followed by pneumococcal polysaccharide vaccine (PPSV23) at least 8 weeks later, meningococcal conjugate vaccine (MenACWY) with a booster every 5 years, meningococcal serogroup B vaccine, and Haemophilus influenzae type b conjugate vaccine. For elective splenectomy, all vaccines should be administered at least 14 days preoperatively; for emergency splenectomy, vaccination is given 14 days postoperatively when the immune response is adequate. Lifelong antibiotic prophylaxis with daily oral penicillin V (or amoxicillin) is recommended for all children under age 5 following splenectomy and should be considered for at least 1–2 years in adults. All asplenic patients should carry a medical alert card or bracelet identifying their asplenic status, maintain a standby supply of empiric antibiotics (amoxicillin-clavulanate) for self-administration at the first sign of febrile illness before reaching medical care, and receive annual influenza vaccination to reduce the risk of secondary bacterial pneumonia.

Thrombocytosis and Thromboembolic Risk

Reactive thrombocytosis following splenectomy is nearly universal, with platelet counts peaking at 1–3 weeks postoperatively and occasionally exceeding 1,000 × 10^9/L. While reactive thrombocytosis is generally considered a benign and self-limited phenomenon, it contributes to a postsplenectomy thromboembolic risk that is two to three times higher than the baseline population risk. Portal vein thrombosis is the most characteristic postsplenectomy venous complication, occurring in 5–10% of patients within the first month — presentation includes vague abdominal pain, fever, and unexpectedly prolonged ileus. Deep vein thrombosis and pulmonary embolism also occur at increased rates. Pharmacologic thromboprophylaxis with low-molecular-weight heparin is maintained throughout hospitalization and extended for 2–4 weeks after discharge in high-risk patients, including those with myeloproliferative disorders, splenomegaly, or a platelet count exceeding 800 × 10^9/L.

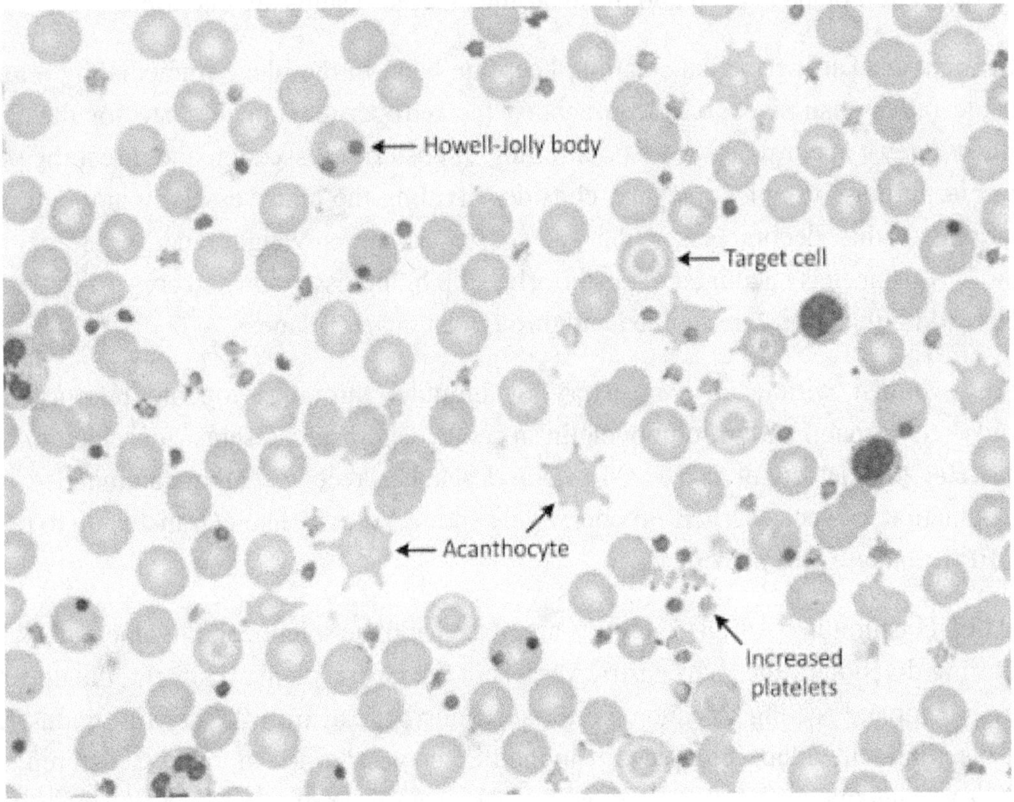

THE OPERATIVE DANGER ZONE ATLAS — Left Kidney Capsular Injury During Posterolateral Splenic Mobilization

The Zone: The splenorenal ligament and the posterolateral plane between the splenic hilum and the anterior surface of the left kidney. During medial rotation of the spleen for open splenectomy, the surgeon's hand sweeps behind the spleen to divide the posterior attachments — this blind maneuver passes directly over the upper pole and anterior capsule of the left kidney, which lies immediately behind the splenic hilum with only Gerota fascia and the splenorenal ligament separating the two organs.

The Structure at Risk: The renal capsule and anterior cortex of the left kidney, particularly the upper pole. Forceful blunt dissection or instrument-assisted mobilization against resistance can strip or tear the renal capsule, producing subcapsular hematoma and parenchymal contusion. In patients with splenomegaly, the enlarged spleen compresses and displaces the left kidney inferiorly, making the renal capsule even more vulnerable during mobilization because the surgeon encounters the kidney earlier and deeper than expected.

The Consequence: Renal capsular injury ranges from minor subcapsular hematoma (managed conservatively) to parenchymal laceration requiring partial nephrectomy or nephrorrhaphy. Even minor injuries produce retroperitoneal hemorrhage that may not be immediately apparent in the peritoneal cavity, presenting postoperatively as unexplained hemoglobin decline, flank pain, or perirenal hematoma on imaging. The incidence is higher with massive splenomegaly (spleen weight exceeding 1,500 g), where the posterior dissection plane is deep and the anatomical relationships are distorted.

The Safe Maneuver: During medial rotation, keep the hand in the plane immediately on the posterior splenic capsule rather than sweeping deep against the retroperitoneum. Palpate for the firm, rounded contour of the kidney's upper pole before committing to posterior dissection and direct the plane anterior to Gerota fascia. In massive splenomegaly, consider dividing the hilar vessels in situ before attempting medial rotation — this decompresses the spleen, reducing its weight and the force required for mobilization. If resistance is encountered posteriorly, stop blunt dissection and convert to sharp dissection under direct vision rather than forcing the hand through an unseen plane.

A 34-year-old woman with a 3-year history of immune thrombocytopenic purpura refractory to corticosteroids, rituximab, and thrombopoietin receptor agonists presents for elective laparoscopic splenectomy. Her platelet count is 18 × 10^9/L and she has received all recommended encapsulated organism vaccinations 3 weeks earlier. Preoperatively she receives a platelet transfusion to raise the count above 50 × 10^9/L for safe port placement.

In the right lateral decubitus position, four ports are placed and the splenocolic ligament is divided without difficulty. During division of the short gastric vessels in the gastrosplenic ligament, the uppermost vessel retracts after incomplete sealing, producing arterial hemorrhage against the gastric fundus. The surgeon controls the bleeding with a laparoscopic clip applied to the gastric side of the vessel stump and confirms no fundal injury. The splenic hilum is approached from the inferior pole after full mobilization, and a single firing of the endovascular stapler divides the hilar pedicle. Before firing, the pancreatic tail is confirmed to be clear of the stapler jaws by lifting the device and visualizing the posterior tissues. The specimen is retrieved in a bag, morcellated, and extracted through the enlarged camera port site. A systematic search identifies a 1.5-cm accessory spleen in the gastrosplenic ligament, which is excised. Postoperatively, the platelet count rises to 150 × 10^9/L by day 2, and the patient is discharged on postoperative day 1 with instructions for lifelong infection awareness and a medical alert bracelet.

This case illustrates several critical principles of laparoscopic splenectomy for hematologic indications. The short gastric vessel bleeding episode demonstrates the importance of the inferior-to-superior division sequence — the uppermost vessels are shortest and most prone to avulsion, and handling them last gives the surgeon maximum experience with the tissue planes before addressing the highest-risk structures. The preoperative platelet transfusion addresses the paradox of operating for thrombocytopenia in a patient whose low platelet count creates a hemorrhagic risk from the surgery itself. The accessory spleen found in the gastrosplenic ligament underscores the importance of a systematic search in all patients undergoing splenectomy for immune thrombocytopenic purpura, because a missed accessory spleen is the most common cause of persistent or recurrent thrombocytopenia after otherwise technically successful splenectomy.

THE OPERATIVE DANGER ZONE ATLAS — Splenic Surgery Danger Zones

Pancreatic Tail at the Splenic Hilum: The pancreatic tail lies within the splenorenal ligament in intimate contact with the splenic hilar vessels. Palpate the tail before clamping; ligate vessels individually in the distributed hilar pattern. Place closed suction drainage near the pancreatic tail if any capsular disruption is suspected.

Short Gastric Vessels at the Upper Pole: The highest short gastric vessels in the gastrosplenic ligament are shortest and most prone to avulsion under traction. Divide from inferior to superior; minimize cephalad traction on the upper pole while handling the final vessels.

Splenic Flexure During Inferior Pole Mobilization: The colonic splenic flexure may be adherent to the splenic inferior pole. Identify the colon before dividing the splenocolic ligament; develop the plane from the colonic side through any inflammatory adhesions.

Left Kidney During Posterolateral Mobilization: The anterior capsule of the left kidney lies immediately behind the splenic hilum. Keep the dissection plane on the posterior splenic capsule; palpate for the kidney before committing to deep mobilization, especially in massive splenomegaly.

Summary and Key Concepts

The spleen is suspended by four ligamentous attachments — gastrosplenic, splenorenal, splenocolic, and splenophrenic — that define the planes of surgical mobilization. The splenic artery follows a tortuous course along the superior pancreatic border and divides at the hilum in either a distributed (70%) or magistral (30%) pattern.

Open splenectomy proceeds through systematic ligament division, early splenic artery ligation to reduce congestion, individual hilar vessel ligation with visualization of the pancreatic tail, and a systematic search for accessory spleens when performed for hematologic indications.

Laparoscopic splenectomy in the right lateral decubitus position is the standard approach for normal to moderately enlarged spleens, utilizing gravity-assisted retraction and endovascular stapler division of the hilar pedicle.

Partial splenectomy exploits the segmental blood supply to resect diseased or injured parenchyma while preserving immunologic function, guided by a demarcation line that appears after segmental vessel ligation.

The four principal danger zones of splenic surgery are the pancreatic tail at the hilum, the short gastric vessels at the upper pole, the splenic flexure at the inferior pole, and the left kidney during posterolateral mobilization.

Overwhelming postsplenectomy infection is a fulminant bacteremia with mortality exceeding 50% that can progress from nonspecific symptoms to irreversible shock within hours, driven by the loss of marginal zone B-cell and macrophage function against encapsulated organisms.

Prevention of OPSI requires preoperative or early postoperative vaccination, lifelong infection awareness education, medical alert identification, standby antibiotics, and consideration of prophylactic penicillin — particularly in children under age 5 and patients with hematologic malignancy.

CHAPTER 23 PEDIATRIC SURGICAL OPERATIONS

Principles of Pediatric Surgical Anatomy and Physiology

Anatomical Differences Relevant to Operative Planning

The pediatric patient is not a scaled-down adult. The infant abdominal wall is thinner, more compliant, and carries less subcutaneous fat than the adult wall, which means that port-site and incision closure requires finer technique to avoid fascial dehiscence. The peritoneal cavity is proportionally smaller, and the omentum — the surgeon's ally in walling off contamination in adults — is thin, poorly developed, and functionally immature in neonates and infants. The inguinal canal is shorter and more oblique, with the internal ring positioned more medially than in adults, which alters the approach to hernia repair. The bladder in infants and young children is an intra-abdominal organ that rises well above the pubic symphysis when distended, placing it at risk during lower abdominal incisions unless decompressed preoperatively with a urethral catheter.

Physiologic Considerations and Fluid Management

Neonates and infants have a higher metabolic rate per kilogram than adults, a larger body surface area-to-mass ratio that increases insensible fluid and heat losses, and limited glycogen stores that make them vulnerable to hypoglycemia during even brief periods of fasting. Thermoregulation is immature — the operating room must be warmed, forced-air warming blankets applied, and intravenous fluids warmed before infusion to prevent hypothermia, which compounds coagulopathy and metabolic acidosis. Maintenance fluid requirements are calculated by the Holliday-Segar formula (4 mL/kg/h for the first 10 kg, 2 mL/kg/h for the next 10 kg, 1 mL/kg/h thereafter), and intraoperative replacement of third-space and blood losses must be meticulous because the margin between euvolemia and hypovolemia is narrow. Blood volume estimation follows weight-based norms: approximately 80 mL/kg in the neonate and 70 mL/kg in the older child, meaning that a 3-kg neonate has a total blood volume of only 240 mL and can tolerate minimal absolute blood loss before requiring transfusion.

Anesthetic and Airway Considerations

The pediatric airway differs from the adult in several ways that directly affect operative planning and emergency management. The larynx is positioned higher (C3–C4 in neonates versus C5–C6 in adults), the epiglottis is omega-shaped and floppy, and the subglottic region — rather than the glottis — is the narrowest point of the airway, making subglottic edema from traumatic intubation a significant concern. Uncuffed endotracheal tubes have traditionally been used in children under 8 years of age to minimize subglottic pressure injury, though modern low-pressure cuffed tubes are increasingly accepted. Pediatric patients are more susceptible to rapid oxygen desaturation during apneic periods because of their higher oxygen consumption relative to functional residual capacity, which leaves less oxygen reserve. These considerations do not change the fundamental surgical technique but influence the urgency of the operation — procedures that can safely wait until the child is optimized (such as elective pyloromyotomy after fluid and electrolyte correction) should not be rushed to the operating room before the anesthesia team has addressed the airway and metabolic status.

Pyloromyotomy for Hypertrophic Pyloric Stenosis

Clinical Presentation and Diagnosis

Hypertrophic pyloric stenosis presents classically between 2 and 8 weeks of age with progressive, nonbilious, projectile vomiting that occurs immediately after feeding. The infant is characteristically hungry after vomiting and feeds eagerly, distinguishing pyloric stenosis from conditions that cause feeding intolerance (such as necrotizing enterocolitis or sepsis). Prolonged vomiting produces a characteristic hypochloremic, hypokalemic metabolic alkalosis because the infant loses hydrochloric acid in the vomitus. The diagnosis is confirmed by abdominal ultrasound, which demonstrates a pyloric muscle thickness of 3 mm or greater and a pyloric channel length of 15 mm or greater. Palpation of the hypertrophied pylorus — the classic olive-shaped mass in the epigastrium — is diagnostic when present but is identified in fewer than 50% of cases in the era of early ultrasound diagnosis.

Preoperative Resuscitation

Pyloromyotomy is never an emergency operation. The critical preoperative step is correction of the metabolic alkalosis and dehydration, which may take 24–48 hours of intravenous fluid resuscitation with normal saline supplemented with potassium chloride. Surgery should not proceed until the serum bicarbonate is below 30 mEq/L and the chloride is above 100 mEq/L, because residual alkalosis increases the risk of postoperative apnea — a potentially fatal complication in an infant who may not be continuously monitored after transfer to a standard ward.

KEY POINT: Pyloromyotomy is a medical urgency, not a surgical emergency. The operation must wait until the metabolic alkalosis is fully corrected. Proceeding with residual alkalosis (serum bicarbonate above 30 mEq/L) increases the risk of postoperative apnea, particularly in neonates and premature infants, because alkalosis shifts the oxyhemoglobin dissociation curve leftward and depresses the central respiratory drive.

Operative Technique — Open (Ramstedt) Pyloromyotomy

The standard open approach uses a right upper quadrant transverse incision placed over the palpable pyloric mass, or a supraumbilical curvilinear incision that provides excellent cosmesis. The pylorus is delivered into the wound, and the surgeon identifies the avascular anterior surface of the hypertrophied muscle. A longitudinal seromuscular incision is made along the anterior pylorus, beginning on the duodenal side and extending to the gastric antrum. The hypertrophied circular muscle fibers are then spread — not cut — using a pyloric spreader or the blunt handle of a scalpel, opening the myotomy until the intact submucosa bulges freely into the gap. The myotomy must extend the full length of the hypertrophied muscle; an incomplete myotomy at the gastric end is the most common cause of persistent vomiting postoperatively. The integrity of the mucosa is confirmed by insufflating air through the nasogastric tube while the surgeon inspects the myotomy site under saline — any air bubbles indicate a perforation that must be repaired immediately.

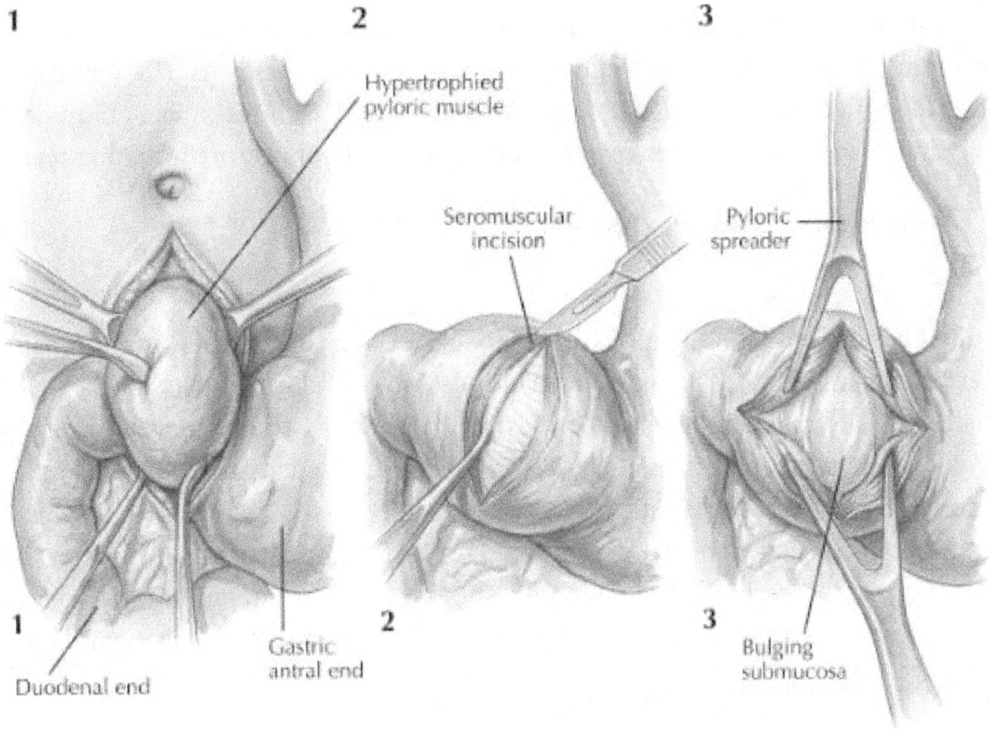

THE OPERATIVE DANGER ZONE ATLAS — Duodenal Mucosal Perforation During Pyloromyotomy

The Zone: The duodenal end of the pyloromyotomy, where the hypertrophied pyloric muscle transitions abruptly to the thin, normal-caliber duodenal wall. The muscle at this junction is thinnest and the underlying submucosa is most tightly adherent to the overlying serosa, because the gradual thickening of the pyloric muscle creates a shoulder where the transition from hypertrophied to normal tissue occurs over just a few millimeters.

The Structure at Risk: The duodenal mucosa and submucosa at the pyloric-duodenal junction. Perforation at this point creates a communication between the duodenal lumen and the peritoneal cavity.

The Consequence: Duodenal perforation occurs in 1–4% of pyloromyotomies and is the most serious intraoperative complication. An unrecognized perforation produces bilious peritonitis within 12–24 hours, manifesting as feeding intolerance, abdominal distension, and clinical deterioration. Even when recognized and repaired intraoperatively, perforation may require conversion from a laparoscopic to an open approach, prolongs the period of nil per os, and increases the length of hospitalization.

The Safe Maneuver: Begin the myotomy incision at the duodenal end, where the muscle is thinnest and the risk of perforation is highest, so the surgeon can apply maximum visual attention to the most dangerous zone first. Use the blunt spreading technique rather than sharp dissection — the muscle fibers separate along natural planes when spread, but cutting risks traversing the submucosa. Stop the myotomy at the first sign of the submucosa bulging freely at the duodenal end; do not extend beyond the pyloric-duodenal junction onto normal duodenum. Confirm mucosal integrity with the air-insufflation test before closing. If perforation is identified, repair with interrupted fine absorbable sutures, rotate an omental pedicle flap over the repair, and keep the nasogastric tube on suction for 24 hours before initiating feeds.

Inguinal Hernia Repair and Orchiopexy in Children

Pathophysiology and Indications

Pediatric inguinal hernias are virtually all indirect, arising from a patent processus vaginalis that failed to obliterate after testicular descent. The incidence is highest in premature infants (up to 30%) and in males (male-to-female ratio of 6:1). Unlike adult hernias, which develop from acquired fascial weakness, the pediatric indirect hernia is a congenital defect that will not resolve spontaneously and carries a significant risk of incarceration — particularly in infants under 6 months of age, where the incarceration rate approaches 30%. For this reason, pediatric inguinal hernias are repaired promptly after diagnosis rather than observed. In girls, the hernia sac may contain the ovary and fallopian tube (hernia of the canal of Nuck), and incarceration can compromise ovarian blood supply, making timely repair equally important.

Operative Technique — High Ligation of the Hernia Sac

The standard pediatric inguinal hernia repair is high ligation of the hernia sac at the internal ring — no mesh is used and no floor reconstruction is performed, because the transversalis fascia and inguinal floor are normal in children. A skin-crease incision is made over the inguinal canal, the external oblique aponeurosis is opened, and the hernia sac (processus vaginalis) is identified on the anterolateral surface of the spermatic cord. The sac is dissected free from the cord structures — vas deferens and testicular vessels — using gentle blunt and sharp dissection, grasping only the sac and never the cord. The dissection is carried to the level of the internal ring, where the sac is twisted, transfixed with an absorbable suture, and excised. The distal sac is left open in males to prevent hydrocele formation. The testis is returned to the scrotum and confirmed to be in a dependent position with intact blood supply. In premature infants, the tissues are thin and friable, and the vas deferens may be difficult to distinguish from the hernia sac — magnification loupes are recommended for this dissection.

THE OPERATIVE DANGER ZONE ATLAS — Vas Deferens Injury During Pediatric Inguinal Hernia Repair

The Zone: The posterolateral aspect of the hernia sac where the vas deferens and testicular vessels are adherent to the peritoneal surface of the processus vaginalis. In premature and very young infants, the vas deferens is a thread-like structure less than 1 mm in diameter that is easily mistaken for a fibrous band or incorporated into the hernia sac during dissection. The danger is greatest when the sac is densely adherent to the cord structures — a situation more common after previous incarceration episodes.

The Structure at Risk: The vas deferens and its accompanying deferential artery. The vas deferens in a neonate is gossamer-thin and virtually transparent; forceful traction, electrocautery near the cord, or inadvertent inclusion in a suture ligature can transect it. Because the vas deferens is a single structure on each side with no collateral duct, injury produces permanent ipsilateral obstruction to sperm transport.

The Consequence: Unilateral vas deferens injury reduces fertility potential, and bilateral injury causes obstructive azoospermia and infertility. The injury is rarely recognized intraoperatively because the vas is so small in infants. It is typically diagnosed years later when the patient presents with infertility in adulthood and imaging reveals absence of the vas. The reported incidence is 0.5–2% in high-volume pediatric centers but may be higher in general surgical practice, where familiarity with the infant inguinal anatomy is less routine.

The Safe Maneuver: Identify the vas deferens before any dissection begins by gently palpating the cord structures between thumb and forefinger — the vas has a characteristic gritty, cord-like feel even in neonates. Dissect only the hernia sac, not the cord en bloc. Grasp the sac with fine forceps and use blunt spreading dissection to peel the sac away from the cord structures, keeping the dissection plane on the peritoneal surface. Never apply electrocautery directly to the cord or within 2 mm of the vas. If the sac is densely adherent to the vas after previous incarceration, leave a strip of sac wall on the vas rather than risking avulsion — this retained peritoneal strip is harmless, while a divided vas is irreparable in a neonate.

Orchiopexy for Undescended Testis

Cryptorchidism affects approximately 3% of full-term male neonates, with spontaneous descent occurring in most by 6 months of age. Orchiopexy is recommended between 6 and 12 months of age for testes that remain undescended, because early fixation preserves the germ cell population — which begins to decline after the first year of life — and reduces the long-term risk of testicular malignancy. The standard inguinal orchiopexy involves mobilizing the testis through an inguinal incision, dividing the gubernacular attachments, ligating the associated processus vaginalis (present in virtually all cryptorchid testes), and creating a dartos pouch in the ipsilateral hemiscrotum. The testicular vessels must be mobilized to sufficient length to reach the scrotum without tension — this requires retroperitoneal dissection of the spermatic cord to the level of the internal ring and occasionally division of the lateral spermatic fascia. A testis fixed under tension will retract to its original position.

Appendectomy in the Pediatric Patient

Diagnostic Challenges in Children

Acute appendicitis is the most common surgical emergency in children, with a peak incidence between 10 and 12 years of age. The diagnosis is more challenging in children than in adults because younger children cannot reliably localize or describe their pain, and the classic migratory pain pattern (periumbilical to right lower quadrant) is present in fewer than 60% of pediatric cases. The differential diagnosis is broader in children, encompassing mesenteric lymphadenitis, Meckel diverticulitis, intussusception, and ovarian pathology in adolescent girls. The Pediatric Appendicitis Score and the Alvarado score provide structured clinical assessment tools, but imaging — typically ultrasound as the first-line modality to avoid ionizing radiation — remains essential when the clinical picture is equivocal. CT is reserved for cases where ultrasound is nondiagnostic and clinical suspicion remains moderate.

Operative Technique and Perforation Management

Laparoscopic appendectomy has become the standard approach in children, offering lower wound infection rates, shorter hospital stays, and better cosmesis compared with open McBurney incision. The technique is analogous to adult laparoscopic appendectomy, though port sizes are smaller (3-mm or 5-mm instruments) and the working space is more limited. The mesoappendix is divided with an energy device, and the base of the appendix is secured with an endoloop or a linear stapler depending on the width and inflammation of the base. Perforated appendicitis, which occurs in up to 30% of children under 5 years of age because the shorter omentum provides less effective containment, is managed with appendectomy, peritoneal irrigation, and postoperative antibiotics. Interval appendectomy following initial nonoperative management of a periappendiceal abscess is debated — contemporary evidence supports immediate appendectomy even in the presence of abscess, with acceptably low complication rates and the advantage of definitive single-stage treatment.

CLINICAL PEARL: In children under 5 years, the perforation rate at presentation exceeds 30% because the omentum is short and thin, limiting its ability to contain inflammation. The surgeon should have a low threshold for broadening antibiotic coverage and extending the postoperative antibiotic course when operating on young children with appendicitis of more than 48 hours duration.

Repair of Congenital Abdominal Wall Defects (Omphalocele and Gastroschisis)

Embryology and Distinguishing Features

Omphalocele and gastroschisis are the two principal congenital abdominal wall defects, each arising from a distinct embryologic failure. Omphalocele results from failure of the lateral body folds to fuse at the umbilical ring during the fourth week of gestation, producing a midline defect covered by a membrane of peritoneum and amnion through which the abdominal viscera herniate. The defect is centrally located at the umbilicus, and the umbilical cord inserts directly into the sac membrane. Gastroschisis, by contrast, is a full-thickness paraumbilical defect — almost always to the right of a normally inserted umbilical cord — through which bowel herniates directly into the amniotic cavity without a covering membrane. Because the exposed bowel in gastroschisis is bathed in amniotic fluid throughout gestation, it develops a characteristic inflammatory peel that thickens the bowel wall, shortens the mesentery, and impairs intestinal motility and absorption for weeks to months after repair.

Operative Management of Gastroschisis

The initial management priority in gastroschisis is protecting the exposed bowel from desiccation and heat loss. The bowel is wrapped in warm, saline-moistened gauze and covered with a sterile plastic bag or silo immediately after delivery. Primary fascial closure is attempted when the eviscerated bowel can be reduced into the abdomen without producing intra-abdominal hypertension — assessed by monitoring intragastric or intravesical pressure, with a target below 20 mmHg. When primary closure is not feasible because of visceroabdominal disproportion, a preformed spring-loaded silo is placed at the bedside in the neonatal intensive care unit without general anesthesia. The silo is serially reduced over 3–7 days by gently tucking bowel into the abdominal cavity at each reduction, and definitive fascial closure is performed in the operating room when all bowel has been reduced. Complications of gastroschisis repair include abdominal compartment syndrome from overly aggressive primary closure, intestinal atresia (present in 10–15% of cases and requiring a second-stage repair), and prolonged intestinal dysmotility requiring weeks of parenteral nutrition.

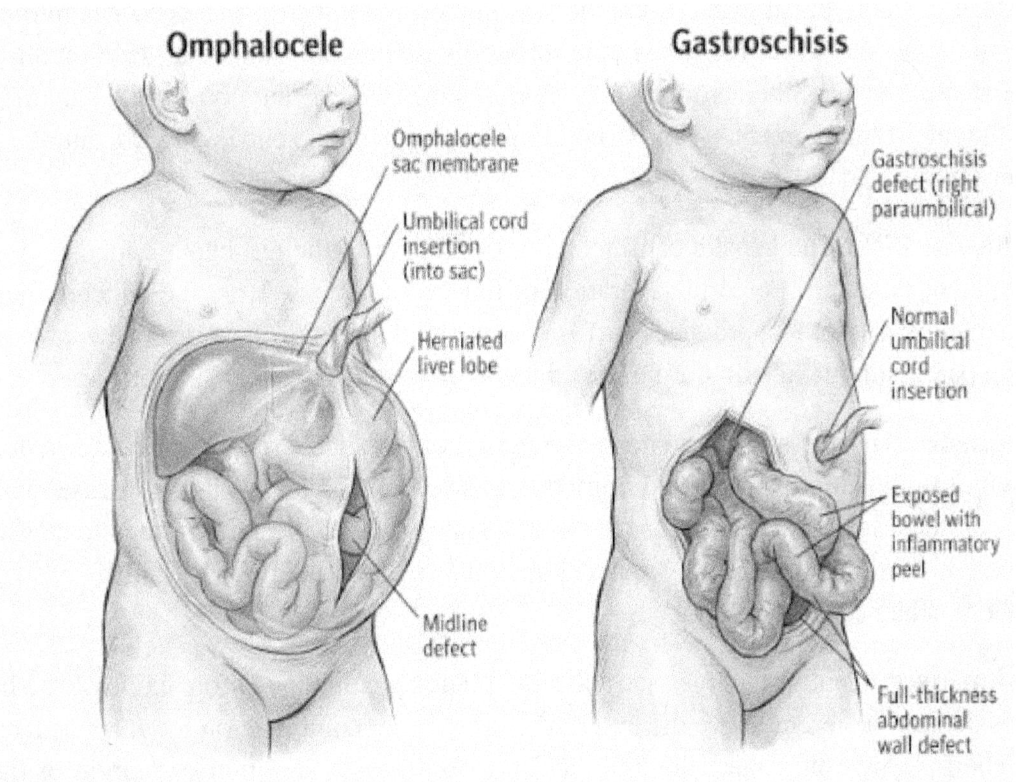

Operative Management of Omphalocele

Small omphaloceles (defect diameter less than 4 cm) are amenable to primary fascial closure in the newborn period. The sac membrane is excised, the viscera are reduced, and the fascia is closed in layers. Giant omphaloceles (defect diameter exceeding 6–8 cm), which may contain the liver and a substantial portion of the intestine, pose a greater challenge because the abdominal cavity has failed to develop sufficient volume to accommodate the herniated viscera. Forced closure produces abdominal compartment syndrome, respiratory compromise from diaphragmatic splinting, and inferior vena cava compression. The staged approach for giant omphalocele uses a silo or prosthetic mesh to cover the defect initially, with gradual reduction over days to weeks as the abdominal domain expands. An alternative strategy — the paint-and-wait technique — applies topical antiseptic agents (silver sulfadiazine or povidone-iodine) to the intact omphalocele sac, which epithelializes over weeks to months, creating a ventral hernia that is repaired electively at 6–12 months of age when the child has grown and the abdominal domain has expanded naturally.

THE OPERATIVE DANGER ZONE ATLAS — Umbilical Vein and Hepatic Injury During Omphalocele Sac Excision

---

The Zone: The superior aspect of the omphalocele sac where the membrane is in direct contact with the inferior surface of the liver. In giant omphaloceles, the left lobe of the liver herniates into the sac and is adherent to the inner surface of the membrane through vascular adhesions that develop during fetal life. The umbilical vein (or its obliterated remnant) traverses the inferior margin of the sac membrane to enter the liver at the falciform ligament — this structure is often patent and carries significant blood flow in the newborn period.

The Structure at Risk: The hepatic capsule and parenchyma of the left hepatic lobe, and the umbilical vein (or its patent remnant). Forceful separation of the sac membrane from the adherent hepatic surface strips the hepatic capsule and produces diffuse parenchymal hemorrhage from the raw liver surface. Division of a patent umbilical vein during sac excision causes brisk venous hemorrhage.

The Consequence: Hepatic surface hemorrhage during omphalocele repair can be difficult to control in a neonate with limited blood volume and immature coagulation. The bleeding is diffuse rather than from a single vessel, making suture ligation ineffective. Combined blood loss from hepatic capsular stripping and umbilical vein division can rapidly exhaust a neonate's blood volume (240 mL in a 3-kg infant) and precipitate hemorrhagic shock.

The Safe Maneuver: Identify the liver-sac adhesion plane by palpation before excising the membrane — if the liver is densely adherent, leave the inner layer of the sac membrane on the liver surface rather than attempting sharp separation. Ligate the umbilical vein remnant at the inferior margin of the sac before dividing it, and confirm it is not patent with gentle traction and inspection before transection. For giant omphaloceles where the liver is extensively adherent, the paint-and-wait approach avoids sac excision entirely and eliminates the risk of hepatic injury.

Surgical Management of Intestinal Malrotation and Volvulus

Embryology and Pathophysiology of Malrotation

Normal intestinal rotation occurs during weeks 5–12 of gestation as the midgut herniates into the umbilical coelom, undergoes a 270-degree counterclockwise rotation around the axis of the superior mesenteric artery, and returns to the abdominal cavity with the duodenojejunal junction fixed at the ligament of Treitz in the left upper quadrant and the cecum fixed in the right lower quadrant. This rotation creates a broad-based mesenteric root that extends from the duodenojejunal junction to the ileocecal region — a distance of approximately 15–20 cm — which prevents the midgut from twisting on its vascular pedicle. Malrotation occurs when this process is interrupted, leaving the duodenojejunal junction displaced to the right and the cecum abnormally positioned. The mesenteric root is narrowed from its normal 15–20 cm to a narrow pedicle of 2–3 cm, creating the anatomical substrate for midgut volvulus — a catastrophic clockwise torsion of the entire midgut around the superior mesenteric artery.

Clinical Presentation and Emergent Evaluation

Midgut volvulus presents most commonly in the first month of life with sudden onset of bilious vomiting — a clinical sign that must always be considered a surgical emergency until proven otherwise. The vomiting is bilious because the obstruction occurs distal to the ampulla of Vater, and it is abrupt in onset because volvulus produces acute, complete duodenal obstruction. If the volvulus is not relieved, progressive torsion occludes first the mesenteric veins (producing intestinal congestion and bloody stools) and then the superior mesenteric artery (producing transmural intestinal ischemia and necrosis). The entire midgut — from the duodenojejunal junction to the mid-transverse colon — may infarct within hours, producing short bowel syndrome or death. An upper gastrointestinal contrast study is the diagnostic study of choice, demonstrating an abnormally positioned duodenojejunal junction (to the right of the left vertebral pedicle) with a corkscrew appearance of the distal duodenum and proximal jejunum when volvulus is present. When volvulus is clinically suspected and the child is deteriorating, operative exploration should not be delayed for imaging.

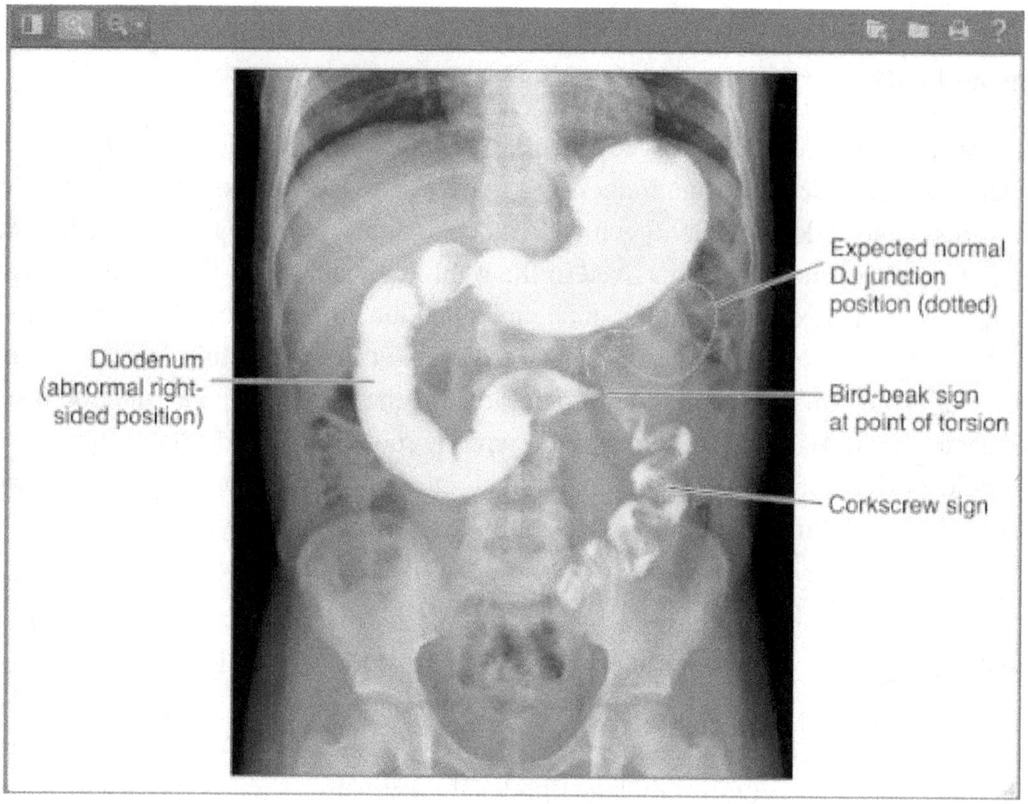

The Ladd Procedure

The Ladd procedure is the definitive operation for malrotation with or without volvulus. The operation has four components performed in sequence. First, the volvulus is detorsed by rotating the midgut counterclockwise (the opposite direction of the torsion). The surgeon lifts the small bowel out of the abdomen and rotates it counterclockwise until the mesentery lies flat and untwisted — typically requiring two to three full turns. The bowel is then inspected for viability; frankly necrotic segments are resected, while segments of questionable viability are left in situ for a planned second-look laparotomy at 24–48 hours. Second, the Ladd bands — peritoneal attachments that cross the duodenum to fix the abnormally positioned cecum — are divided, which relieves extrinsic duodenal obstruction. Third, the mesenteric root is broadened by lysing the adhesions between the duodenum and the proximal jejunum, fanning the mesentery out to widen its base and reduce the risk of recurrent volvulus. Fourth, an appendectomy is performed because the cecum is repositioned to the left upper quadrant, where a future appendicitis would present with atypical symptoms and be diagnostically misleading.

THE OPERATIVE DANGER ZONE ATLAS — Superior Mesenteric Vessel Injury During Ladd Band Division

The Zone: The peritoneal bands (Ladd bands) that cross the second and third portions of the duodenum to reach the abnormally positioned cecum. These bands pass in close proximity to the superior mesenteric artery and vein, which run within or immediately behind the narrowed mesenteric root. In the setting of acute volvulus with edematous, congested mesentery, the vascular anatomy is distorted and the landmarks that normally distinguish band from vessel are obscured.

The Structure at Risk: The superior mesenteric artery and vein, and the marginal arterial arcade supplying the duodenum. The superior mesenteric artery is the sole blood supply to the entire midgut, and injury during Ladd band division threatens the viability of the small bowel and right colon. The duodenal branches are small and easily avulsed during band division, producing hemorrhage from the duodenal wall.

The Consequence: Injury to the superior mesenteric artery during the Ladd procedure is rare but devastating — partial laceration or intimal dissection can produce mesenteric thrombosis and total midgut infarction, which is uniformly fatal or results in permanent total parenteral nutrition dependence. Even minor duodenal arterial injury produces a duodenal wall hematoma that may obstruct the lumen and necessitate prolonged nasogastric decompression.

The Safe Maneuver: Divide Ladd bands with scissors under direct vision, cutting only tissue that can be clearly identified as avascular peritoneal membrane. Palpate the mesenteric root before beginning band division to identify the pulsation of the superior mesenteric artery and confirm its position. Retract the duodenum gently while dividing the bands, maintaining the plane of dissection on the duodenal serosal surface. If the bands are thick, edematous, or cannot be distinguished from mesenteric tissue, ligate them individually rather than dividing with electrocautery — the thermal spread from cautery near the mesenteric vessels risks delayed vessel wall necrosis and thrombosis.

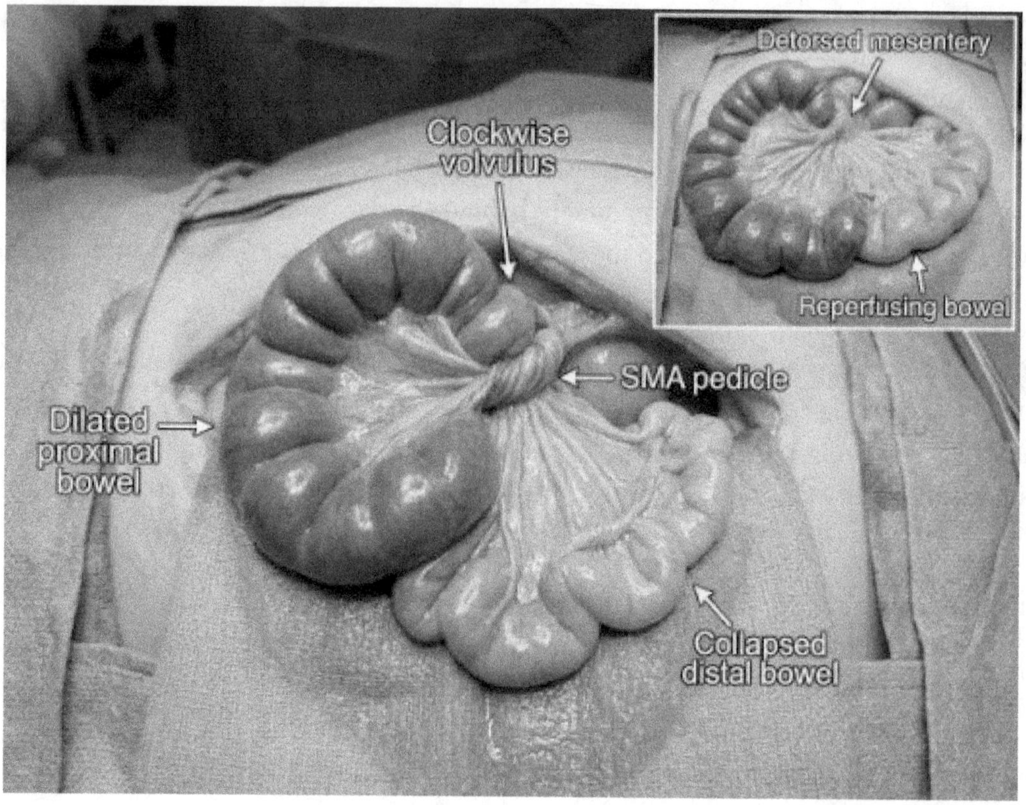

A 3-week-old male neonate presents to the emergency department with sudden onset of bilious vomiting and irritability of 4 hours duration. On examination, the abdomen is mildly distended with diffuse tenderness. A nasogastric tube returns 40 mL of bile-stained fluid. An upper GI series demonstrates the duodenojejunal junction to the right of midline with a corkscrew pattern confirming midgut volvulus. The infant is taken emergently to the operating room.

At laparotomy, the entire midgut is twisted 540 degrees clockwise around the superior mesenteric artery pedicle. The bowel is deeply congested but no segments are frankly necrotic. Counterclockwise detorsion is performed in two stages (270 degrees each), and the bowel is returned to the abdomen and observed for 10 minutes. All segments gradually reperfuse from purple to pink. Ladd bands crossing the duodenum are divided with scissors, the mesenteric root is broadened, and an incidental appendectomy is performed. The cecum is positioned in the left upper quadrant. The infant tolerates enteral feeding by postoperative day 3 and is discharged on day 5 with no complications. This case illustrates the urgency of bilious vomiting in a neonate — the 4-hour symptom-to-operating-room interval prevented the progression from venous congestion to arterial ischemia and midgut infarction.

THE OPERATIVE DANGER ZONE ATLAS — Pediatric Operative Danger Zones

Duodenal Mucosa at the Pyloric-Duodenal Junction: The thinnest point of the hypertrophied pyloric muscle overlies the most vulnerable segment of the duodenal mucosa. Begin the myotomy at the duodenal end under maximum visual attention; use blunt spreading only; confirm integrity with air insufflation.

Vas Deferens During Pediatric Inguinal Hernia Repair: The thread-like vas deferens in neonates is easily incorporated into the hernia sac dissection. Palpate the cord to identify the vas before dissection; dissect only the sac, never the cord en bloc; leave sac wall on the vas rather than risking avulsion.

Umbilical Vein and Hepatic Surface During Omphalocele Repair: The liver adheres to the inner omphalocele sac membrane, and the umbilical vein may remain patent. Ligate the umbilical vein before division; leave sac membrane on the hepatic surface if densely adherent; consider paint-and-wait for giant omphaloceles.

Superior Mesenteric Vessels During Ladd Band Division: Ladd bands pass in close proximity to the SMA and SMV within the narrowed malrotation mesenteric root. Divide bands with scissors under direct vision; palpate for arterial pulsation; ligate thick bands individually rather than dividing with electrocautery.

Summary and Key Concepts

The pediatric patient presents unique anatomical and physiological challenges: a thinner abdominal wall, underdeveloped omentum, higher metabolic rate, limited glycogen reserves, smaller blood volume (80 mL/kg in neonates), and an immature airway positioned higher in the neck.

Pyloromyotomy for hypertrophic pyloric stenosis requires preoperative correction of hypochloremic, hypokalemic metabolic alkalosis before operative intervention, and demands meticulous blunt spreading technique to avoid duodenal mucosal perforation at the pyloric-duodenal junction.

Pediatric inguinal hernias are congenital (patent processus vaginalis), repaired by high ligation without mesh, and require careful identification of the thread-like vas deferens to prevent inadvertent transection.

Gastroschisis is managed by primary closure when visceroabdominal disproportion allows, or staged silo reduction over 3–7 days when primary closure would produce abdominal compartment syndrome.

Giant omphaloceles containing liver require cautious sac management to avoid hepatic capsular stripping and umbilical vein hemorrhage; the paint-and-wait approach provides a safe alternative to primary closure.

Bilious vomiting in a neonate is midgut volvulus until proven otherwise. The Ladd procedure detorses the volvulus, divides the Ladd bands, broadens the mesenteric root, and includes appendectomy.

The four principal danger zones of pediatric operations are the duodenal mucosa during pyloromyotomy, the vas deferens during inguinal hernia repair, the hepatic surface during omphalocele sac excision, and the superior mesenteric vessels during Ladd band division.

CHAPTER 24 VASCULAR ACCESS AND CENTRAL LINE PROCEDURES

Surgical Anatomy of Central Venous Access Sites

Internal Jugular Vein Anatomy

The internal jugular vein (IJV) emerges from the jugular foramen at the skull base and descends through the neck within the carotid sheath, lateral and slightly anterior to the internal carotid artery in the upper neck and lateral to the common carotid artery in the lower neck. The vein runs deep to the sternocleidomastoid muscle throughout its course and is most accessible for percutaneous cannulation at the apex of the triangle formed by the two heads of the sternocleidomastoid, where it lies superficially — typically 1.0–1.5 cm beneath the skin. At the base of the neck the IJV joins the subclavian vein behind the sternoclavicular joint to form the brachiocephalic (innominate) vein. The right IJV is preferred for central venous access because it provides a straight path into the superior vena cava without the acute angulation required by the left-sided approach, and because the thoracic duct — which drains into the venous system at the junction of the left IJV and left subclavian vein — is avoided. The phrenic nerve descends on the anterior surface of the anterior scalene muscle, medial to the IJV in the lower neck; it is at risk only during surgical cutdown or excessively deep needle passes.

Subclavian Vein Anatomy

The subclavian vein is a continuation of the axillary vein, beginning at the lateral border of the first rib and passing over the first rib anterior to the insertion of the anterior scalene muscle. The vein lies in the costoclavicular space — the triangular interval between the clavicle anteriorly, the first rib posteroinferiorly, and the anterior scalene muscle medially. Immediately behind the subclavian vein, separated only by the anterior scalene muscle, lies the subclavian artery; the brachial plexus trunks pass between and behind these vessels. The cupola of the lung (pleural dome) rises 2–3 cm above the medial third of the clavicle, and the apex of the lung is in direct contact with the floor of the costoclavicular space. This intimate relationship between the subclavian vein and the lung apex is the anatomical basis for pneumothorax during subclavian catheterization — the most characteristic and potentially life-threatening mechanical complication of central venous access.

Femoral Vein Anatomy

The femoral vein lies medial to the femoral artery in the femoral triangle, with the mnemonic NAVEL (Nerve, Artery, Vein, Empty space, Lymphatics) describing the lateral-to-medial arrangement of structures beneath the inguinal ligament. The femoral vein is readily accessible by palpating the femoral artery and inserting the needle 1–2 cm medially, though ultrasound guidance has become standard to account for anatomical variation. The femoral site avoids the risks of pneumothorax and thoracic duct injury associated with internal jugular and subclavian approaches, but carries higher rates of catheter-related infection and deep vein thrombosis, which limit its use to emergent situations or patients in whom cervical and subclavian access is contraindicated.

Access Site	Landmark / Position	Adjacent Structure at Risk	Primary Complication
Right IJV	Apex of SCM triangle; lateral to carotid pulsation	Common carotid artery (medial)	Carotid artery puncture
Subclavian	Infraclavicular; junction of medial and middle thirds of clavicle	Lung apex (posterior-inferior)	Pneumothorax
Femoral	2 cm below inguinal ligament; medial to arterial pulse	Femoral artery (lateral)	Arterial puncture, DVT
Left IJV	Same as right IJV (left side)	Thoracic duct (at venous confluence)	Chylothorax (left-sided)

Internal Jugular Vein Catheterization (Ultrasound-Guided)

Indications and Preparation

Internal jugular vein catheterization is indicated for central venous pressure monitoring, administration of vasoactive medications and hyperosmolar solutions (parenteral nutrition, hypertonic saline), rapid volume resuscitation through large-bore access, and temporary hemodialysis catheter placement. The patient is positioned supine in 15 degrees of Trendelenburg to distend the IJV and reduce the risk of air embolism. The head is turned slightly to the contralateral side — excessive rotation compresses the IJV against the carotid artery and makes cannulation more difficult. The neck, chest, and ipsilateral shoulder are prepared with chlorhexidine-alcohol antiseptic using a scrubbing motion for at least 30 seconds, followed by full sterile draping. A high-frequency linear ultrasound probe (7.5–12 MHz) in a sterile sheath is used for real-time guidance throughout the procedure.

Ultrasound-Guided Technique — Seldinger Method

The ultrasound probe is placed transversely over the apex of the sternocleidomastoid triangle to obtain a short-axis view of the IJV and carotid artery. The IJV is identified as a thin-walled, compressible, anechoic structure lateral to the round, pulsatile, non-compressible carotid artery. The skin entry point is chosen so that the needle approaches the IJV at a 30–45-degree angle, with the needle tip visible on the ultrasound image throughout its advance — this real-time visualization is what distinguishes ultrasound-guided from landmark-based technique and reduces the rate of carotid artery puncture from 6–9% to less than 1%. When the needle tip is seen entering the anterior wall of the IJV and dark venous blood is aspirated freely, a J-tipped guidewire is advanced through the needle into the vein. The needle is withdrawn over the wire, a small skin incision is made at the wire entry site to facilitate dilator passage, and the tract is dilated before the central venous catheter is advanced over the wire to the desired depth (typically 15–17 cm from the right IJV to position the catheter tip at the cavoatrial junction). The wire is removed, all ports are aspirated and flushed, and catheter position is confirmed with chest radiography or point-of-care echocardiography.

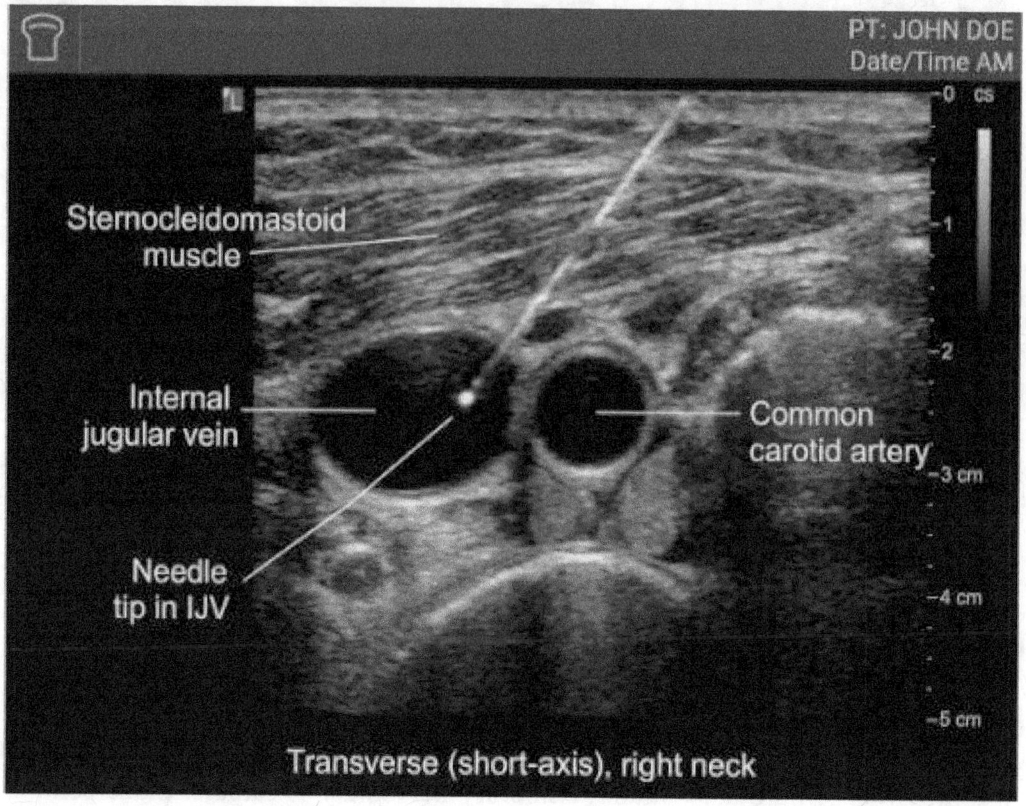

THE OPERATIVE DANGER ZONE ATLAS — Carotid Artery Puncture During Internal Jugular Vein Catheterization

---

The Zone: The medial aspect of the internal jugular vein where it overlies or lies immediately lateral to the common carotid artery in the carotid sheath. In up to 54% of patients, the IJV overlaps the carotid artery to some degree when the head is rotated, meaning that a needle directed medially during IJV cannulation will traverse the IJV and enter the carotid artery. Without ultrasound guidance, the landmark-based approach relies on palpation of the carotid pulse and insertion of the needle lateral to it, but this method has a carotid puncture rate of 6–9%.

The Structure at Risk: The common carotid artery and, in the event of catheter or dilator advancement through an unrecognized arterial puncture, the arterial wall itself. A small-gauge needle puncture of the carotid artery is usually self-limited with direct pressure. However, advancement of a large-bore dilator (7–9 French) through an arterial puncture creates a tract that cannot be controlled with external compression alone and may produce an arteriovenous fistula, pseudoaneurysm, carotid dissection, or stroke from thrombus or air entry into the arterial system.

The Consequence: Simple needle puncture of the carotid artery occurs in fewer than 1% of ultrasound-guided procedures and is managed with 5 minutes of direct pressure. Unrecognized arterial cannulation with dilator or catheter advancement — a never event under real-time ultrasound guidance but still reported when the guidewire position is not confirmed before dilation — can produce hemorrhagic stroke, carotid dissection, or exsanguinating hemorrhage requiring emergent surgical repair.

The Safe Maneuver: Use real-time ultrasound guidance for every IJV catheterization, with the needle tip visualized at all times during advancement. Before dilating, confirm venous (not arterial) wire placement by one of the following methods: transduction of the wire-port showing a venous waveform, ultrasound confirmation of the wire within the IJV lumen, or aspiration of dark non-pulsatile blood through the needle with the syringe off. If bright red pulsatile blood is aspirated, remove the needle immediately and hold direct pressure for 5 minutes; do not advance the wire. Limit the head rotation to 30 degrees or less to minimize IJV-carotid overlap.

Subclavian Vein Catheterization

Infraclavicular Approach and Technique

The infraclavicular approach remains the most common technique for subclavian vein catheterization. The needle entry point is at the junction of the medial and middle thirds of the clavicle, directed toward the sternal notch. The needle is advanced beneath the clavicle, hugging the posterior surface of the bone to remain anterior to the subclavian artery and above the lung apex. The needle is kept parallel to the floor (not angled posteriorly or inferiorly) to reduce the risk of pleural puncture. When venous blood is freely aspirated, the Seldinger technique proceeds as for IJV catheterization. Ultrasound guidance for subclavian catheterization is technically more challenging than for IJV because the clavicle creates an acoustic shadow, but supraclavicular and lateral approaches using ultrasound have been described and may reduce complication rates. The left subclavian vein is generally avoided for long-term catheters because of the risk of thoracic duct injury and the higher incidence of catheter malposition into the left IJV rather than the SVC.

Complications and Management

Pneumothorax is the signature complication of subclavian vein catheterization, occurring in 1–6% of procedures in large series. It results from the needle traversing the subclavian vein and puncturing the pleural dome, which lies immediately beneath and behind the vein in the costoclavicular space. A small pneumothorax (less than 20% of the hemithorax) in an asymptomatic patient may be managed with observation, serial chest radiography, and supplemental oxygen. A larger or symptomatic pneumothorax requires tube thoracostomy. Tension pneumothorax — though rare — can develop rapidly in mechanically ventilated patients and demands immediate needle decompression followed by chest tube placement. Subclavian artery puncture occurs in 1–4% of attempts and is more difficult to manage than carotid puncture because the subclavian artery lies behind the clavicle and cannot be effectively compressed externally. Direct pressure from above the clavicle against the first rib may tamponade the artery, but large-bore arterial injuries from dilator advancement may require endovascular stent-graft repair or open surgical exploration.

THE OPERATIVE DANGER ZONE ATLAS — Pneumothorax from Subclavian Vein Catheterization

The Zone: The costoclavicular space, where the subclavian vein passes over the first rib anterior to the anterior scalene muscle. The pleural dome rises 2–3 cm above the medial clavicle, and the lung apex fills this space during inspiration. The needle must pass through this confined corridor to enter the subclavian vein, and any deviation posteriorly or inferiorly from the plane immediately beneath the clavicle brings the needle tip into contact with the pleura.

The Structure at Risk: The parietal pleura and the apex of the lung. Needle puncture of the lung parenchyma allows air to enter the pleural space through the visceral pleural defect, producing a pneumothorax that enlarges with each breath cycle. In patients receiving positive-pressure ventilation, the injured lung is subjected to continuous insufflation pressure that drives air through the defect, accelerating pneumothorax development and increasing the risk of tension physiology.

The Consequence: Pneumothorax complicates 1–6% of subclavian catheterizations and may not be apparent on the immediate post-procedure chest radiograph — a delayed pneumothorax can evolve over 24–48 hours as the pleural defect expands. Tension pneumothorax in a ventilated patient produces rapid cardiovascular collapse with hypotension, tracheal deviation, and absent breath sounds on the affected side. The bilateral subclavian catheterization attempt — left side after right-sided failure — carries the risk of bilateral pneumothorax, which is immediately life-threatening.

The Safe Maneuver: Keep the needle parallel to the floor and in continuous contact with the posterior surface of the clavicle during advancement — the clavicle acts as a bony rail that prevents posterior deviation toward the pleura. Never redirect the needle inferiorly if the initial pass does not find the vein; withdraw and redirect with the same flat trajectory. Obtain a post-procedure chest radiograph (upright PA preferred) within 1 hour and recheck at 4–6 hours to detect delayed pneumothorax. If the first subclavian attempt fails, switch to the ipsilateral IJV rather than attempting the contralateral subclavian, to avoid the risk of bilateral pneumothorax. In patients on positive-pressure ventilation, perform the puncture during end-expiration when the pleural dome is at its lowest.

Peripherally Inserted Central Catheters and Midline Catheters

Indications and Insertion Technique

Peripherally inserted central catheters (PICCs) provide central venous access through a peripheral upper extremity vein — typically the basilic, brachial, or cephalic vein at the mid-upper arm level. The basilic vein is the preferred insertion site because it is the largest and most medially positioned upper arm vein, providing the straightest path to the axillary and subclavian veins and into the superior vena cava. PICCs are indicated for medium-duration venous access (weeks to months) requiring central tip position — parenteral nutrition, prolonged antibiotic courses, chemotherapy, and frequent blood sampling. Insertion is performed under ultrasound guidance at the bedside using a modified Seldinger or micro-introducer technique, with fluoroscopic or electrocardiographic confirmation of tip position at the cavoatrial junction. Midline catheters, by contrast, are shorter catheters (8–20 cm) whose tip terminates in the axillary vein — not the central circulation — and are therefore classified as peripheral rather than central catheters. They are suitable for medications compatible with peripheral infusion but of longer duration than a standard peripheral IV (up to 4 weeks).

Complications and Maintenance

PICC-related complications include catheter-related thrombosis (upper extremity deep vein thrombosis in 2–5% of patients, higher in oncology and ICU populations), catheter-related bloodstream infection, mechanical phlebitis, catheter malposition, and catheter fracture with embolization. Upper extremity DVT presents as arm swelling, pain, and difficulty flushing the catheter; duplex ultrasound confirms the diagnosis. Management includes therapeutic anticoagulation and catheter removal when the catheter is no longer needed, though some guidelines permit retention if the catheter remains functional and the patient is anticoagulated. Catheter-related bloodstream infection (CRBSI) is diagnosed by differential time-to-positivity of blood cultures drawn simultaneously from the catheter and a peripheral vein. Prevention follows standard central line bundle practices: maximal sterile barrier precautions at insertion, chlorhexidine skin antisepsis, daily assessment of catheter necessity, and prompt removal when no longer indicated. PICCs should not be placed in arms with existing arteriovenous fistulas, planned fistula creation, lymphedema, or prior axillary lymph node dissection.

KEY POINT: PICCs placed in the upper arm should never be inserted into the arm ipsilateral to a functioning or planned arteriovenous fistula for hemodialysis. Central venous stenosis from PICC-related thrombosis can render the ipsilateral arm unusable for future fistula creation — a devastating consequence for a patient with end-stage renal disease whose long-term survival depends on reliable vascular access.

Tunneled Central Venous Catheter and Implantable Port Placement

Tunneled Catheter Placement

Tunneled central venous catheters (Hickman, Broviac, Groshong types) are designed for long-term venous access (months to years) and differ from non-tunneled catheters in two critical ways: a subcutaneous tunnel separates the venous entry site from the skin exit site, reducing the path for bacterial migration, and a Dacron cuff positioned within the tunnel incites a fibrotic reaction that anchors the catheter and creates a mechanical barrier against ascending infection. The catheter is typically inserted via the right IJV using the Seldinger technique. The tunnel is created by passing a tunneling device from a chest wall exit site (usually below the ipsilateral clavicle) subcutaneously to the venotomy, threading the catheter through the tunnel in a retrograde fashion, and positioning the Dacron cuff at least 2 cm inside the tunnel entrance. The catheter tip is positioned at the cavoatrial junction under fluoroscopic guidance. The venous entry site is closed with absorbable suture, and the skin exit site is dressed with a transparent sterile dressing.

Implantable Port Placement

An implantable port consists of a subcutaneous reservoir (port body) connected to a central venous catheter whose tip sits at the cavoatrial junction. The port is accessed percutaneously through the intact skin using a non-coring (Huber) needle, and is completely internalized when not in use — eliminating the infection risk associated with a percutaneous exit site. Ports are preferred for intermittent central venous access (cyclic chemotherapy, periodic infusions) where the catheter is accessed for days at a time with intervals of non-use. The port body is implanted in a subcutaneous pocket created over the anterior chest wall, lateral to the sternum and inferior to the clavicle. The pocket must be sufficiently deep to prevent skin erosion but superficial enough to allow reliable needle access. The catheter is inserted via the IJV or subclavian vein and tunneled subcutaneously to the pocket, where it is connected to the port body and locked into place. The incision is closed in layers, and the port is accessed immediately to confirm function and flush with heparinized saline.

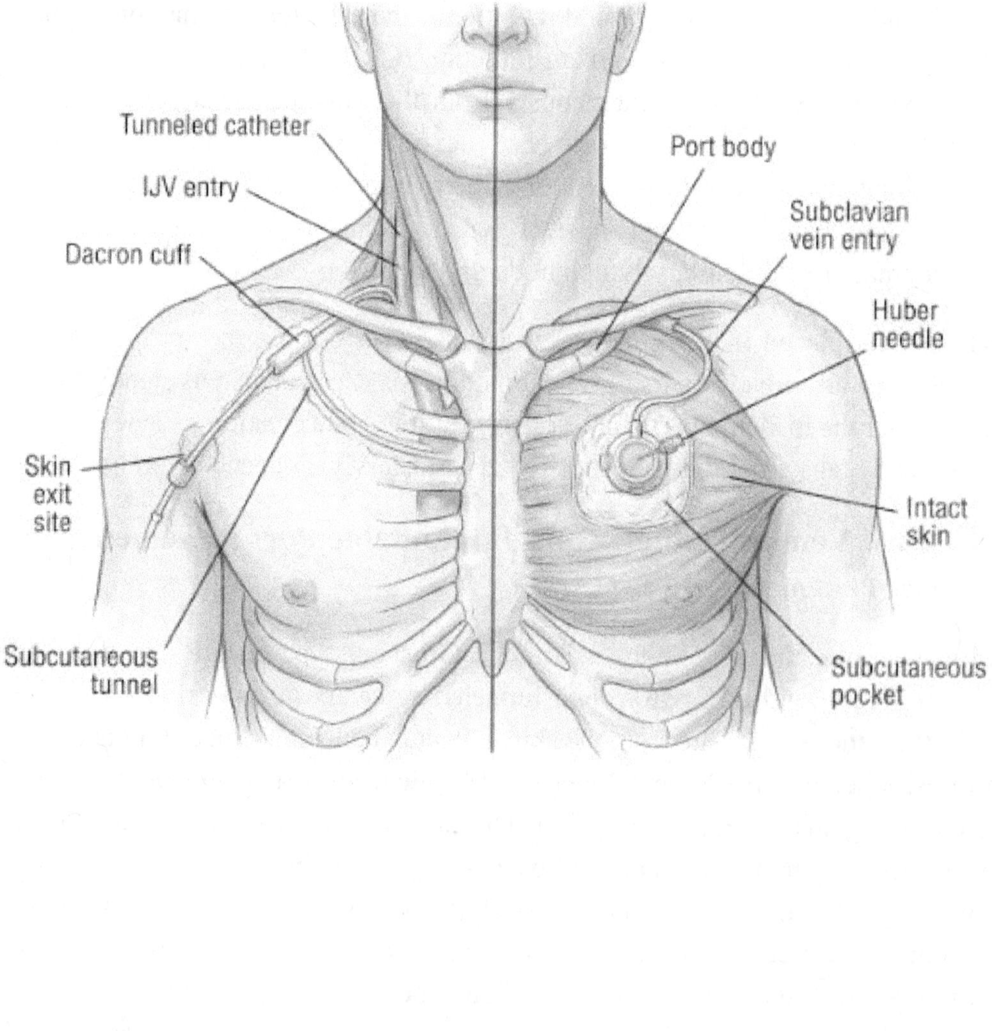

THE OPERATIVE DANGER ZONE ATLAS — Air Embolism During Central Venous Catheter Insertion or Removal

The Zone: Any moment during central venous catheterization when the venous lumen is open to atmospheric air — needle hub disconnection, catheter port left open during connection, wire exchange, or catheter removal. The central veins operate at subatmospheric pressure during spontaneous inspiration, generating a pressure gradient that draws air into the venous system through any open tract. The risk is highest when the patient is upright or in reverse Trendelenburg, which maximizes the negative intrathoracic pressure.

The Structure at Risk: The right ventricle and pulmonary vasculature. Air entering the venous system travels to the right heart, where a large bolus (3–5 mL/kg) creates an air lock in the right ventricular outflow tract that obstructs pulmonary blood flow. Even smaller volumes of air embolize to the pulmonary arterioles, producing ventilation-perfusion mismatch and hypoxemia. In patients with a patent foramen ovale (present in 25% of the population), venous air can cross to the arterial circulation, producing paradoxical air embolism with stroke or coronary air embolism.

The Consequence: Clinically significant venous air embolism is rare (estimated at 0.1–0.2% of central line procedures) but carries mortality of up to 30% when a large volume is entrained. The classic presentation is sudden cardiovascular collapse with hypotension, tachycardia, and a characteristic mill-wheel murmur on auscultation. Smaller volumes produce dyspnea, chest pain, and oxygen desaturation without hemodynamic collapse.

The Safe Maneuver: Position the patient in Trendelenburg during insertion and removal of central venous catheters — this raises the central venous pressure above atmospheric and reverses the gradient that draws air into the veins. Never disconnect any catheter hub or leave any port open to air without first occluding the tract with a finger or clamp. During catheter removal, have the patient exhale and hold the breath (Valsalva maneuver) or time the removal with positive-pressure ventilation in intubated patients to maintain positive intrathoracic pressure. Apply an occlusive dressing immediately after catheter removal and maintain it for 24 hours, because the subcutaneous tract may persist and serve as an air entry point even after the cathcter is removed.

Arteriovenous Fistula and Graft Creation for Hemodialysis

Principles of Hemodialysis Access Planning

The arteriovenous fistula (AVF) is the preferred form of permanent hemodialysis access because it offers the lowest rates of infection, thrombosis, and interventional maintenance compared with arteriovenous grafts (AVGs) and tunneled dialysis catheters. The Fistula First initiative and KDOQI guidelines recommend autogenous AVF creation as the first-line access, with AVG reserved for patients with inadequate native veins and tunneled catheters used only as a bridge to permanent access or when all surgical options are exhausted. Preoperative vein mapping with duplex ultrasound is mandatory to assess vein diameter (minimum 2.5 mm for AVF), continuity, compressibility, and the absence of stenosis or thrombosis. Arterial assessment confirms adequate inflow by documenting a normal Allen test and radial or ulnar artery diameter of at least 2.0 mm. The preferred order of access site selection proceeds from distal to proximal: radiocephalic (wrist) AVF first, then brachiocephalic (elbow) AVF, then brachiobasilic AVF with transposition, then prosthetic AVG (forearm loop or upper arm straight configuration).

Operative Technique — Radiocephalic Arteriovenous Fistula

The radiocephalic AVF (Brescia-Cimino fistula) is created at the wrist through a transverse or longitudinal incision over the anatomical snuffbox or the volar wrist. The cephalic vein and radial artery are isolated, and the vein is mobilized for sufficient length to allow a tension-free anastomosis. The vein is ligated distally, spatulated, and anastomosed end-to-side to the radial artery using a continuous 7-0 polypropylene suture. The anastomosis length should be 5–7 mm — shorter anastomoses restrict inflow and delay maturation, while longer anastomoses produce excessive flow that can lead to steal syndrome. After releasing the clamps, a palpable thrill at the anastomosis and an audible continuous bruit along the outflow vein confirm fistula patency. The fistula requires 6–12 weeks of maturation before first cannulation, during which the arterialized vein dilates and its wall thickens in response to arterial pressure and shear stress. A mature fistula suitable for cannulation has a flow rate exceeding 600 mL/min, a diameter of at least 6 mm, and a depth of less than 6 mm from the skin surface — the rule of sixes.

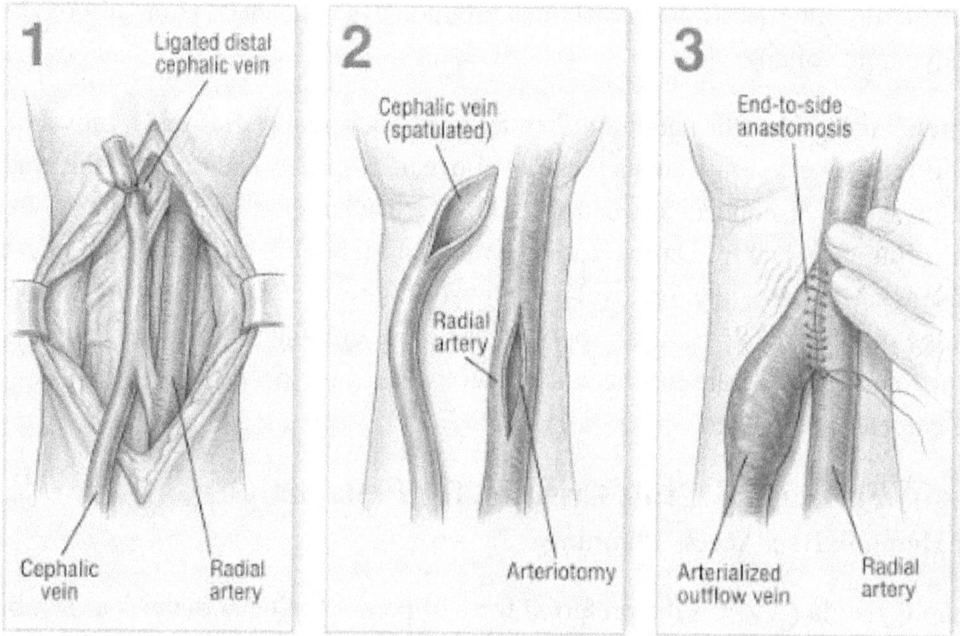

Arteriovenous Graft and Access Complications

When native veins are inadequate for autogenous AVF creation, a prosthetic arteriovenous graft (typically expanded polytetrafluoroethylene, ePTFE) is placed as a conduit between an artery and a vein. The most common configurations are the forearm loop graft (radial artery to antecubital vein) and the upper arm straight graft (brachial artery to axillary vein). Grafts can be cannulated as early as 2 weeks after placement (some immediately-use grafts within 24–72 hours), but have higher rates of thrombosis (annual primary patency of 40–50% compared with 60–70% for AVF) and infection (because the prosthetic material lacks the native vein's resistance to bacterial colonization). Thrombotic graft occlusion presents as loss of the palpable thrill and audible bruit, and is treated with surgical or percutaneous thrombectomy combined with angioplasty of any underlying venous stenosis. Graft infection presents as erythema, warmth, tenderness, and purulent drainage at the graft site, and typically requires complete graft excision with ligation of the arterial and venous anastomoses — partial graft salvage is attempted only when infection is clearly limited to a segment distant from both anastomoses.

THE OPERATIVE DANGER ZONE ATLAS — Steal Syndrome After Arteriovenous Fistula Creation

The Zone: The arterial segment distal to the AVF anastomosis, where blood flow is diverted into the low-resistance venous outflow of the fistula rather than continuing distally through the native arterial bed. The risk is greatest with proximal (brachial artery) fistulas that have large anastomoses (greater than 7 mm) producing high flow rates, in patients with peripheral arterial disease, diabetes, or calcified non-compliant arteries that cannot augment collateral flow to compensate for the fistula steal.

The Structure at Risk: The hand and digits distal to the fistula. Arterial steal diverts blood away from the palmar arches and digital arteries, producing ischemia that ranges from mild coolness and numbness during dialysis sessions (access-related hand ischemia, Grade 1) to rest pain (Grade 2), tissue loss with ulceration or gangrene of the fingers (Grade 3), and acute hand ischemia with limb-threatening motor and sensory deficits (Grade 4).

The Consequence: Symptomatic steal syndrome occurs in 5–10% of upper arm fistulas and 1–2% of forearm fistulas. Grade 3–4 steal requires urgent intervention to prevent permanent hand ischemia. If untreated, digital gangrene progresses to autoamputation or necessitates surgical amputation.

The Safe Maneuver: Assess the palmar arch integrity with the Allen test and measure digital pressures before and after temporary fistula occlusion at the time of creation. Limit the anastomosis length to 5–7 mm to control fistula flow. If steal symptoms develop postoperatively, initial management includes hand elevation and warming. For persistent or progressive steal, the DRIL procedure (Distal Revascularization-Interval Ligation) restores distal perfusion by creating a bypass from the brachial artery proximal to the fistula to a point distal to it, then ligating the native artery between the fistula and the bypass origin — this maintains fistula flow while redirecting blood to the hand through the bypass conduit.

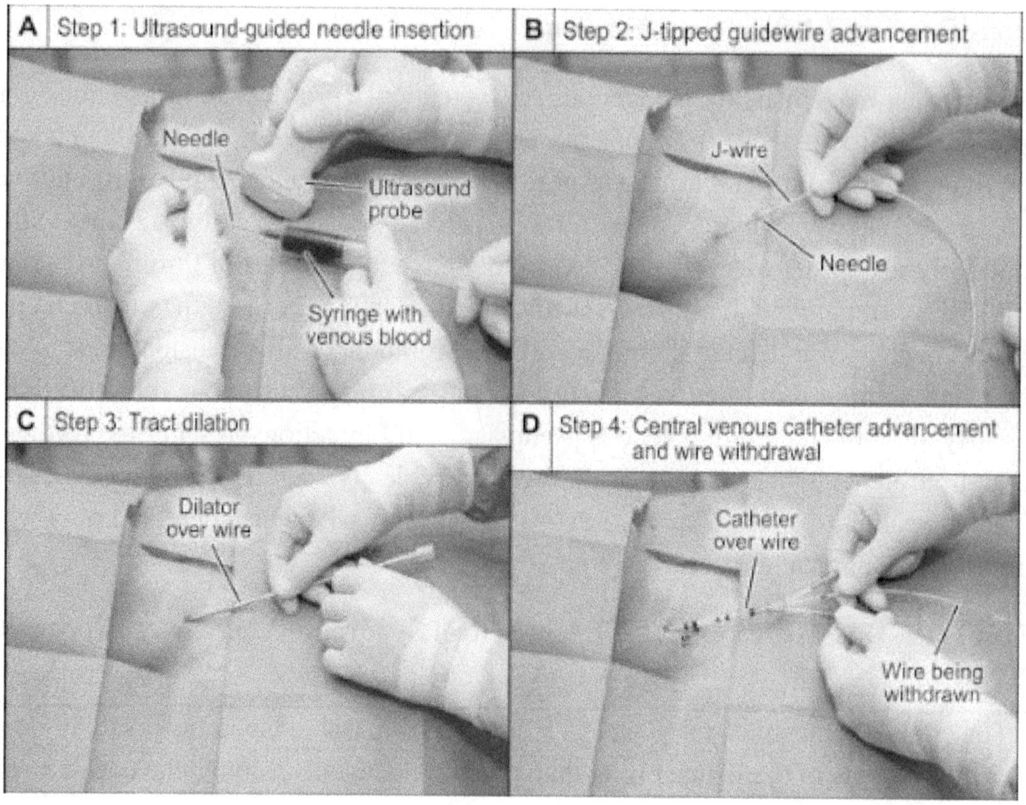

A 58-year-old man with end-stage renal disease secondary to diabetic nephropathy is referred for hemodialysis access creation. He has a functioning right-sided tunneled dialysis catheter placed emergently 3 months ago when he developed uremic pericarditis. Preoperative vein mapping demonstrates a 3.0-mm cephalic vein at the left wrist with good distensibility and no stenosis, and a 2.5-mm radial artery with a normal Allen test. A left radiocephalic AVF is created through a volar wrist incision using a 6-mm end-to-side anastomosis with 7-0 polypropylene continuous suture. A palpable thrill is present at the anastomosis immediately after clamp release. The patient is instructed to perform daily fistula exercises (repeated hand squeezing with a soft ball) to promote maturation. At 8 weeks, duplex ultrasound demonstrates a flow rate of 850 mL/min and a vein diameter of 7 mm at the mid-forearm, meeting the rule-of-sixes criteria for cannulation. The tunneled catheter is removed after successful first dialysis through the mature fistula.

This case illustrates the staged approach to hemodialysis access: emergent catheter placement for immediate dialysis followed by definitive AVF creation as soon as the patient is medically optimized. The 8-week maturation period is typical for radiocephalic fistulas. The fistula exercises promote arterialization by increasing flow-mediated shear stress on the vein wall, accelerating the dilation and wall-thickening that define maturation. The removal of the tunneled catheter after successful fistula cannulation eliminates the ongoing risks of catheter-related bloodstream infection and central venous stenosis.

Carotid Artery During IJV Catheterization: The internal jugular vein overlaps the carotid artery in up to 54% of patients when the head is rotated. Use real-time ultrasound guidance with continuous needle tip visualization; confirm venous placement before dilation; limit head rotation to 30 degrees.

Pleural Dome During Subclavian Catheterization: The lung apex rises 2–3 cm above the clavicle, directly beneath the subclavian vein. Keep the needle parallel to the floor and against the posterior clavicle; never redirect inferiorly; obtain chest radiography post-procedure and at 4–6 hours.

Venous System During Catheter Insertion or Removal (Air Embolism): Any open communication between the central veins and atmospheric air generates a pressure gradient that entrains air during inspiration. Position the patient in Trendelenburg; occlude all open hubs; time catheter removal with exhalation or positive-pressure ventilation.

Distal Hand After Arteriovenous Fistula Creation (Steal Syndrome): Proximal fistulas divert arterial flow from the hand, producing ischemia in susceptible patients. Assess palmar arch integrity preoperatively; limit anastomosis length to 5–7 mm; perform the DRIL procedure for persistent Grade 2 or higher steal.

Summary and Key Concepts

The internal jugular, subclavian, and femoral veins each have characteristic anatomical relationships to adjacent structures — the carotid artery, lung apex, and femoral artery respectively — that define the danger zones and complication profiles of central venous catheterization at each site.

Ultrasound-guided internal jugular vein catheterization using the Seldinger technique reduces carotid artery puncture from 6–9% (landmark-based) to less than 1% and is the standard of care for elective and emergent central venous access.

Subclavian vein catheterization carries a 1–6% pneumothorax risk because the needle traverses the costoclavicular space in close proximity to the pleural dome, and subclavian artery puncture is difficult to manage externally because thc vessel lies behind the clavicle.

Peripherally inserted central catheters provide medium-duration central access through upper arm veins but carry a 2–5% risk of upper extremity deep vein thrombosis and should never be placed ipsilateral to a functioning or planned hemodialysis fistula.

Tunneled catheters and implantable ports are designed for long-term access — tunneled catheters maintain a percutaneous exit site with a Dacron cuff barrier, while ports are fully internalized and accessed only through the intact skin.

The radiocephalic arteriovenous fistula is the gold standard for hemodialysis access, requiring 6–12 weeks of maturation to achieve the rule-of-sixes criteria (flow exceeding 600 mL/min, diameter at least 6 mm, depth less than 6 mm).

The four principal danger zones of vascular access procedures are carotid artery puncture during IJV catheterization, pneumothorax during subclavian catheterization, air embolism during any central line insertion or removal, and steal syndrome after arteriovenous fistula creation.

CHAPTER 25 MISCELLANEOUS OPERATIVE PROCEDURES

Tracheostomy (Open and Percutaneous)

Indications and Timing

Tracheostomy is indicated when prolonged mechanical ventilation is anticipated (typically beyond 10–14 days of translaryngeal intubation), when upper airway obstruction cannot be relieved by less invasive means, and when pulmonary toilet requires direct tracheal access in patients with copious secretions or impaired cough. The advantages of tracheostomy over prolonged translaryngeal intubation include reduced laryngeal injury, improved patient comfort and communication, facilitated weaning from mechanical ventilation, and secure airway access that is less prone to inadvertent dislodgement than an endotracheal tube. The timing of tracheostomy in critically ill patients remains debated; current evidence suggests that early tracheostomy (within 7 days of intubation) reduces the duration of mechanical ventilation and ICU stay in selected populations, though it does not consistently reduce mortality.

Open Surgical Tracheostomy — Technique

The patient is positioned supine with the neck extended using a shoulder roll. A horizontal skin incision is made midway between the cricoid cartilage and the sternal notch, centered on the midline. The platysma is divided, and the strap muscles (sternohyoid and sternothyroid) are separated in the midline raphe to expose the pretracheal fascia. The thyroid isthmus, which crosses the trachea at the second and third tracheal rings, is identified; it is either retracted superiorly or divided between clamps and suture-ligated to provide access to the anterior tracheal wall. A window is created in the anterior trachea, typically between the second and third or third and fourth tracheal rings, by removing a rectangular segment of cartilage or by creating an inferiorly-based Bjork flap (a U-shaped flap that is sutured to the skin to facilitate tube reinsertion in the event of accidental decannulation in the early postoperative period). The endotracheal tube is withdrawn under direct vision by the anesthesiologist until the tip is above the tracheostomy site, and the tracheostomy tube is inserted under direct vision. Correct position is confirmed by end-tidal CO_2 detection, bilateral breath sounds, and flexible bronchoscopy through the tracheostomy tube.

Percutaneous Dilational Tracheostomy

Percutaneous dilational tracheostomy (PDT) is performed at the bedside in the ICU, avoiding the risks and logistical burden of operating room transport. Under bronchoscopic guidance, a needle is inserted into the trachea between the first and second or second and third tracheal rings, a guidewire is advanced through the needle, and the tract is serially dilated using a tapered dilator (Ciaglia technique) or a forceps-based dilator (Griggs technique) until a tracheostomy tube can be passed over the dilator into the trachea. Bronchoscopic visualization throughout the procedure confirms midline needle entry, prevents posterior tracheal wall injury by the needle or dilator, and confirms correct tube placement. PDT has equivalent or lower rates of peristomal infection and bleeding compared with open tracheostomy, and produces smaller scars. It is contraindicated in patients with difficult cervical anatomy (short thick neck, cervical spine immobilization, prior neck surgery with distorted landmarks), pediatric patients, and those with coagulopathy that cannot be corrected.

Early and Late Complications of Tracheostomy

Early complications include hemorrhage from the thyroid isthmus or anterior jugular veins (controlled with electrocautery or suture ligation), pneumothorax or pneumomediastinum from dissection below the tracheal entry site into the mediastinum, subcutaneous emphysema from air tracking along the pretracheal fascial planes, and accidental decannulation before the tract matures (particularly dangerous in the first 5–7 days when the stoma has not yet epithelialized and tube reinsertion may create a false passage into the pretracheal soft tissues rather than the tracheal lumen). Late complications include tracheal stenosis at the stoma site or at the cuff site from pressure necrosis of the tracheal cartilage (minimized by maintaining cuff pressures below 25 cmH_2O), tracheo-innominate artery fistula (a rare but catastrophic hemorrhagic complication caused by erosion of the tracheostomy tube tip or cuff into the innominate artery, which crosses the trachea at rings 7–9), tracheomalacia, and persistent tracheocutaneous fistula after decannulation. Tracheo-innominate fistula presents as a sentinel bleed — a brief self-limited hemorrhage from the tracheostomy site — followed hours to days later by massive hemorrhage. Any bleeding from a mature tracheostomy site that is not explained by local granulation tissue must be investigated urgently with bronchoscopy to evaluate for tracheo-innominate erosion.

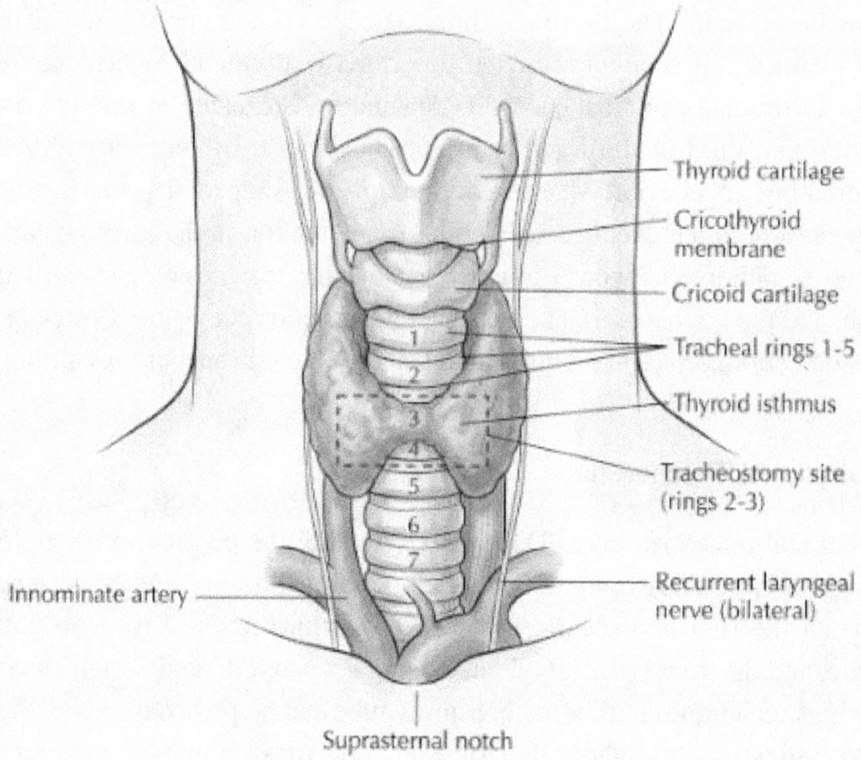

THE OPERATIVE DANGER ZONE ATLAS — Posterior Tracheal Wall Perforation During Percutaneous Tracheostomy

---

The Zone: The membranous posterior wall of the trachea, which is directly anterior to the esophagus. Unlike the cartilaginous anterior and lateral tracheal walls, the posterior wall is composed of the thin trachealis muscle with no cartilaginous support. During percutaneous tracheostomy, the introducing needle and guidewire pass through the anterior wall and traverse the tracheal lumen; if advanced too far, they perforate the posterior wall and enter the preesophageal space or the esophagus itself.

The Structure at Risk: The posterior tracheal wall membrane and the anterior esophageal wall. Perforation creates a tracheoesophageal fistula that allows oral and gastric contents to enter the airway, producing aspiration pneumonia and compromising ventilation. The posterior wall is only 3–4 mm thick, and in patients with prolonged intubation it may be thinned further by pressure necrosis from the endotracheal tube cuff.

The Consequence: Posterior tracheal wall injury during PDT occurs in 0.5–1% of procedures and ranges from superficial mucosal laceration (managed conservatively) to full-thickness perforation creating a tracheoesophageal fistula. A tracheoesophageal fistula requires surgical repair — typically through a cervical approach with interposition of a strap muscle flap between the tracheal and esophageal repairs to prevent recurrence.

The Safe Maneuver: Perform PDT under continuous bronchoscopic guidance with the bronchoscope positioned above the insertion site to visualize the needle entering the anterior tracheal wall in real time. Withdraw the endotracheal tube cuff above the puncture site before needle insertion so the posterior wall is visible to the bronchoscopist. Direct the needle at a 45-degree angle toward the carina (not perpendicular to the skin) so that the needle tip tends to glide along the anterior wall rather than traversing the lumen and striking the posterior wall. Stop needle advancement immediately when air is aspirated or when the bronchoscopist confirms the needle tip in the tracheal lumen.

Feeding Access Procedures (Gastrostomy and Jejunostomy)

Indications and Approach Selection

Gastrostomy provides enteral feeding access when oral intake is inadequate and prolonged tube feeding (exceeding 4–6 weeks) is anticipated. Common indications include neurologic dysphagia from stroke or traumatic brain injury, head and neck malignancy obstructing the oropharynx or esophagus, and supplemental feeding in failure to thrive. Three approaches are used: percutaneous endoscopic gastrostomy (PEG), laparoscopic gastrostomy, and open surgical gastrostomy. PEG is the most common and least invasive, performed at the bedside or in the endoscopy suite under conscious sedation. Jejunostomy bypasses the stomach entirely and is indicated when gastric feeding is contraindicated — severe gastroparesis, gastric outlet obstruction, recurrent aspiration despite postpyloric feeding, or after major upper gastrointestinal surgery where the stomach is excluded from the alimentary tract (such as after esophagectomy or total gastrectomy). Jejunostomy tubes deliver feeds directly into the proximal jejunum, but require continuous rather than bolus infusion because the small bowel lacks the reservoir capacity of the stomach.

Percutaneous Endoscopic Gastrostomy Technique

The PEG technique uses transillumination and finger indentation to identify the point of closest apposition between the anterior gastric wall and the anterior abdominal wall, ensuring that no intervening viscera (colon, small bowel, liver) are interposed. After local anesthesia and a small skin incision, a needle and sheath are advanced through the abdominal wall into the gastric lumen under endoscopic visualization. A guidewire or snare is passed through the sheath and captured endoscopically, and the PEG tube is pulled retrograde through the mouth, esophagus, and stomach, exiting through the abdominal wall at the puncture site (pull technique). An internal bumper on the gastric side and an external bumper on the abdominal wall maintain apposition of the gastric and abdominal walls, which promotes tract maturation over 7–10 days. Alternatively, the push or introducer (Russell) technique places the tube directly through the abdominal wall over a guidewire without the oropharyngeal passage, reducing the theoretical risk of peristomal wound infection from pharyngeal flora.

CAUTION: Before PEG placement, transillumination — the endoscopic light visible through the abdominal wall — and finger indentation — the endoscopic visualization of the abdominal wall being depressed into the gastric lumen by external palpation — must BOTH be confirmed. Absence of either sign suggests interposition of the colon or omentum between the stomach and abdominal wall, and the procedure should be aborted or converted to a laparoscopic or open approach.

Open Surgical Gastrostomy — Stamm Technique

Open surgical gastrostomy is indicated when PEG cannot be performed — prior gastric surgery, esophageal obstruction preventing endoscope passage, absence of transillumination, or the need for concomitant abdominal surgery. The Stamm gastrostomy is the most widely used open technique. Through a small left upper quadrant or upper midline incision, the anterior wall of the gastric body is identified and two concentric purse-string sutures of absorbable material are placed. A gastrotomy is made in the center of the inner purse-string, the gastrostomy tube (balloon-tipped or mushroom-tipped) is inserted into the stomach, and both purse-strings are tightened and tied sequentially to invaginate the gastric wall around the tube, creating a seal that prevents leakage. The gastric wall at the tube site is then sutured to the anterior abdominal wall (gastropexy) with four cardinal sutures to maintain apposition of the gastric and parietal peritoneal surfaces, which prevents peritoneal contamination if the tube is inadvertently dislodged before the tract matures. The tube is brought through a separate stab incision in the left upper quadrant — never through the primary incision — to reduce wound infection risk. Tract maturation requires 7–10 days; premature tube dislodgement before maturation allows free gastric contents to spill into the peritoneal cavity, producing chemical peritonitis.

Surgical Jejunostomy — Witzel Technique

When jejunal feeding access is required — typically during upper gastrointestinal cancer surgery or after esophagectomy — a Witzel jejunostomy is constructed. A loop of proximal jejunum 20–30 cm distal to the ligament of Treitz is selected, and a small enterotomy is made on the antimesenteric border. A feeding tube (typically 10–14 French) is inserted into the jejunal lumen and directed distally. The Witzel tunnel is created by folding the jejunal serosa over the tube with a series of interrupted seromuscular sutures extending 5–6 cm proximally from the enterotomy, burying the extraluminal portion of the tube within the serosal tunnel. This tunnel creates a valve mechanism that prevents reflux of jejunal contents along the tube tract after tube removal. The jejunum at the tube site is sutured to the anterior abdominal wall (jejunopexy) with the same rationale as gastropexy — to prevent peritoneal contamination from premature dislodgement. Jejunostomy tubes are smaller caliber than gastrostomy tubes and clog more easily; continuous rather than bolus feeds are mandatory because the jejunum lacks the reservoir capacity of the stomach, and bolus delivery produces cramping, diarrhea, and dumping physiology.

THE OPERATIVE DANGER ZONE ATLAS — Colonic Interposition Injury During Percutaneous Endoscopic Gastrostomy

The Zone: The space between the anterior gastric wall and the anterior abdominal wall in the left upper quadrant, where the transverse colon or splenic flexure may interpose — particularly in patients with prior abdominal surgery, colonic distension, or hepatomegaly that displaces the stomach inferiorly and allows the colon to occupy the space between the stomach and the abdominal wall.

The Structure at Risk: The transverse colon or splenic flexure. The PEG trocar and tube traverse the interposed colon during placement, creating a gastrocolic fistula that may not be immediately apparent because the tube passes through both walls of the colon and functions normally for feeding. The diagnosis is often delayed weeks to months until the tube is replaced or dislodged, at which point the colonic perforation becomes evident.

The Consequence: Colonic interposition injury during PEG occurs in 0.5–3% of placements and may produce peritonitis from colonic perforation, gastrocolic fistula with diarrhea and malabsorption from gastric contents entering the colon, or colo-cutaneous fistula after tube removal. The delayed presentation makes this complication particularly dangerous because it may not be recognized during the initial procedure.

The Safe Maneuver: Confirm both transillumination and finger indentation before advancing the trocar. If either sign is absent, do not proceed with PEG — convert to laparoscopic gastrostomy, which allows direct visualization of the gastric-abdominal wall interface and identification of interposed viscera. In patients with prior abdominal surgery or known colonic redundancy, consider CT abdomen to evaluate the spatial relationship between the stomach, colon, and abdominal wall before planning the approach. Insufflate the stomach adequately to displace the transverse colon inferiorly before selecting the puncture site.

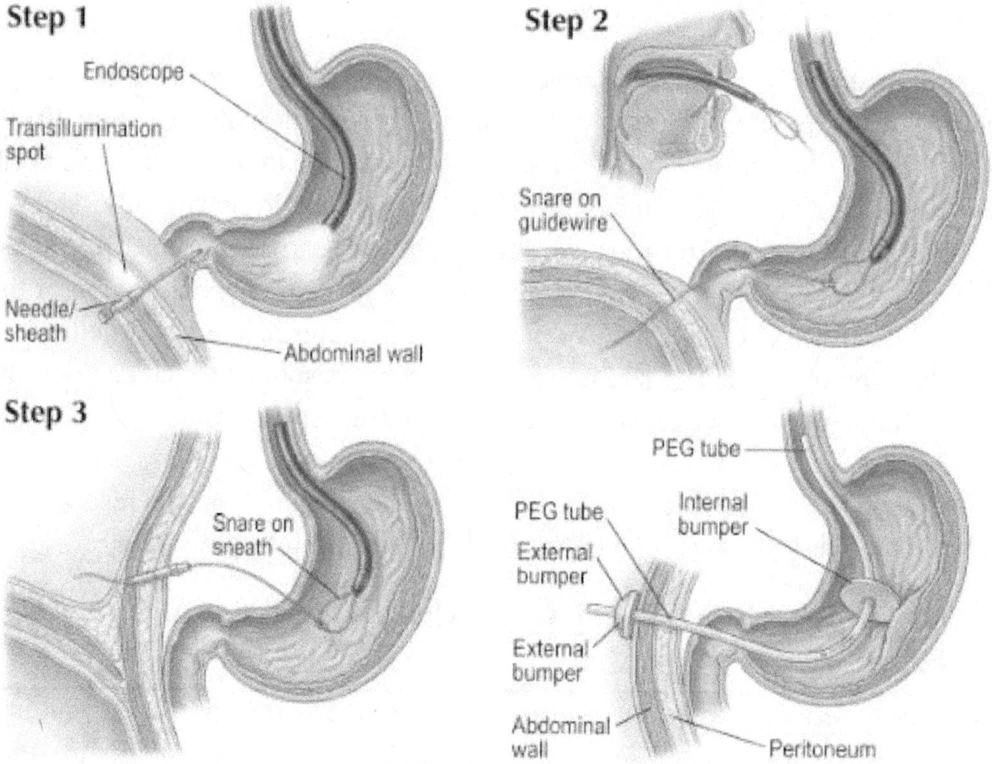

Surgical Management of Pilonidal Disease

Pathophysiology and Clinical Presentation

Pilonidal disease is an acquired condition of the natal cleft caused by loose hair shafts penetrating the skin of the intergluteal fold, inciting a chronic foreign-body inflammatory reaction and abscess formation. The disease predominantly affects young adults (peak incidence 15–30 years), males more than females, and individuals with coarse body hair, deep natal clefts, sedentary occupations, and obesity. Acute presentation is a painful, fluctuant abscess lateral to the midline in the natal cleft; chronic presentation includes one or more draining sinuses with intermittent purulent discharge, often with visible tufts of hair protruding from the sinus openings. The differential diagnosis includes perianal abscess, hidradenitis suppurativa, and sacrococcygeal dermoid cyst. Recurrence is common regardless of treatment modality, affecting 10–30% of patients overall, and is more likely in patients who continue to have hair growth in the natal cleft without hair removal maintenance. Postoperative measures to reduce recurrence include regular depilation of the natal cleft using laser hair removal, shaving, or depilatory creams for at least 6–12 months following surgical treatment.

Surgical Treatment Options

Acute pilonidal abscess is treated with incision and drainage as the initial procedure — definitive excision during the acute inflammatory phase carries higher wound complication rates and is not recommended. Definitive treatment of chronic pilonidal disease requires excision of all sinus tracts and the chronic inflammatory tissue. Excision with primary midline closure has historically been the most common approach but carries wound dehiscence and recurrence rates of 10–25%, because the midline closure places the suture line directly in the deepest part of the natal cleft, where shearing forces and moisture promote wound breakdown. Off-midline closure techniques — particularly the Limberg (rhomboid) flap and the Karydakis flap — shift the wound away from the midline crease, producing significantly lower recurrence rates (2–5%) and faster wound healing. The Limberg flap excises the disease as a rhomboid defect and rotates a fasciocutaneous flap from the adjacent gluteal skin to fill the defect, flattening the natal cleft and eliminating the deep midline groove that perpetuates hair penetration. The Karydakis technique creates an asymmetric, off-midline, tension-free closure by advancing a thick fasciocutaneous flap across the midline.

Minimally Invasive Approaches

Minimally invasive techniques have gained acceptance for chronic pilonidal disease in selected patients. The endoscopic pilonidal sinus treatment (EPSiT) uses a fistuloscope to visualize the sinus tract, ablate its lining with electrocautery or laser, and extract hair and debris under direct vision — preserving the overlying skin and gluteal tissue. Pit-picking (Bascom procedure) involves excising only the midline pits (the hair entry points) through tiny incisions and draining any lateral abscess cavity through a separate incision. These techniques offer faster recovery and lower wound complication rates than wide excision, but recurrence rates remain higher than with flap-based repairs, and patient selection is critical — extensive branching sinuses and prior failed excisions are better served by formal excision and flap reconstruction.

Excision of Sebaceous and Dermoid Cysts

Clinical Features and Surgical Principles

Epidermal inclusion cysts (commonly called sebaceous cysts, though true sebaceous cysts are uncommon) are the most frequent subcutaneous cysts encountered in surgical practice. They present as firm, mobile, subcutaneous nodules with a visible central punctum representing the obstructed pilosebaceous unit. The cyst is lined by stratified squamous epithelium and contains laminated keratinous material with a characteristic odor. Excision is indicated for symptomatic, enlarging, or recurrently infected cysts. The standard technique involves an elliptical skin incision encompassing the punctum, careful dissection of the cyst wall from the surrounding tissue in the plane between the cyst capsule and the subcutaneous fat, and delivery of the intact cyst. The critical technical principle is complete excision of the cyst wall — any residual epithelial lining left in the wound serves as a nidus for recurrence. If the cyst ruptures during dissection and keratinous contents spill into the wound, the wound must be copiously irrigated and any visible cyst wall fragments excised. Infected cysts should be incised and drained first, with definitive excision deferred until the inflammation has resolved, because acute inflammation obscures the tissue planes and increases the risk of incomplete excision.

Dermoid Cysts

Dermoid cysts are congenital inclusion cysts that arise from epithelial elements trapped along embryonic fusion lines. They are most commonly located at the lateral eyebrow (external angular dermoid), the anterior fontanelle, the nose, and the sacrococcygeal region. Unlike epidermal inclusion cysts, dermoid cysts may contain hair follicles, sebaceous glands, sweat glands, and occasionally bone or cartilage. External angular dermoid cysts are excised through an eyebrow incision with careful dissection of the cyst from the underlying periosteum of the lateral orbital rim — the cyst may extend through a bony defect into the orbit, and preoperative imaging (CT or MRI) is recommended for any cyst fixed to the periosteum to rule out intracranial extension. Sacrococcygeal dermoid cysts in neonates require evaluation for connection to the spinal canal (dermal sinus tract) and may require MRI before excision to exclude a tethered cord.

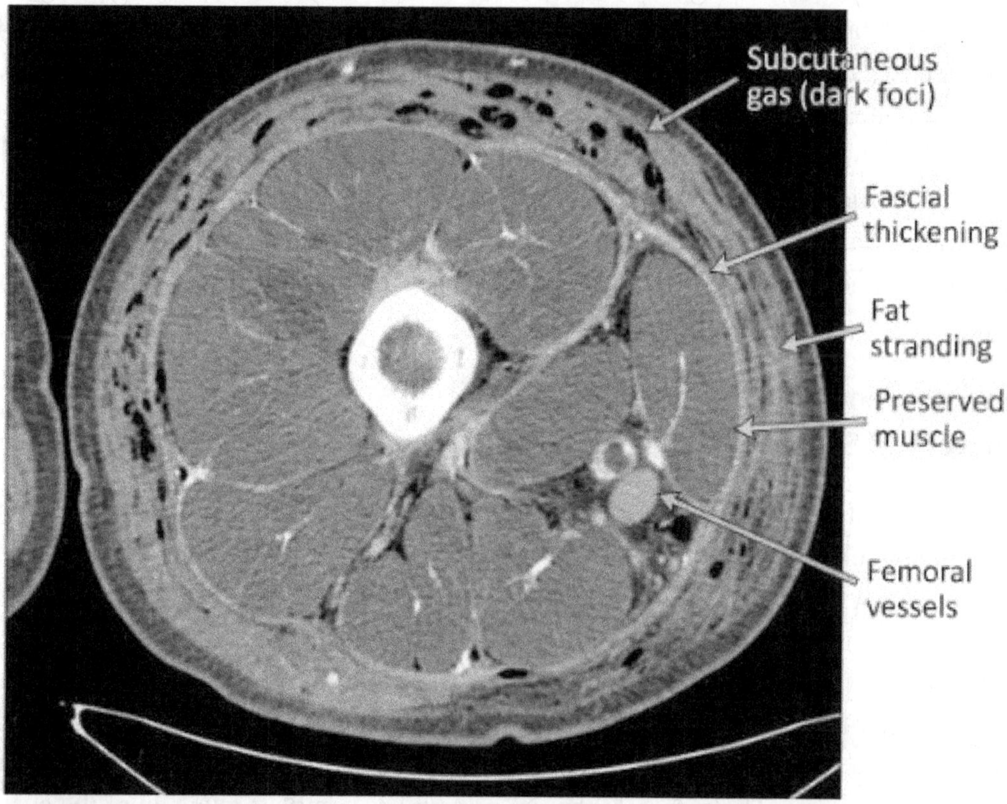

Surgical Drainage of Abscesses and Debridement of Necrotizing Soft Tissue Infections

Principles of Abscess Drainage

Incision and drainage is the definitive treatment for soft tissue abscesses — antibiotics alone cannot sterilize a walled-off collection of pus because the abscess cavity is avascular and antibiotic penetration into the cavity is negligible. The incision should be placed over the point of maximal fluctuance, made long enough to allow complete evacuation of pus and disruption of loculations, and oriented along the natural skin tension lines when feasible to optimize cosmesis. After incision, the cavity is explored with a finger or blunt instrument to break up internal septations, irrigated with saline, and packed loosely with gauze or fitted with a loop drain to maintain drainage. The packing is removed in 24–48 hours and the wound is allowed to close by secondary intention. Complex or deep-seated abscesses — perianal, breast, psoas, subphrenic — may require imaging-guided percutaneous drainage or operative drainage under general anesthesia because the anatomy requires controlled dissection near structures that blind incision could damage.

Recognition of Necrotizing Soft Tissue Infections

Necrotizing soft tissue infections (NSTIs) are surgical emergencies that demand immediate wide debridement. The clinical challenge is distinguishing necrotizing from non-necrotizing infection in the early stages, when the cutaneous signs may be subtle. Features that should raise suspicion for NSTI include: pain disproportionate to the visible skin findings, rapidly progressive erythema with indistinct borders, crepitus on palpation (indicating subcutaneous gas from anaerobic organisms), hemorrhagic bullae, skin necrosis with violaceous discoloration, systemic toxicity (fever, tachycardia, hypotension, altered mental status) out of proportion to the local wound, and failure to improve with appropriate antibiotic therapy within 24–48 hours. Laboratory findings supporting the diagnosis include markedly elevated white blood cell count, elevated C-reactive protein and creatine kinase, hyponatremia, and elevated serum lactate. CT imaging may demonstrate subcutaneous gas, fascial thickening, and fluid tracking along fascial planes, but imaging must not delay operative exploration when clinical suspicion is high — the diagnosis is ultimately confirmed in the operating room.

KEY POINT: Necrotizing fasciitis is a clinical and operative diagnosis, not an imaging diagnosis. CT or MRI findings of subcutaneous gas, fascial thickening, or fluid tracking support the diagnosis, but normal imaging does NOT exclude it. When clinical suspicion is high — pain out of proportion, systemic toxicity, crepitus, skin necrosis — proceed directly to the operating room for exploration. Every hour of delay in surgical debridement increases mortality.

Operative Debridement Technique

The initial incision is placed through the area of maximal skin involvement and extended into the subcutaneous tissue and fascia. The hallmark intraoperative finding of necrotizing fasciitis is dishwater-gray, non-bleeding fascia that separates from the underlying muscle with gentle finger dissection — in healthy tissue, the fascia adheres firmly to the muscle and does not separate without sharp dissection. The necrotic tissue produces a characteristic foul-smelling, thin, grayish exudate (dishwater pus) that is distinct from the thick, creamy pus of a simple abscess. Once the diagnosis is confirmed, debridement must be aggressive: all necrotic skin, subcutaneous tissue, and fascia are excised back to healthy, bleeding tissue in all directions. The debridement should not stop at the visible margin of skin necrosis because fascial necrosis typically extends well beyond the cutaneous changes — the excision continues until the fascia is firmly adherent to the underlying muscle and bleeds normally when cut. The resulting wounds are large and left open, packed with moist gauze, and dressed with negative-pressure wound therapy when feasible.

Planned re-exploration at 24–48 hours is mandatory because the infection may continue to advance despite the initial debridement, and additional tissue may require excision at the second look.

THE OPERATIVE DANGER ZONE ATLAS — Inadvertent Deep Structure Injury During Necrotizing Fasciitis Debridement

The Zone: The plane between the deep fascia and the underlying muscle, tendons, and neurovascular bundles — the plane of surgical debridement in NSTI. Because necrotizing fasciitis destroys the normal tissue architecture, the surgeon cannot rely on standard anatomical landmarks to identify and protect deep structures. The tissue planes are distorted by edema, necrosis, and inflammatory exudate, and structures that would normally be visible and identifiable are obscured by the grayish necrotic tissue that replaces the fascia.

The Structure at Risk: Major neurovascular bundles, tendons, and exposed joint capsules that lie deep to the fascia. In extremity NSTI, the femoral vessels, brachial vessels, median nerve, peroneal nerve, and extensor and flexor tendons are vulnerable. In perineal Fournier gangrene, the spermatic cord structures, urethra, and anal sphincter complex are at risk.

The Consequence: Neurovascular injury during debridement produces distal ischemia, motor and sensory deficits, or hemorrhage that complicates an already critically ill patient. Tendon transection compromises limb function and requires later reconstruction. Urethral injury during Fournier gangrene debridement necessitates suprapubic catheterization and staged urethral repair.

The Safe Maneuver: Debride fascia aggressively but muscle only when frankly necrotic — the goal is to remove all dead fascia and subcutaneous tissue while preserving viable muscle and all identifiable deep structures. When the plane of necrosis approaches a known neurovascular bundle, slow the debridement, identify the structure by its anatomical position and visual characteristics, and dissect around it with scissors rather than continuing blunt finger debridement. In Fournier gangrene, identify and protect the urethra with a Foley catheter placed before debridement begins, and identify the external sphincter before debriding perianal tissue. Accept that the debridement wound will be large and disfiguring — the alternative is progressive sepsis and death.

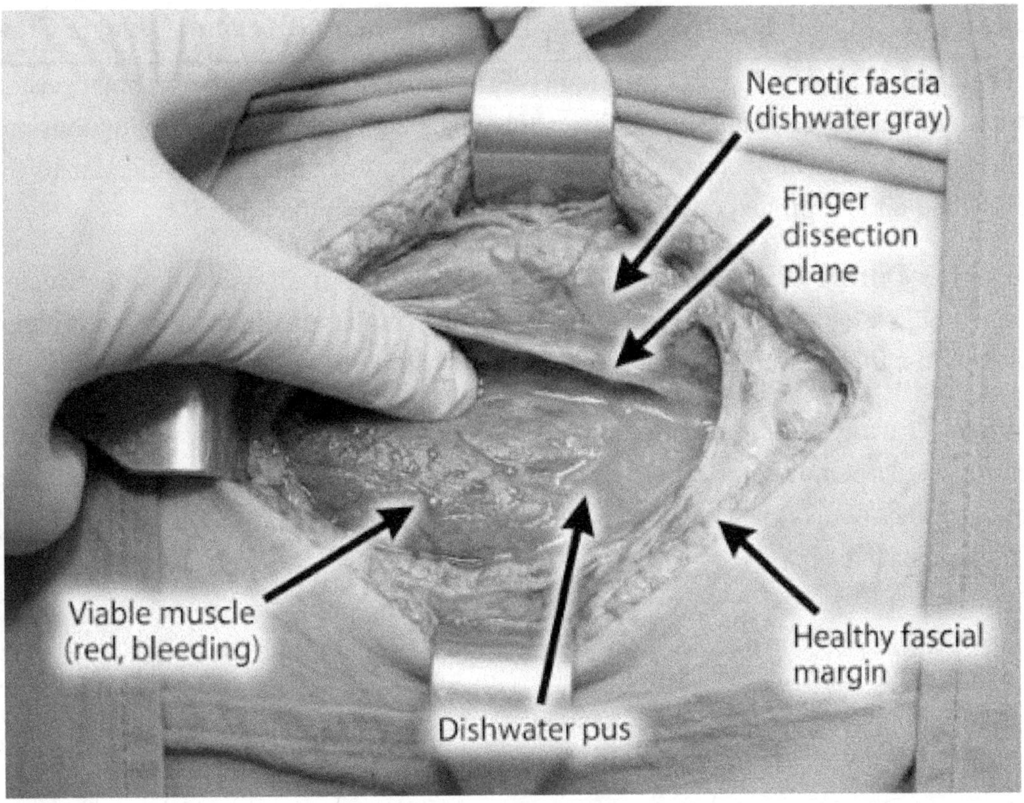

A 52-year-old man with poorly controlled type 2 diabetes presents with 2 days of progressive left thigh pain, fever of 39.5°C, and tachycardia. Physical examination reveals diffuse left thigh erythema with indistinct borders, tense swelling, and pain that extends well beyond the area of visible redness. Crepitus is palpable over the medial thigh. White blood cell count is 24×10^9/L with a left shift, serum sodium is 131 mEq/L, and lactate is 4.2 mmol/L. CT demonstrates extensive subcutaneous gas tracking along the fascial planes of the medial and anterior compartments.

The patient is taken emergently to the operating room after initiation of broad-spectrum antibiotics (vancomycin, piperacillin-tazobactam, and clindamycin for toxin suppression). A longitudinal incision over the medial thigh reveals dishwater-gray fascia with easy finger-plane separation from the underlying adductor muscles, confirming necrotizing fasciitis. Wide debridement is performed, excising all necrotic skin, subcutaneous tissue, and fascia from the mid-thigh to the inguinal crease, extending laterally to healthy bleeding margins. The femoral vessels and saphenous nerve are identified in the adductor canal and preserved. The wound is packed with saline-moistened gauze and a negative-pressure wound therapy device is applied. At re-exploration 36 hours later, the wound margins are healthy with no further necrosis, and the wound is managed with serial dressing changes until granulation tissue is sufficient for split-thickness skin grafting at 3 weeks.

Posterior Tracheal Wall During Percutaneous Tracheostomy: The membranous posterior tracheal wall (3–4 mm thick) lies directly anterior to the esophagus. Perform PDT under continuous bronchoscopic guidance; direct the needle at 45 degrees toward the carina rather than perpendicular to the skin; stop advancement when air is aspirated or the needle tip is visualized in the lumen.

Transverse Colon During PEG Placement: The transverse colon may interpose between the stomach and abdominal wall, particularly after prior surgery. Confirm both transillumination and finger indentation before advancing the trocar; convert to laparoscopic gastrostomy if either sign is absent.

Deep Structures During NSTI Debridement: Necrotizing infection destroys normal tissue planes and obscures neurovascular bundles, tendons, and the urethra. Debride fascia aggressively but preserve viable muscle; slow the debridement near known neurovascular structures; protect the urethra with a catheter before Fournier debridement.

Summary and Key Concepts

Open tracheostomy creates a tracheal window between rings 2-3 under direct vision, while percutaneous dilational tracheostomy uses bronchoscopic guidance for bedside serial dilation — both require awareness of the posterior tracheal wall and its proximity to the esophagus.

Percutaneous endoscopic gastrostomy relies on transillumination and finger indentation to confirm safe puncture without colonic interposition; both signs must be present before trocar advancement.

Pilonidal disease is an acquired condition of the natal cleft treated definitively by excision with off-midline flap closure (Limberg or Karydakis), which produces lower recurrence rates (2–5%) than midline primary closure (10–25%).

Epidermal inclusion cysts require complete capsule excision including the punctum to prevent recurrence; infected cysts should be drained first with definitive excision deferred until inflammation resolves.

Necrotizing soft tissue infections demand emergent wide debridement back to healthy, adherent, bleeding fascia in all directions, with mandatory planned re-exploration at 24–48 hours to assess for progressive necrosis.

The hallmark intraoperative finding of necrotizing fasciitis is dishwater-gray fascia that separates from underlying muscle with gentle finger dissection — this finding is pathognomonic and distinguishes necrotizing from non-necrotizing infection.

The four principal danger zones of miscellaneous operative procedures are the posterior tracheal wall during PDT, the interposed transverse colon during PEG, the deep neurovascular structures during NSTI debridement, and the cyst-periosteum interface during dermoid excision near the orbit.

THE OPERATIVE DANGER ZONE MASTER ATLAS

Introduction and How to Use This Atlas

The Operative Danger Zone Master Atlas consolidates every Danger Zone identified throughout this textbook into a single, indexed reference that can be consulted rapidly during preoperative planning, intraoperative decision-making, and case preparation. Each entry in this Atlas corresponds to a fully developed Danger Zone block in its parent chapter, where the clinical context, mechanism of injury, consequence, and safe maneuver are presented in detail. The Atlas distills each Danger Zone to its essential elements: the zone itself, the structure at risk, and the safe maneuver — sufficient for quick reference when the full chapter treatment is not needed.

The Atlas is organized in three complementary indexes that allow the surgeon to find the relevant Danger Zone from any starting point. The **Anatomical Region Index** groups Danger Zones by the body region where the hazard is located — Head and Neck, Thorax, Abdomen and Pelvis, Extremities, and General/Systemic. The **Procedure Index** groups Danger Zones by the operation during which they are encountered, matching the chapter structure of the textbook. The **Structure at Risk Index** groups Danger Zones by the specific anatomical structure that may be injured — arteries, veins, nerves, viscera, and other structures — allowing the surgeon to quickly identify every operation that threatens a given structure. A Cross-Reference Table at the end links every Danger Zone to its chapter location, anatomical region, and structure at risk in a single scannable format.

Danger Zone Index by Anatomical Region

Head and Neck

Danger Zone	Structure at Risk	Safe Maneuver Summary	Ch
Facial Nerve Branch Injury During Facial Skin Excision	Temporal and marginal mandibular branches of CN VII	Dissect above the parotid fascia; identify nerve branches before excising deep lesions	21
Spinal Accessory Nerve Injury During Posterior Triangle Resection	Spinal accessory nerve (CN XI)	Identify CN XI at Erb point before dissection; trace it across the posterior triangle	21
Recurrent Laryngeal Nerve Injury at the Ligament of Berry	Recurrent laryngeal nerve	Identify the RLN in the tracheoesophageal	15

		groove before dividing the ligament of Berry	
Parathyroid Devascularization During Thyroidectomy	Parathyroid glands and their vascular pedicles	Ligate the thyroid artery branches on the thyroid capsule, not the main trunk	15
Cranial Nerve Injury During Carotid Endarterectomy	Hypoglossal, vagus, superior laryngeal nerves	Identify each nerve before clamping; maintain dissection on the carotid adventitia	17
Posterior Tracheal Wall Perforation During Percutaneous Tracheostomy	Posterior tracheal membrane and esophagus	Perform PDT under bronchoscopic guidance; angle needle 45° toward carina	25
Thoracic Duct Injury During Left Cervical Lymph Node Biopsy	Thoracic duct at the left jugulosubclavian venous confluence	Avoid dissection inferior to the omohyoid on the left side; ligate any lymphatic duct	18
Esophageal Injury Missed During Neck Exploration	Cervical esophagus	Perform intraoperative esophagoscopy or methylene blue swallow for all Zone II penetrating injuries	20
Carotid Artery Puncture During IJV Catheterization	Common carotid artery	Real-time ultrasound guidance with continuous needle tip visualization; limit head rotation	24

Thorax

Danger Zone	Structure at Risk	Safe Maneuver Summary	Ch
Long Thoracic Nerve Injury During Axillary Dissection	Long thoracic nerve (serratus anterior)	Identify the nerve on the chest wall medial to the axillary vein; dissect lateral to it	14

Pulmonary Artery Injury During Hilar Dissection	Main or lobar pulmonary artery branches	Dissect the PA branches individually in the fissure; have vascular clamp ready	19
Intercostal Artery Hemorrhage During Chest Wall Resection	Posterior intercostal arteries	Ligate or cauterize intercostal vessels at the rib's inferior border before division	19
Innominate Artery Injury During Cervical Mediastinoscopy	Innominate (brachiocephalic) artery	Maintain scope in the pretracheal plane; biopsy only tissue that can be clearly identified	19
Vagal Trunk Injury During Esophageal Mobilization	Anterior and posterior vagal trunks	Identify the vagal trunks on the esophageal surface before circumferential mobilization	5
Esophageal Perforation During Paraesophageal Hernia Sac Dissection	Esophageal wall	Dissect on the sac, not on the esophagus; use a bougie for esophageal identification	5
Thoracic Duct Injury During Esophageal Mobilization	Thoracic duct in the posterior mediastinum	Mass-ligate all tissue between the aorta and azygos vein above the diaphragm	5
Pneumothorax from Subclavian Vein Catheterization	Parietal pleura and lung apex	Keep needle parallel to floor, against posterior clavicle; never redirect inferiorly	24
Air Embolism During Central Venous Catheter Insertion or Removal	Right ventricle and pulmonary vasculature	Trendelenburg position; occlude all open hubs; time removal with Valsalva	24
Missed Diaphragmatic Injury Progressing to Strangulated Hernia	Diaphragm (left hemidiaphragm)	Explore the diaphragm in all left thoracoabdominal penetrating injuries	20

Abdomen and Pelvis

Danger Zone	Structure at Risk	Safe Maneuver Summary	Ch
Common Bile Duct Misidentification and Transection	Common bile duct / common hepatic duct	Achieve the critical view of safety before clipping or dividing any structure	7
Right Hepatic Artery Injury in Calot Triangle	Right hepatic artery (especially replaced or aberrant)	Identify the cystic artery origin; maintain dissection within Calot triangle	7
Unrecognized Bile Duct Injury — Delayed Presentation	Common bile duct	Obtain intraoperative cholangiogram for anatomical uncertainty	7
Hepatic Vein Injury During Parenchymal Transection	Hepatic veins (right, middle, left)	Identify veins on preoperative imaging; maintain transection plane 1 cm from vein	8
Portal Pedicle Injury During Hilar Dissection	Portal vein, hepatic artery, bile duct at hilum	Use hilar Glissonian approach; confirm portal structures before ligation	8
Retrohepatic IVC Injury (Liver Surgery)	Retrohepatic inferior vena cava	Maintain anterior plane during caudate mobilization; prepare for total vascular exclusion	8
Inadvertent Rupture of Hydatid Cyst Contents	Peritoneal cavity (anaphylaxis, dissemination)	Aspirate before opening; pack with hypertonic saline-soaked sponges	8
SMV-Portal Vein Hemorrhage During Uncinate Dissection	Superior mesenteric vein and portal vein confluence	Identify SMV early; divide uncinate in small pedicles close to the specimen	9
Splenic Vein Avulsion During Distal Pancreatectomy	Splenic vein	Ligate the splenic vein before the artery during distal pancreatectomy	9

CBD Injury During Puestow Procedure	Intrapancreatic common bile duct	Palpate and probe the CBD before opening the pancreatic duct	9
Mesenteric Vascular Injury During Adhesiolysis	Mesenteric vessels	Dissect on the bowel wall; use sharp dissection under direct vision	10
Enterotomy During Adhesiolysis	Small bowel wall	Run the bowel from ligament of Treitz to ileocecal valve; inspect all serosal injuries	10
Parastomal Vascular Compromise During Ileostomy Maturation	Mesenteric arcade feeding stoma segment	Confirm pulsatile mesenteric flow before maturation; avoid tension	10
Cecal Wall Injury During Appendiceal Base Stapling	Cecal wall	Confirm appendiceal-cecal junction; fire stapler on appendix, not cecum	11
Ileal and Cecal Injury During Appendectomy in a Phlegmon	Ileum and cecum wall	Consider nonoperative management with interval appendectomy for phlegmon	11
Appendicular Artery Hemorrhage	Appendicular artery in mesoappendix	Secure mesoappendix with energy device or clips before division	11
Duodenal Injury During Right Hemicolectomy	Second and third portions of duodenum	Identify the duodenum before dividing the right mesocolon; use medial-to-lateral approach	12
Splenic Injury During Splenic Flexure Mobilization	Splenic capsule	Begin mobilization at the omentum, not the splenic attachments; avoid traction on spleen	12

Left Ureteral Injury During Sigmoid Resection	Left ureter at pelvic brim crossing	Identify the ureter on the left pelvic brim before dividing the inferior mesenteric pedicle	12
Parastomal Vascular Compromise During Colostomy Creation	Mesenteric arcade to colostomy segment	Ensure tension-free delivery with pulsatile mesenteric flow	12
Autonomic Nerve Injury During TME	Hypogastric and pelvic splanchnic nerves	Maintain the holy plane of TME; identify and preserve the hypogastric nerves	13
Sphincter Injury During Fistulotomy	Internal and external anal sphincter	Classify fistula (Parks) before division; never divide muscle above the dentate line	13
Incomplete Vagotomy and the Criminal Nerve of Grassi	Criminal nerve of Grassi (posterior branch)	Mobilize the gastric fundus to expose the posterior vagal trunk completely	6
Duodenal Stump Blowout After Subtotal Gastrectomy	Duodenal stump closure	Reinforce the stump with omental patch; place drain adjacent to the stump	6
GDA Hemorrhage from Posterior Duodenal Ulcer	Gastroduodenal artery	Three-point suture ligation: proximal, distal, and transverse on the ulcer bed	6
Internal Hernia Through Petersen Space After Gastric Bypass	Petersen space defect	Close Petersen space and jejunojejunal mesenteric defect with running nonabsorbable suture	6
Ilioinguinal Nerve Injury During Anterior Hernia Repair	Ilioinguinal nerve	Identify the nerve on the external oblique; mobilize and protect it during repair	3
Triangle of Doom — Vascular Injury	External iliac artery and vein	Never place tacks, staples, or dissection	3

		below the iliopubic tract lateral to the vas	
Femoral Vein Injury During Femoral Ring Closure	Femoral vein (medial wall)	Identify the vein at the femoral ring before placing sutures; use Cooper ligament repair	3
Cord Devascularization During Reoperative Hernia Repair	Testicular artery and pampiniform plexus	If cord cannot be safely separated, consider inguinal orchiectomy or cord lipoma acceptance	3
Segmental Neurovascular Injury During Retrorectus Dissection	Segmental intercostal neurovascular bundles	Identify and preserve the neurovascular bundles at the lateral edge of the posterior rectus sheath	4
Inadvertent Enterotomy During Adhesiolysis for Ventral Hernia	Bowel wall adherent to mesh or fascia	Use sharp dissection under direct vision; accept a small serosal defect over a full-thickness injury	4
Neurovascular Bundle Injury During TAR	Segmental intercostal nerves in the TAR plane	Enter the TAR plane lateral to the semilunar line; stay posterior to the transversus abdominis	4
Abdominal Compartment Syndrome After Hernia Reduction	Intra-abdominal viscera and diaphragm	Monitor bladder pressure; use component separation rather than forced closure	4
Pancreatic Tail Injury During Splenic Hilar Dissection	Pancreatic tail and main pancreatic duct	Palpate the pancreatic tail before clamping; ligate hilar vessels individually	22
Short Gastric Vessel Avulsion	Short gastric vessels and gastric fundal wall	Divide gastrosplenic ligament from inferior to superior; minimize upper pole traction	22

Splenic Flexure Injury During Inferior Pole Mobilization	Splenic flexure of colon	Identify the colon before inferior pole dissection; develop the plane from thc colonic side	22
Left Kidney Capsular Injury During Posterolateral Splenic Mobilization	Left kidney capsule and cortex	Keep dissection on the posterior splenic capsule; palpate for kidney before deep mobilization	22
Colonic Interposition Injury During PEG Placement	Transverse colon	Confirm transillumination and finger indentation before trocar advancement	25
Pelvic Hematoma Exploration in Blunt Trauma	Pelvic venous plexus	Do not open a stable pelvic hematoma; use preperitoneal packing or angioembolization	20
Retrohepatic IVC Injury in Major Hepatic Trauma	Retrohepatic IVC and hepatic veins	Pack and compress; avoid blind clamping; consider atriocaval shunt for exsanguination	20

Extremities and Vascular

Danger Zone	Structure at Risk	Safe Maneuver Summary	Ch
Left Renal Vein Injury During Infrarenal Aortic Cross-Clamping	Left renal vein	Identify the left renal vein crossing the aorta before applying the cross-clamp	17
Popliteal Vein Injury During Below-Knee Popliteal Artery Exposure	Popliteal vein	Retract the vein gently; maintain the dissection plane on the arterial adventitia	17
Popliteal Artery Disruption in Posterior Knee Dislocation	Popliteal artery	Assess ABI in all knee dislocations; proceed to angiography if ABI is less than 0.9	17

Iliac Vein Perforation During Venous Thrombectomy	Common iliac vein at IVC confluence	Use fluoroscopic guidance for balloon catheter passage; stop at first resistance	18
Common Femoral Vein Injury During SFJ Ligation	Common femoral vein	Identify the SFJ by duplex before ligation; never ligate below the SFJ	18
Saphenous Nerve Injury During STSG Harvest from the Thigh	Saphenous nerve (medial thigh)	Harvest the graft from the lateral or anterior thigh, avoiding the medial compartment	21
Steal Syndrome After Arteriovenous Fistula Creation	Hand and digits distal to the fistula	Limit anastomosis length to 5–7 mm; perform DRIL procedure for Grade 2+ steal	24
Inadvertent Deep Structure Injury During NSTI Debridement	Neurovascular bundles, tendons, urethra	Debride fascia aggressively but preserve viable muscle; identify structures before debridement	25

General and Systemic

Danger Zone	Structure at Risk	Safe Maneuver Summary	Ch
Instrument-Related Tissue Injury	Adjacent organs and vessels	Use atraumatic technique; never apply force blindly; convert when exposure is inadequate	1
Blind Clamping in a Bloody Field	Unidentified nerves, vessels, and ducts	Apply pressure to control hemorrhage; identify structures before clamping	1
Thermal Spread from Energy Devices	Adjacent bowel, nerves, bile duct	Maintain safe distance (5–10 mm) from critical structures; allow	1

		cooling between activations	
Positioning-Related Nerve Injury	Brachial plexus, ulnar nerve, peroneal nerve	Pad all pressure points; limit arm abduction to 90 degrees; document positioning	1
Unrecognized Perioperative Cardiac Risk	Myocardium	Apply RCRI or ACS-NSQIP calculator; obtain preoperative ECG and troponin in high-risk patients	2
Prophylactic Antibiotic Timing Failure	Surgical site (infection risk)	Administer within 60 minutes of incision; redose for prolonged cases	2
Nutritional Depletion and Anastomotic Failure	Intestinal anastomosis (leak)	Screen with albumin and prealbumin; optimize nutrition 7–14 days preoperatively	2
Failure to Rescue from Postoperative Complications	Any organ system	Establish escalation protocols; monitor vital sign trends and laboratory markers	2
Positive Margin After Lumpectomy Due to Inadequate Specimen Orientation	Tumor margin status	Orient the specimen with clips or sutures; obtain intraoperative margin assessment	14
Right Adrenal Vein Avulsion from the IVC	Right adrenal vein and IVC wall	Identify the vein early; ligate close to the adrenal gland; have vascular suture ready	16
Tumor Capsule Rupture During Adrenocortical Carcinoma Resection	Peritoneal cavity (tumor spillage)	Avoid grasping the mass; perform en bloc resection with intact capsule	16
Catecholamine Crisis During Pheochromocytoma Resection	Cardiovascular system	Alpha-blockade 10–14 days preoperatively; volume expand; have	16

		IV phentolamine available	
Adrenal Cortical Insufficiency After Cortisol-Producing Adenoma Resection	Contralateral adrenal cortex (atrophied)	Begin perioperative stress-dose hydrocortisone; taper over weeks to months	16
Circumferential Eschar Producing Compartment Syndrome	Extremity vasculature and muscles	Monitor compartment pressures; perform escharotomy within 6 hours of burn	21
Duodenal Mucosal Perforation During Pyloromyotomy	Duodenal mucosa at the pyloric-duodenal junction	Begin myotomy at duodenal end; use blunt spreading only; air-insufflation test before closing	23
Vas Deferens Injury During Pediatric Inguinal Hernia Repair	Vas deferens	Palpate the cord to identify the vas; dissect only the sac; leave sac on vas if adherent	23
Umbilical Vein and Hepatic Injury During Omphalocele Sac Excision	Hepatic capsule and umbilical vein	Ligate umbilical vein before division; leave sac membrane on adherent liver surface	23
Superior Mesenteric Vessel Injury During Ladd Band Division	Superior mesenteric artery and vein	Divide bands under direct vision; palpate for arterial pulsation before cutting	23

Danger Zone Index by Procedure

This index organizes every Danger Zone by the procedure during which it is encountered, following the chapter structure of the textbook. Within each chapter heading, the Danger Zones are listed in the order they appear in the chapter text.

Chapter	Danger Zone	Structure at Risk
Ch 1 — Principles of Surgical Technique	Instrument-Related Tissue Injury	Adjacent organs and vessels
Ch 1	Blind Clamping in a Bloody Field	Unidentified structures

Ch 1	Thermal Spread from Energy Devices	Adjacent bowel, nerves, bile duct
Ch 1	Positioning-Related Nerve Injury	Brachial plexus, ulnar, peroneal nerves
Ch 2 — Perioperative Care	Unrecognized Perioperative Cardiac Risk	Myocardium
Ch 2	Prophylactic Antibiotic Timing Failure	Surgical site
Ch 2	Nutritional Depletion and Anastomotic Failure	Anastomosis
Ch 2	Failure to Rescue	Any organ system
Ch 3 — Inguinal and Femoral Hernia	Ilioinguinal Nerve Injury	Ilioinguinal nerve
Ch 3	Triangle of Doom — Vascular Injury	External iliac vessels
Ch 3	Femoral Vein Injury During Femoral Ring Closure	Femoral vein
Ch 3	Cord Devascularization	Testicular artery and plexus
Ch 4 — Ventral and Incisional Hernia	Segmental Neurovascular Injury (Retrorectus)	Intercostal neurovascular bundles
Ch 4	Inadvertent Enterotomy (Adhesiolysis)	Bowel wall
Ch 4	Neurovascular Bundle Injury (TAR)	Intercostal nerves
Ch 4	Abdominal Compartment Syndrome (Reduction)	Intra-abdominal viscera
Ch 5 — Esophagus	Vagal Trunk Injury	Anterior and posterior vagal trunks
Ch 5	Esophageal Perforation (Paraesophageal Hernia)	Esophageal wall
Ch 5	Mucosal Perforation (Heller Myotomy)	Esophageal mucosa
Ch 5	Thoracic Duct Injury (Esophageal Mobilization)	Thoracic duct
Ch 6 — Stomach and Duodenum	Incomplete Vagotomy (Criminal Nerve of Grassi)	Criminal nerve of Grassi
Ch 6	Duodenal Stump Blowout	Duodenal stump
Ch 6	GDA Hemorrhage (Posterior Ulcer)	Gastroduodenal artery

Ch 6	Internal Hernia (Petersen Space)	Small bowel through mesenteric defect
Ch 7 — Gallbladder and Biliary System	CBD Misidentification and Transection	Common bile duct
Ch 7	Right Hepatic Artery Injury	Right hepatic artery
Ch 7	Unrecognized Bile Duct Injury	Common bile duct
Ch 8 — Liver	Hepatic Vein Injury (Transection)	Hepatic veins
Ch 8	Portal Pedicle Injury (Hilar Dissection)	Portal triad structures
Ch 8	Hydatid Cyst Rupture	Peritoneal cavity
Ch 8	Retrohepatic IVC Injury	Inferior vena cava
Ch 9 — Pancreas	SMV-Portal Vein Hemorrhage (Uncinate)	SMV-portal vein confluence
Ch 9	Splenic Vein Avulsion (Distal Pancreatectomy)	Splenic vein
Ch 9	CBD Injury (Puestow Procedure)	Intrapancreatic CBD
Ch 10 — Small Intestine	Mesenteric Vascular Injury (Adhesiolysis)	Mesenteric vessels
Ch 10	Enterotomy (Adhesiolysis)	Small bowel
Ch 10	Parastomal Vascular Compromise (Ileostomy)	Mesenteric arcade
Ch 11 — Appendectomy	Cecal Wall Injury (Base Stapling)	Cecal wall
Ch 11	Ileal/Cecal Injury (Phlegmon)	Ileum and cecum
Ch 11	Appendicular Artery Hemorrhage	Appendicular artery
Ch 12 — Colon	Duodenal Injury (Right Hemicolectomy)	Duodenum
Ch 12	Splenic Injury (Flexure Mobilization)	Splenic capsule
Ch 12	Left Ureteral Injury (Sigmoid Resection)	Left ureter
Ch 12	Parastomal Vascular Compromise (Colostomy)	Mesenteric arcade

Ch 13 — Rectum and Anus	Autonomic Nerve Injury (TME)	Hypogastric nerves
Ch 13	Sphincter Injury (Fistulotomy)	Anal sphincter complex
Ch 14 — Breast	Positive Margin (Lumpectomy)	Tumor margin
Ch 14	Long Thoracic Nerve Injury (Axillary Dissection)	Long thoracic nerve
Ch 15 — Thyroid and Parathyroid	RLN Injury (Ligament of Berry)	Recurrent laryngeal nerve
Ch 15	Parathyroid Devascularization	Parathyroid glands
Ch 16 — Adrenal Gland	Right Adrenal Vein Avulsion from IVC	Right adrenal vein and IVC
Ch 16	Tumor Capsule Rupture (Adrenocortical Carcinoma)	Peritoneal cavity
Ch 16	Catecholamine Crisis (Pheochromocytoma)	Cardiovascular system
Ch 16	Adrenal Cortical Insufficiency (Cushing Adenoma)	Contralateral adrenal
Ch 17 — Arteries	Cranial Nerve Injury (Carotid Endarterectomy)	CN XII, X, superior laryngeal
Ch 17	Left Renal Vein Injury (Aortic Cross-Clamp)	Left renal vein
Ch 17	Popliteal Vein Injury (Below-Knee Exposure)	Popliteal vein
Ch 17	Popliteal Artery Disruption (Knee Dislocation)	Popliteal artery
Ch 18 — Veins and Lymphatics	Iliac Vein Perforation (Thrombectomy)	Common iliac vein
Ch 18	CFV Injury (SFJ Ligation)	Common femoral vein
Ch 18	Thoracic Duct Injury (Left Neck Biopsy)	Thoracic duct
Ch 19 — Chest	PA Injury (Lobectomy Hilar Dissection)	Pulmonary artery
Ch 19	Intercostal Artery Hemorrhage (Chest Wall)	Posterior intercostal arteries
Ch 19	Innominate Artery Injury (Mediastinoscopy)	Innominate artery

Ch 20 — Trauma Surgery	Pelvic Hematoma Exploration (Blunt Trauma)	Pelvic venous plexus
Ch 20	Retrohepatic IVC Injury (Hepatic Trauma)	Retrohepatic IVC
Ch 20	Missed Diaphragmatic Injury	Left hemidiaphragm
Ch 20	Esophageal Injury Missed (Neck Exploration)	Cervical esophagus
Ch 21 — Skin and Soft Tissue	Facial Nerve Branch Injury (Facial Excision)	CN VII branches
Ch 21	Spinal Accessory Nerve Injury (Posterior Triangle)	CN XI
Ch 21	Saphenous Nerve Injury (STSG Harvest)	Saphenous nerve
Ch 21	Circumferential Eschar — Compartment Syndrome	Extremity vasculature
Ch 22 — Spleen	Pancreatic Tail Injury (Hilar Dissection)	Pancreatic tail
Ch 22	Short Gastric Vessel Avulsion	Short gastric vessels, gastric fundus
Ch 22	Splenic Flexure Injury (Inferior Pole)	Splenic flexure of colon
Ch 22	Left Kidney Capsular Injury (Posterolateral Mobilization)	Left kidney capsule
Ch 23 — Pediatric Surgery	Duodenal Mucosal Perforation (Pyloromyotomy)	Duodenal mucosa
Ch 23	Vas Deferens Injury (Pediatric Hernia Repair)	Vas deferens
Ch 23	Umbilical Vein and Hepatic Injury (Omphalocele)	Hepatic capsule, umbilical vein
Ch 23	SMA/SMV Injury (Ladd Band Division)	Superior mesenteric artery and vein
Ch 24 — Vascular Access	Carotid Artery Puncture (IJV Catheterization)	Common carotid artery
Ch 24	Pneumothorax (Subclavian Catheterization)	Lung apex and pleura
Ch 24	Air Embolism (Central Line Insertion/Removal)	Right ventricle, pulmonary vasculature
Ch 24	Steal Syndrome (AVF Creation)	Hand and digits

Ch 25 — Miscellaneous Procedures	Posterior Tracheal Wall Perforation (PDT)	Posterior trachea, esophagus
Ch 25	Colonic Interposition Injury (PEG)	Transverse colon
Ch 25	Deep Structure Injury (NSTI Debridement)	Neurovascular bundles, tendons

Danger Zone Index by Structure at Risk

This index allows the surgeon to quickly identify every operation in the textbook that threatens a given anatomical structure. Structures are grouped by category: arteries, veins, nerves, hollow viscera, solid organs, and other.

Arteries

Structure at Risk	Danger Zone	Ch
Carotid artery (common)	Carotid Artery Puncture During IJV Catheterization	24
Gastroduodenal artery	GDA Hemorrhage from Posterior Duodenal Ulcer	6
Hepatic artery (right)	Right Hepatic Artery Injury in Calot Triangle	7
Innominate artery	Innominate Artery Injury During Mediastinoscopy	19
Popliteal artery	Popliteal Artery Disruption in Posterior Knee Dislocation	17
Pulmonary artery	PA Injury During Hilar Dissection for Lobectomy	19
Superior mesenteric artery	SMA Injury During Ladd Band Division	23
Testicular artery	Cord Devascularization During Reoperative Hernia Repair	3
Appendicular artery	Appendicular Artery Hemorrhage	11
Intercostal arteries	Intercostal Artery Hemorrhage During Chest Wall Resection	19

Veins

Structure at Risk	Danger Zone	Ch
Adrenal vein (right)	Right Adrenal Vein Avulsion from IVC	16
Common femoral vein	CFV Injury During SFJ Ligation	18
External iliac vessels	Triangle of Doom — Vascular Injury	3
Femoral vein	Femoral Vein Injury During Femoral Ring Closure	3
Hepatic veins	Hepatic Vein Injury During Parenchymal Transection	8
Iliac vein (common)	Iliac Vein Perforation During Thrombectomy	18
Inferior vena cava (retrohepatic)	Retrohepatic IVC Injury (Liver Surgery and Trauma)	8, 20
Left renal vein	Left Renal Vein Injury During Aortic Cross-Clamping	17
Pelvic venous plexus	Pelvic Hematoma Exploration in Blunt Trauma	20
Popliteal vein	Popliteal Vein Injury During Below-Knee Exposure	17
Portal vein / SMV	SMV-Portal Vein Hemorrhage During Uncinate Dissection	9
Short gastric vessels	Short Gastric Vessel Avulsion	22
Splenic vein	Splenic Vein Avulsion During Distal Pancreatectomy	9
Umbilical vein	Umbilical Vein and Hepatic Injury During Omphalocele Repair	23

Nerves

Structure at Risk	Danger Zone	Ch
Autonomic nerves (pelvic)	Autonomic Nerve Injury During TME	13

Brachial plexus	Positioning-Related Nerve Injury	1
Cranial nerves (XII, X, SLN)	Cranial Nerve Injury During Carotid Endarterectomy	17
Facial nerve (CN VII)	Facial Nerve Branch Injury During Facial Skin Excision	21
Ilioinguinal nerve	Ilioinguinal Nerve Injury During Anterior Hernia Repair	3
Long thoracic nerve	Long Thoracic Nerve Injury During Axillary Dissection	14
Recurrent laryngeal nerve	RLN Injury at the Ligament of Berry	15
Saphenous nerve	Saphenous Nerve Injury During STSG Harvest	21
Segmental intercostal nerves	Neurovascular Injury During Retrorectus/TAR Dissection	4
Spinal accessory nerve (CN XI)	CN XI Injury During Posterior Triangle Resection	21
Vagal trunks	Vagal Trunk Injury During Esophageal Mobilization	5
Vas deferens	Vas Deferens Injury During Pediatric Hernia Repair	23

Hollow Viscera and Ducts

Structure at Risk	Danger Zone	Ch
Bile duct (common)	CBD Misidentification and Transection; CBD Injury (Puestow)	7, 9
Cecum	Cecal Wall Injury During Base Stapling; Ileal/Cecal Injury (Phlegmon)	11
Colon (splenic flexure)	Splenic Flexure Injury During Inferior Pole Mobilization	22
Colon (transverse)	Colonic Interposition Injury During PEG	25
Duodenum	Duodenal Injury (Right Hemicolectomy); Duodenal	12, 6, 23

	Stump Blowout; Duodenal Mucosal Perforation (Pyloromyotomy)	
Esophagus	Esophageal Perforation (Paraesophageal Hernia); Mucosal Perforation (Heller Myotomy); Esophageal Injury (Neck Exploration)	5, 20
Small bowel	Enterotomy and Mesenteric Vascular Injury During Adhesiolysis	10
Trachea (posterior wall)	Posterior Tracheal Wall Perforation During PDT	25
Ureter (left)	Left Ureteral Injury During Sigmoid Resection	12

Solid Organs and Other

Structure at Risk	Danger Zone	Ch
Adrenal cortex (contralateral)	Adrenal Cortical Insufficiency After Cushing Adenoma Resection	16
Anal sphincter complex	Sphincter Injury During Fistulotomy	13
Diaphragm	Missed Diaphragmatic Injury (Trauma)	20
Hand and digits	Steal Syndrome After AVF Creation	24
Hepatic capsule / parenchyma	Hepatic Injury During Omphalocele Repair; Hydatid Cyst Rupture	23, 8
Kidney (left)	Left Kidney Capsular Injury During Splenic Mobilization	22
Lung apex / pleura	Pneumothorax from Subclavian Catheterization	24
Myocardium	Unrecognized Perioperative Cardiac Risk	2
Pancreatic tail	Pancreatic Tail Injury During Splenic Hilar Dissection	22

Parathyroid glands	Parathyroid Devascularization During Thyroidectomy	15
Right ventricle / pulmonary vasculature	Air Embolism During Central Line Insertion or Removal	24
Spleen	Splenic Injury During Splenic Flexure Mobilization	12
Tumor capsule / margins	Tumor Capsule Rupture (Adrenocortical Carcinoma); Positive Margin (Lumpectomy)	16, 14

Cross-Reference Tables Linking Danger Zones to Chapters

The following master table provides a single-row entry for every Danger Zone in the textbook, listing its chapter number, anatomical region, structure at risk, and page reference. This table is designed for rapid lookup — the surgeon scans the structure or region column to find the entry, then turns to the corresponding chapter for the full Danger Zone block with detailed mechanism, consequence, and safe maneuver.

#	Danger Zone	Region	Structure at Risk	Ch
1	Instrument-Related Tissue Injury	General	Adjacent organs/vessels	1
2	Blind Clamping in a Bloody Field	General	Unidentified structures	1
3	Thermal Spread from Energy Devices	General	Adjacent structures	1
4	Positioning-Related Nerve Injury	General	Peripheral nerves	1
5	Unrecognized Perioperative Cardiac Risk	General	Myocardium	2
6	Prophylactic Antibiotic Timing Failure	General	Surgical site	2

7	Nutritional Depletion / Anastomotic Failure	General	Anastomosis	2
8	Failure to Rescue	General	Any organ system	2
9	Ilioinguinal Nerve Injury	Abdomen	Ilioinguinal nerve	3
10	Triangle of Doom	Abdomen	External iliac vessels	3
11	Femoral Vein Injury (Femoral Ring)	Abdomen	Femoral vein	3
12	Cord Devascularizatio n	Abdomen	Testicular artery	3
13	Segmental Neurovascular Injury (Retrorectus)	Abdomen	Intercostal bundles	4
14	Inadvertent Enterotomy (Ventral Hernia)	Abdomen	Bowel wall	4
15	Neurovascular Injury (TAR)	Abdomen	Intercostal nerves	4
16	Abdominal Compartment Syndrome	Abdomen	Intra-abdominal viscera	4
17	Vagal Trunk Injury	Thorax	Vagal trunks	5
18	Esophageal Perforation (PEH Sac)	Thorax	Esophageal wall	5
19	Mucosal Perforation (Heller Myotomy)	Thorax	Esophageal mucosa	5
20	Thoracic Duct Injury (Esophageal)	Thorax	Thoracic duct	5
21	Criminal Nerve of Grassi	Abdomen	Criminal nerve	6

22	Duodenal Stump Blowout	Abdomen	Duodenal stump	6
23	GDA Hemorrhage	Abdomen	Gastroduodenal artery	6
24	Internal Hernia (Petersen Space)	Abdomen	Small bowel	6
25	CBD Misidentificatio n	Abdomen	Common bile duct	7
26	Right Hepatic Artery Injury	Abdomen	Right hepatic artery	7
27	Unrecognized Bile Duct Injury	Abdomen	Common bile duct	7
28	Hepatic Vein Injury	Abdomen	Hepatic veins	8
29	Portal Pedicle Injury	Abdomen	Portal triad	8
30	Hydatid Cyst Rupture	Abdomen	Peritoneal cavity	8
31	Retrohepatic IVC Injury (Liver)	Abdomen	IVC	8
32	SMV-Portal Vein Hemorrhage	Abdomen	SMV-PV confluence	9
33	Splenic Vein Avulsion	Abdomen	Splenic vein	9
34	CBD Injury (Puestow)	Abdomen	Intrapancreatic CBD	9
35	Mesenteric Vascular Injury	Abdomen	Mesenteric vessels	10
36	Enterotomy (Adhesiolysis)	Abdomen	Small bowel	10
37	Parastomal Vascular Compromise (Ileostomy)	Abdomen	Mesenteric arcade	10
38	Cecal Wall Injury	Abdomen	Cecum	11

39	Ileal/Cecal Injury (Phlegmon)	Abdomen	Ileum/Cecum	11
40	Appendicular Artery Hemorrhage	Abdomen	Appendicular artery	11
41	Duodenal Injury (Right Hemicolectomy)	Abdomen	Duodenum	12
42	Splenic Injury (Flexure)	Abdomen	Splenic capsule	12
43	Left Ureteral Injury	Abdomen/Pelvis	Left ureter	12
44	Parastomal Vascular Compromise (Colostomy)	Abdomen	Mesenteric arcade	12
45	Autonomic Nerve Injury (TME)	Pelvis	Hypogastric nerves	13
46	Sphincter Injury (Fistulotomy)	Pelvis	Anal sphincter	13
47	Positive Margin (Lumpectomy)	Thorax	Tumor margin	14
48	Long Thoracic Nerve Injury	Thorax	Long thoracic nerve	14
49	RLN Injury (Ligament of Berry)	Head/Neck	RLN	15
50	Parathyroid Devascularizatio n	Head/Neck	Parathyroid glands	15
51	Right Adrenal Vein Avulsion	Abdomen	Right adrenal vein/IVC	16
52	Tumor Capsule Rupture (ACC)	Abdomen	Peritoneal cavity	16
53	Catecholamine Crisis (Pheochromocyt oma)	General	Cardiovascular system	16

54	Adrenal Cortical Insufficiency	General	Contralateral adrenal	16
55	Cranial Nerve Injury (CEA)	Head/Neck	CN XII, X, SLN	17
56	Left Renal Vein Injury	Abdomen	Left renal vein	17
57	Popliteal Vein Injury	Extremity	Popliteal vein	17
58	Popliteal Artery Disruption	Extremity	Popliteal artery	17
59	Iliac Vein Perforation	Abdomen	Common iliac vein	18
60	CFV Injury (SFJ Ligation)	Extremity	Common femoral vein	18
61	Thoracic Duct Injury (Left Neck)	Head/Neck	Thoracic duct	18
62	PA Injury (Lobectomy)	Thorax	Pulmonary artery	19
63	Intercostal Artery Hemorrhage	Thorax	Intercostal arteries	19
64	Innominate Artery Injury	Thorax	Innominate artery	19
65	Pelvic Hematoma Exploration	Pelvis	Pelvic venous plexus	20
66	Retrohepatic IVC Injury (Trauma)	Abdomen	IVC/Hepatic veins	20
67	Missed Diaphragmatic Injury	Thorax	Diaphragm	20
68	Esophageal Injury (Neck)	Head/Neck	Cervical esophagus	20
69	Facial Nerve Branch Injury	Head/Neck	CN VII branches	21
70	Spinal Accessory Nerve Injury	Head/Neck	CN XI	21

71	Saphenous Nerve Injury (STSG)	Extremity	Saphenous nerve	21
72	Circumferential Eschar	Extremity	Extremity vasculature	21
73	Pancreatic Tail Injury	Abdomen	Pancreatic tail	22
74	Short Gastric Vessel Avulsion	Abdomen	Short gastric vessels	22
75	Splenic Flexure Injury	Abdomen	Splenic flexure	22
76	Left Kidney Capsular Injury	Abdomen	Left kidney	22
77	Duodenal Mucosal Perforation (Pyloromyotomy)	Abdomen	Duodenal mucosa	23
78	Vas Deferens Injury	Abdomen	Vas deferens	23
79	Umbilical Vein/Hepatic Injury	Abdomen	Hepatic capsule	23
80	SMA/SMV Injury (Ladd Bands)	Abdomen	SMA/SMV	23
81	Carotid Artery Puncture	Head/Neck	Common carotid artery	24
82	Pneumothorax (Subclavian)	Thorax	Lung apex/pleura	24
83	Air Embolism (Central Line)	General	Right ventricle	24
84	Steal Syndrome (AVF)	Extremity	Hand/digits	24
85	Posterior Tracheal Wall Perforation	Head/Neck	Trachea/esophagus	25
86	Colonic Interposition (PEG)	Abdomen	Transverse colon	25

87	Deep Structure Injury (NSTI)	Extremity	Neurovascular bundles	25

CONCLUSION

Surgery is, at its core, a discipline of disciplined action — the convergence of anatomical knowledge, technical skill, and clinical judgment applied under conditions that rarely afford the luxury of deliberation. The chapters in this textbook have walked through the operative landscape systematically, from the foundational principles of surgical technique and perioperative care through the full breadth of general surgical procedures, and into the specialized domains of pediatric, vascular access, and miscellaneous operative work. What remains is to draw together the threads that bind these diverse operations into a coherent surgical practice.

The Primacy of Anatomy

Every operation described in this book returns, sooner or later, to the same imperative: know what lies beneath the blade before it moves. The Operative Danger Zone Atlas that accompanies each chapter was designed to make this principle concrete rather than aspirational. Danger zones are not abstract hazards — they are specific anatomical spaces where specific structures face predictable risk from specific maneuvers. The recurrent laryngeal nerve in the tracheoesophageal groove, the common bile duct at the hepatocystic triangle, the left renal vein behind the neck of the pancreas, the thoracodorsal nerve along the lateral border of the latissimus dorsi — these are not complications waiting to happen. They are anatomical facts that, once internalized, transform a technically competent surgeon into a safe one. The reader who has worked through all twenty-five chapters and the Master Atlas now carries a mental map of operative danger that no single rotation or fellowship can replicate in isolation. That map must be maintained. Anatomy does not change, but a surgeon's awareness of it can erode if not actively reinforced.

Technical Skill and Clinical Reasoning

Operative surgery is often reduced, in casual discussion, to manual dexterity — the steadiness of the hand, the precision of the knot, the economy of the dissection. These matter, but they are not what distinguishes the surgeon who consistently achieves good outcomes from the one who intermittently achieves excellent ones. The distinguishing factor is clinical reasoning applied in real time: the decision to convert a laparoscopic cholecystectomy to an open procedure when the critical view of safety cannot be achieved, the judgment to perform a damage-control laparotomy rather than a definitive repair in a hemodynamically unstable trauma patient, the recognition that a planned right hemicolectomy requires proximal diversion because the bowel is too edematous to tolerate a primary anastomosis. These decisions are not made in the operating room alone — they are prepared for in the kind of structured study this textbook supports.

Each chapter has paired step-by-step operative technique with the pathophysiological reasoning that governs when and why each operation is performed. Indications and contraindications are not checklists to memorize but clinical scenarios to understand. The management of a perforated duodenal ulcer, for instance, depends not only on the size and location of the perforation but on the duration of peritoneal contamination, the patient's hemodynamic reserve, and the presence or absence of downstream obstruction. A textbook that teaches the Graham patch without teaching these contextual variables has taught only half the operation. The goal throughout has been to teach the complete operation — anatomy, indication, technique, intraoperative decision-making, and postoperative vigilance — as a single integrated act.

Perioperative Care as Operative Care

The boundary between the operating room and the ward is, in practice, far more porous than training structures suggest. Operative outcomes are shaped as much by the quality of preoperative optimization and postoperative surveillance as by the technical conduct of the procedure itself. The chapter on preoperative assessment and perioperative care was placed second in this textbook deliberately, before any specific operation, because the principles it contains — risk stratification, anticoagulation management, nutritional optimization, glycemic control, venous thromboembolism prophylaxis — apply to every procedure that follows. A technically flawless thyroidectomy complicated by an unrecognized postoperative hematoma compressing the airway is not a successful operation. A well-executed pancreaticoduodenectomy followed by a missed postoperative pancreatic fistula is not a successful operation. The chapters on specific procedures have integrated perioperative considerations into each operative description precisely because they cannot be separated in practice.

The Evolving Surgical Landscape

Surgery is not a static discipline. The operations described in this textbook reflect current evidence and established technique as of 2026, but the field continues to evolve. Robotic-assisted approaches are expanding into domains previously dominated by open and conventional laparoscopic techniques. Enhanced recovery protocols are compressing hospital stays and shifting the window of postoperative complications into the ambulatory setting. Immunotherapy and targeted molecular therapy are altering the indications for and timing of oncologic resection. Damage-control resuscitation principles continue to refine the management of the critically injured patient. The surgeon who completed training a decade ago operates in a different technical and physiological landscape than the trainee entering the operating room today.

This textbook has aimed to present the principles that endure across these changes — the anatomy that does not shift, the physiological responses that remain constant, the decision-making frameworks that apply regardless of whether the instrument in the surgeon's hand is a scalpel, a laparoscopic grasper, or a robotic arm. The specific techniques will continue to be refined, and the reader is encouraged to supplement the operative descriptions here with current literature, society guidelines, and hands-on simulation and proctored experience as new approaches mature into standard practice.

A Final Word to the Trainee

The PGY trainee for whom this textbook was written occupies a unique and demanding position in medicine. The surgical resident is simultaneously a student and a practitioner, expected to learn while performing, to study while working clinically, and to develop judgment while still acquiring the knowledge base that judgment depends on. This textbook was structured to support that dual role. The step-by-step operative descriptions provide the technical foundation needed before entering the operating room. The danger zone callouts provide the anatomical safety layer that protects the patient while the trainee is still building pattern recognition. The clinical cases provide the contextual reasoning that transforms rote knowledge into operative judgment. The Master Atlas provides the consolidated reference that a resident can consult rapidly — on call, before a case, during a quiet moment on service — without re-reading entire chapters.

Surgical competence is not achieved by reading alone, and this textbook makes no claim to replace the irreplaceable experience of operating under supervision. What it provides is the structured knowledge that makes supervised experience maximally productive. The trainee who enters the operating room having studied the relevant chapter — having reviewed the anatomy, understood the indications, visualized the steps, and internalized the danger zones — will extract more learning from every case than the trainee who has not. Over the course of a residency, that cumulative advantage compounds into the kind of deep operative fluency that defines a safe, confident, and effective surgeon.

The operations in this book are the foundation. Master them — not merely their steps, but their reasoning, their anatomy, and their hazards — and you will be prepared for whatever the operating room presents.

www.ingramcontent.com/pod-product-compliance
Lightning Source LLC
LaVergne TN
LVHW060441061126
851857LV00016B/1686